Pseudo-Galenica
The Formation of the Galenic Corpus
from Antiquity to the Renaissance

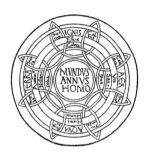

Warburg Institute Colloquia
Edited by Charles Burnett and Jill Kraye

34

Pseudo-Galenica

The Formation of the Galenic Corpus
from Antiquity to the Renaissance

Edited by Caroline Petit, Simon Swain
and Klaus-Dietrich Fischer

The Warburg Institute
London 2021

Published by
The Warburg Institute
School of Advanced Study
University of London
Woburn Square
London WC1H 0AB

© The Warburg Institute 2021
ISBN 9781908590572
ISSN 1352–9986

Typeset by Judith & Juan Acevedo, Cambridge, UK.

Printed by Henry Ling, The Dorset Press, Dorchester, Dorset.

Table of Contents

iii   Contributors

v   Introduction: Muddy Waters: Pseudo-Galenic Texts and the Formation of the Galenic Corpus
Caroline Petit & Simon Swain

1   Three Pseudo-Galenic Texts: Pharmacology and Society in Imperial Rome
Vivian Nutton

13   Is the *Theriac to Piso* Attributed to Galen Authentic?
Véronique Boudon-Millot

31   Easy Remedies – Difficult Texts: the Pseudo-Galenic *Euporista*
Laurence Totelin

47   Les manuscrits grecs des *Definitiones medicae* pseudo-galéniques
Marie Cronier

69   Four Works on Prognostic Attributed to Galen (Kühn vol. 19): New Hypotheses on Their Authorship, Transmission, and Intellectual Milieu
Caroline Petit

83   Pseudonymity and Pseudo-Galen in the Syriac Traditions
Siam Bhayro

98   Pseudo-Galenic Texts on Urines and Pulse in Late Byzantium
Petros Bouras-Vallianatos

129   About the Authenticity of Galen's Περὶ ἀλυπίας in Medieval Hebrew, Compared to the Recently Found Greek Text
Mauro Zonta†

143 Pseudo-Galenic Texts in the Editions of Galen, 1490–1689
Stefania Fortuna

161 Alessandro Achillini and the 1502 Galen *Opera Omnia*: The Influence of Pseudo-Galenic Sources in Early Sixteenth Century Anatomy
R. Allen Shotwell

173 *Commentariis in Hippocratis librum Epidemiarum II uti non licet*: G.B. Rasario and the false 'Galenic' commentary on Epidemics II
Christina Savino

189 La fortune du *De spermate* dans les éditions imprimées de Galien du XVIᵉ au XVIIᵉ
Outi Merisalo

199 *Index codicum manuscriptorum*

201 Index

Contributors

Siam Bhayro, University of Exeter

Véronique Boudon-Millot, CNRS, Paris

Petros Bouras-Vallianatos, University of Edinburgh

Marie Cronier, Institut de Recherche et d'Histoire des Textes, CNRS, Paris

Klaus-Dietrich Fischer, Universität Mainz

Stefania Fortuna, Università Politecnica delle Marche, Ancona

Outi Merisalo, University of Jyväskylä

Vivian Nutton, University College London

Caroline Petit, University of Warwick

Christina Savino, Università degli Studi di Udine

Allen Shotwell, Ivy Tech Community College, Indiana

Simon Swain, University of Warwick

Laurence Totelin, University of Cardiff

Mauro Zonta†, formerly Università La Sapienza, Rome

Introduction
Muddy Waters: Pseudo-Galenic Texts and the Formation of the Galenic Corpus

Caroline Petit & Simon Swain

Rarely has an ancient author taken so much care in establishing the list, purpose, circumstances and contents of each and every work he wrote. Such was Galen's aim in the bio-bibliographical works *On My Own Books* (*De libris propriis*) and *On the Order of My Own Books* (*De ordine librorum propriorum*).[1] Yet his efforts were thwarted. As his reputation rose in imperial Rome, forgeries started circulating under his name in his own lifetime. Twenty centuries on, reading Galen is still a confusing experience for many students and scholars: the standard reference edition (Carl Gottlob Kühn, 1821–1833) offers little help for separating the wheat from the chaff, mixing together authentic, spurious and dubious works – and omitting many others. More importantly, pseudo-Galenic texts do stand as crucial, if often neglected, sources for historians of medicine regardless of authorship: they offer unparalleled evidence on ancient doxography, medical practice and thought, and philosophical debates (such as whether the foetus has a soul). It is hoped that this volume will help all the readers interested in Galen and 'Galenism' from antiquity to the present to navigate the muddy waters of the corpus more confidently.[2]

Galen on his Own Works and the Problem of Pseudepigraphy

The problems of attribution we are facing as scholars began in Galen's own lifetime. In the fierce market of medicine in Antonine and Severan Rome, 'great was the name of Galen'[3] and it could help sell copies. He tells us a (now well-known) anecdote, at the opening of his catalogue, explaining how he was led to

---

[1] About which see also the latest critical edition, by Véronique Boudon-Millot, *Galien. Oeuvres, Tome I,* Collection des Universités de France, Paris, 2007, with abundant notes.

[2] On the (authentic) Galenic corpus and its reception, especially through the medieval period, see P. Bouras-Vallianatos and B. Zipser eds, *Brill Companion to the Reception of Galen,* Leiden, 2019 and to an extent A. Pietrobelli (ed.), *Contre Galien. Critiques d'une autorité médicale de l'antiquité à l'âge moderne,* Paris, 2020. On the early modern period more specifically, see M. Camposampiero-Favaretti & E. Scribano (eds), *Galen and the Early Moderns* (forthcoming with Springer, in the *International Archives of the History of Ideas* series).

[3] Galen, *On prognosis,* 5.4 Nutton (CMG V, 8, 1, p. 95).

write down all the titles of the works he had penned.[4] One day, as he passed through the Sandalarium, the area of Rome dedicated to booksellers, he witnessed an argument between two booklovers over the authenticity of a work on sale, which was attributed to him, bearing the *epigraphè*: *Galènou iatros*. Galen then praises the discerning gentleman who identified the work as a forgery, arguing that it lacked Galen's distinctive stylistic features.

Beyond what this story tells us about Galen's ambitious project and authorial confidence, it reveals a crucial aspect of Galen's (largely retrospective) construction of a 'corpus': responding to critics, but also keeping in check some inconsiderate 'borrowers' of ideas certainly helped shape his writings as we know them, and allow him to write his own works in a way that should prevent any misunderstanding about his thought to occur in the future.[5] It is interesting that, in spite of his effort to shame those who tried to use his name for profit, a text with the very same *epigraphè* has survived among his works and passed as authentic for a long time. The *Introductio sive medicus* (as it is known in Kühn; in Greek, *Galènou iatros. eisagôgè*) was not only preserved but became especially popular: it is found in about forty Greek manuscripts, was translated into Latin in late antiquity, the medieval period, and then again in the Renaissance.[6] The fact that it provides a concise general introduction to 'Galenic' medicine certainly made it valuable teaching and learning material, just like many other inauthentic works. Although we will never know whether the extant text is the one which Galen was discussing, the story is revelatory of many essential problems for the modern scholar: some inauthentic texts date back to Galen's own lifetime and were included in his own works at an early stage; some pseudo-Galenic texts became more successful than genuine, important works by the great Galen; pseudo-Galenic works reflect changing attitudes to the written word and to knowledge more generally – in a way that can find many parallels outside the world of medicine.[7] The main difficulty for historians lies in the fact that we face as many scenarios and case-

[4] Galen, *Libr. propr.* (proem.), p. 134–136 Boudon-Millot (*op. cit.* n. 1).

[5] On Galen's strong authorial voice and concern for posterity, see most recently C. Petit, *Galien de Pergame ou la rhétorique de la Providence*, Leiden, 2018, pp. 12–14; T. Raiola, 'Come si costruisce un corpus: il caso di Galeno', *AION* 39, 2017, pp. 147–167.

[6] See C. Petit, *Galien. Oeuvres, Tome III: Le médecin. Introduction*, Collection des Universités de France, Les Belles Lettres, Paris, 2009a, and C. Petit, 'The fate of a Greek medical handbook in the medieval West: the *Introduction, or the Physician* ascribed to Galen' in B. Zipser (ed.), *Iatrosophia. Byzantine Medical Manuals in Context*, in *Eikasmos online* (2013), pp. 57–78.

[7] See Bhayro's thoughts on pseudepigraphy in this volume. Among various recent projects on forgeries, see for example W. Stephens, E. A. Havens and J. A. Gomez (eds), *Literary Forgery in Early Modern Europe*, Baltimore, 2019.

studies as we have texts: a comprehensive study of pseudepigraphy and the Galenic corpus will only be possible when all the individual stories of pseudo-Galenic texts, in all their variety and complexity, are unfolded and told.

Exploring Pseudo-Galenic Texts

Pseudo-Galenic texts have long suffered a rather widespread lack of interest and understanding, beyond a handful of specialists. There was also confusion, even in scholarly studies, about which text could or could not be authentic. Shifting notions of authenticity (and of the importance of such matters) have had a long-standing effect on the current state of scholarship. Hunayn, for example, was directly concerned with the question of authenticity,[8] but many Renaissance scholars were not – rather, they took in every and any text attributed to Galen as a useful piece of material for study. Such fluid approaches to the written text have favoured blending of 'Galenic' works by theme rather than authorship in early modern printed editions. Texts were read according to the value of their contents, not their perceived authenticity. A shift can be observed: the first two complete editions in Greek, the Aldine and the Basel editions (respectively 1525 and 1538), both set spurious books apart (in volume IV, under the label *notha biblia*); but from the 1550s onwards, editions of the complete works in Latin tend to be more inclusive. The blending of Galenic and Pseudo-Galenic material culminated with the Chartier edition (1639–1679), based on Renaissance erudition; in turn, it formed the basis of the Kühn edition, which, as already mentioned, is still the standard reference edition.[9] As shown below, Kühn made it even worse, by removing hints of inauthenticity that Chartier had included.[10] To this day, historians, physicians, and philologists have thus been struggling to navigate this corpus.[11] The fact that many works are not printed in Kühn makes it all the more confusing.[12]

[8] E. Savage Smith/S. Swain/G. van Gelder, *A Literary History of Medicine*, Chs 5.1.38–40, 8.29.22 nos. 7–8.

[9] On the sources and the making of the Chartier edition, see the studies gathered in G. Cobolet/V. Boudon-Millot (eds), *René Chartier éditeur des oeuvres d'Hippocrate et de Galien. Actes du colloque d'octobre 2010 à Paris*, Paris 2012.

[10] See Petit's contribution in this volume.

[11] Examples of blatant misunderstandings can be found in C. Petit, 'What does Pseudo-Galen tell us that Galen does not? Ancient medical schools in the Roman empire' *in* P. Adamson/R. Hansberger/J. Wilberding (eds), *Philosophical Themes in Galen, BICS supplement 114*, 2014, pp. 269–290 (esp. pp. 269–273).

[12] See, for example, the intriguing commentary to Hippocrates' *Sevens* preserved in Arabic (edited by G. Bergsträsser: CMG XI, 2, 1. Leipzig/Berlin, 1914).

Dissipating some of the most patent misunderstandings about the development of the Galenic corpus is therefore one of the aims of the current volume. Many obstacles prevent us from comprehending the formation of the extant Galenic corpus: the derelict state of the standard edition of Galen's works (Kühn); the scattered nature of the texts, found in multiple languages (esp. Greek, Latin, Arabic), all having an individual story; the multiplicity of patterns of transmission, since texts could be included among authentic texts by accident, through negligence, or deliberately – out of greed (as in the case of Renaissance forgeries,[13] or for lack of a truly Galenic original (for example when the *Compendium pulsuum*, ascribed to Rufus, was translated by Burgundio of Pisa in lieu of the Galenic equivalent text, which he could not find), or yet again because such and such work sounded truly 'Galenic'. The state of scholarship is hardly satisfactory: studies, too, are scattered around and, when they exist, often in need of a tidy up. Last but not least, our reference tools are insufficient: Fichtner's *Corpus Galenicum* is a very useful, but far from perfect instrument. Thankfully, the data available on manuscripts are growing, feeding hopes that the catalogue of Hermann Diels (1905) may be superseded and replaced in the not so distant future. As far as sources in Latin are concerned, the new online catalogue launched by Stefania Fortuna is a precious help.[14] But much remains to be uncovered, in manuscripts (Greek, Latin, Syriac, Arabic, Hebrew, Armenian, and more), of course, but also in the printed editions and the medical works of the Renaissance, in order to understand better who read, copied, bought, and pondered such texts.

There are reasons to be optimistic about the future of scholarship on pseudo-Galenic texts: several have received detailed scrutiny in the past two decades, for example the aforementioned *Introductio sive medicus*, the *De virtute centaureae* (or *De virtutibus centaureae*, the title now favoured by Vivian Nutton), the infamous *Theriac, to Piso*, the *Historia Philosopha*, and the *Ad Gaurum* (now firmly ascribed to Porphyry by James Wilberding). Such studies have raised important methodological and historical questions along the way, and brought much evidence to light in various areas of ancient medicine and thought, even contributing to debates about Galen's biography.[15] They are slowly filling the gaps

---

[13] See the case study by Savino in this volume.

[14] See galenolatino.com.

[15] For the *Introductio sive medicus*, see C. Petit, *Galien. Oeuvres, Tome III*, Paris, 2009; and on various aspects of the text and its transmission, C. Petit, 'L'*Introductio sive medicus* du Pseudo-Galien dans le Haut Moyen Age latin : problèmes d'édition posés par la tradition indirecte', in A. Ferraces Rodríguez (ed.), *Colloquio Internacional Textos medicos latinos*, La Coruña, 2–4 Sept. 2004, La Coruña, 2007, pp. 250–270; C. Petit, 'La place d'Hippocrate dans un manuel médical d'époque romaine : l'*Introductio sive medicus* du Pseudo-Galien', *Les Etudes Classiques* 77, 2009b, pp. 295–312;

left between earlier scholarship and the 21st century.[16] Some prominent 'Galenic' works have been at times considered authentic, at times not: this is notably the case of the *Theriac to Piso*, but also of the *Ars medica* (although it was a cornerstone of Galenic teaching in the middle ages and in the Renaissance).[17] Similar debates have taken place over works attributed to Galen yet lost, such as *On medicine in Homer*.[18]

C. Petit, 'The fate of a Greek medical handbook in the medieval West' in B. Zipser (ed.), *Iatrosophia. Byzantine Medical Manuals in Context*, in *Eikasmos online*, 2013, pp. 57–78; C. Petit, 'What does Pseudo-Galen tell us that Galen does not?' in P. Adamson *et alii* (eds), *Philosophical Themes in Galen*, BICS suppl. 114, 2014, pp. 269–290. On *De virt. cent.*, see V. Nutton, '*De virtutibus centaureae*: a Pseudo-Galenic text on pharmacology', *Galenos*, 8, 2014, pp. 149–75 and V. Nutton, '*De virtute centaureae*: a neglected Methodist text?', in *Body, Disease and Treatment in a Changing World. Latin texts and contexts in ancient and medieval medicine*, eds D. Langslow and B. Maire, Lausanne, 2010, pp. 213–22. On the *De theriaca ad Pisonem*, see V. Boudon-Millot, *Galien. Thériaque à Pison*, Paris, 2017 (see also her contribution in the present volume); R. Leigh, *On Theriac to Piso, Attributed to Galen. A Critical Edition with Translation and Commentary*, Leiden, 2016 (based on the author's thesis). On the *Ad Gaurum an animal sit*, see J. Wilberding, *Porphyry: To Gaurus on How Embryos are Ensouled and On What is in Our Power*, London, 2011; see also L. Brisson, M.-H. Congourdeau et J.-L. Solère, *L'embryon: Formation et Animation. Antiquité grecque et latine, traditions hébraïque, chrétienne et islamique*, Paris, 2008. On the *Historia Philosopha*, see J. Mansfeld and D. T. Runia, *Aëtiana. The method and intellectual context of a doxographer*, Leiden, 1997 (vol. 1: The Sources); 2009 (vol. 2, in two tomes: The Compendium); 2010 (vol. 3: Studies in the doxographical traditions of ancient philosophy); 2018 (vol. 4: Papers of the Melbourne Colloquium on Ancient Doxography); 2020 (vol. 5, forthcoming). See also the recent doctoral thesis of Mareike Jas (Munich) and her paper in Mansfeld and Runia 2018, 'Towards a Better Text of Ps.Plutarch's Placita Philosophorum: Fresh Evidence from the Historia philosopha of Ps.Galen', pp. 130–155. More studies on pseudo-Galenic are cited in C. Petit, 'What does Pseudo-Galen say that Galen does not?', in P. Adamson *et alii* (eds), *Philosophical Themes in Galen*, 2014, and the reader will find much more in the contributions of the present volume.

[16] Earlier scholarship on pseudo-Galenic texts in Greek focuses especially on the *Introductio sive medicus* and the *Definitiones medicae*. See the pioneering work of Emil Issel, *Quaestiones Sextinae et Galenianae*, Phil. Diss., Marburg, 1917; later, F. Kudlien, 'Die Datierung des Sextus Empiricus und des Diogenes Laertius', *Rhein. Mus.* 106, 1963, pp. 251–254; J. Kollesch, *Untersuchungen zu den pseudogalenischen Definitiones medicae*. Berlin 1973; other works studied at an early date include the works attributed to Galen on life of the embryo, for example K. Kalbfleisch, *Die neuplatonische, fälschlich dem Galen zugeschriebene Schrift Pros Gauron Peri Tou Pôs Empsychoutai ta Embrya*, Berlin, 1895. Meanwhile, an edition of the *An animal sit quod in utero est* (reputedly the work of a sophist) was produced in 1914 by Hermann Wagner, but this text, to my knowledge, has not received any detailed study since then. See however the Italian translation by C. M. Colucci: *Se ciò che è nell'utero è un essere vivente*, Roma, 1971 and the pages in K. Kapparis, *Abortion in the Ancient World*, pp. 201–213.

[17] See J. Kollesch, 'Anschauungen von den ἀρχαί in der *Ars medica* und die Seelenlehre Galens' in P. Manuli and M. Vegetti (eds), *Le opere psicologiche di Galeno*, Napoli 1988, pp. 215–229; *contra*, V. Boudon-Millot, 'l'*Ars medica* de Galien est-il un traité authentique?', *REG* 109, 1996, pp. 111–156.

[18] A text once thought to date to the later life of Galen (according to Alexander of Tralles); in favour of authenticity, see A. Guardasole, 'L'héritage de Galien dans l'oeuvre d'Alexandre de Tralles',

Meanwhile, the present volume attempts to contextualise some of these works – especially the pharmacological treatises under scrutiny in Nutton and Boudon-Millot's papers, and those transmitted in the Syriac tradition (Bhayro); it probes the contents and transmission of more neglected works, such as the *Euporista* (Totelin), the *Definitiones medicae* (Cronier), or the group of small texts on uroscopy and sphygmology (*De urinis, De urinis compendium, Ad Antonium de pulsibus*) attributed to Galen (Petit; and, for the shape of such texts in a late Byzantine, manuscript, Bouras-Vallianatos). Among the many medieval misattributions, the astro-medical text *Prognostica de decubitu infirmorum ex mathematica scientia* provides a wonderful example of a complex tradition in Greek, Latin, and the vernacular, and presents enduring readers' ambivalence towards Galenic material (Petit). Later works, like the *De spermate* transmitted in Latin (Merisalo), and many inauthentic works, were in fact very well represented among printed editions of Galen up to the 17th century (as demonstrated by Fortuna). They were read, and pondered by physicians: Shotwell's study illuminates the links between bookish knowledge and practical medicine, with a focus on the pseudo-Galenic *De anatomia vivorum*. Finally, Savino's study reminds us that some 'Galenic' works were forged in the Renaissance to serve a growing market of medical students.

Thus the long history of pseudepigraphy and the Galenic corpus can only help us understand better the paths of the transmission of Galen; it is also naturally a key to comprehending the shifting conceptions of Galenism itself. In the process, of course, we encounter or revisit familiar historical problems about readerships, medical education, theory and practice, the history of the book, and humanism; we rediscover major questions in the history of the transmission, translation, and reception of individual texts and larger bodies of works. This book is therefore a contribution to several areas of intellectual history.

Some topics deserve more work: we did not have the opportunity to dedicate sufficient attention to Pseudo-Galenic texts in Semitic languages, and in the vernacular. In its current, imperfect state, this volume brings together specialists of various periods, languages and cultural areas: it is hoped that it will help

in J. Jouanna & J. Leclant (eds), *La médecine grecque antique*, Paris, 2004, pp. 219–234 (pp. 230–231); J. Jouanna, 'Médecine rationnelle et magie: le statut des amulettes et des incantations chez Galien', *REG* 124, 2011, pp. 47–77 (p. 71); C. Petit, 'Alexandrie, carrefour des traditions médicales au 7e s.' in J.-P. Caillet/ S. Destephen/ B. Dumézil/H. Inglebert (eds.), *Des dieux civiques aux saints patrons*, Paris, 2015, pp. 287–307 (pp. 305–306) and 'Galen, Pharmacology and the Boundaries of Medicine' in, L. Lehmhaus & M. Martelli (eds), *Collecting Recipes. Byzantine and Jewish Pharmacology in Dialogue*, Berlin, 2017, pp. 51–79 (pp. 70–75). *Contra*, F. Kudlien, 'Zum Thema 'Homer und die Medizin'', *Rheinisches Museum* 108, 1965, pp. 193–199.

navigate the meanders of the Galenic corpus, shed new light on neglected texts and manuscripts, and stimulate further research.

*

We owe special thanks to several institutions and individuals for their support. First of all the Warburg Institute, for agreeing to host this conference; especially Jane Ferguson (now retired), for all the administrative burden she took off us in the run up to the conference, and Charles Burnett, for welcoming this volume in the *Colloquia* series. We are especially grateful to Charles for his incredible patience and help throughout the publication process. The Institute of Classical Studies, through Olga Kriskowska and Greg Woolf, awarded a grant to cover travel and accommodation of one European speaker. The Wellcome Trust was enlightened enough to support this conference on Pseudo-Galenic texts (as part of my project on *Medical Prognosis in Late Antiquity*, 2013–2018). This conference is a very old idea that came to life thanks to the opportunity to run this project in the first place.

Our gratitude goes to all the contributors, and to the audience of the Warburg Institute for their enthusiastic engagement with the topic.

It has been quite a journey from the conference to this volume: some adjustments had to be made due to various, sometimes tragic, circumstances. Klaus-Dietrich Fischer had to publish his paper as a matter of urgency in another medium.[19] Mauro Zonta was ill at the time of the conference and could not travel, but sent us a paper, read *in absentia* by Vivian Nutton, and, later, a finalised version for publication. Sadly, he passed away before being able to revise or proof-read his paper.

Finally, we owe very special thanks to Matthew Smith, who provided invaluable assistance in preparing the proceedings for publication.

[19] K.-D. Fischer, 'Drugs to declare. Two pharmaceutical works attributed to Galen', *Cuadernos de Filología Clásica. Estudios griegos e indoeuropeos* 28, 2018, pp. 225–241.

Three Pseudo-Galenic Texts:
Pharmacology and Society in Imperial Rome

Vivian Nutton

An examination of the substantial corpus of Pseudo-Galenic texts has long been a desideratum. Ranging in date from Galen's own lifetime, if not slightly earlier, down to the sixteenth century, and created or translated in a variety of languages, they throw light on the whole process whereby Galen or, more precisely, Galenism came to dominate medicine in the Christian and Islamic worlds at least until the seventeenth century. But they repay attention for many other reasons, not least because some long-suspected writings, like *De motibus dubiis*, may turn out on further examination to be genuine, or, like *De voce*, contain material that goes back directly or indirectly to Galen himself.[1] A second, and perhaps more important reason, is that non-Galenic texts, particularly if, like the *Introductio*, they can be dated to the period from AD 150 to AD 250 may throw light on Galen's context in unsuspected, or at any rate, neglected ways. As Otto Brunfels put it, when justifying his reedition of *De virtutibus centaureae* in 1531, the fact that a treatise is clearly not by Galen should not be a reason for discarding it entirely, for it may contain much that is valuable.[2] Even if we are not, like him, seeking to use these treatises for therapeutic purposes, they are an important resource for many aspects of ancient medicine and for Greek culture in the Roman world. They do not deserve the neglect of historians put off by the mere philological observation that they were not composed by the great doctor from Pergamum.

The three texts discussed here exemplify this neatly. The two treatises on theriac, dedicated respectively to Piso and Pamphilianus, and the short *De virtutibus centaureae* all deal with practical pharmaceutics, an area where Galen's own writings, although substantial, are not as helpful to the average practitioner as they might be, as well as being tedious and expensive to copy by hand.[3] All three tracts were written by Greeks who were living in Rome, or at the very least

---

[1] V. Nutton, 'Galen and the Latin De voce: a new edition and English translation', forthcoming in T. Raiola, ed., *Nell'officina del filologo: studi sui testi e i loro lettori per Ivan Garofalo*, Biblioteca di Galenos, 2021; V. Nutton, with G. Bos, *Galen, On Problematical Movements*, Cambridge, 2011; H. Baumgarten, 'Galen, Über die Stimme.Testimonien der verlorenen Schrift Περὶ Φωνῆς. Pseudo-Galen *De voce et anhelitu*. Kommentar', PhD. diss., University of Göttingen, 1962.

[2] O. Brunfels, *Johannes Serapion, De Simplicibus*, Strasbourg, 1531, pp. 309–12.

[3] Galen, *De theriaca ad Pisonem*, XIV, 210–94 K.; modern editions by V. Boudon-Millot, *Galien. Thériaque à Pison*, Paris, 2017; R. Leigh, *On Theriac to Piso, Attributed to Galen. A Critical Edition with Translation and Commentary*, Leiden, 2016; *De theriaca ad Pamphilianum*, XIV, 295–310 K.; V.

had spent some time there, yet none has attracted much interest or been edited in a modern edition until recently.

Twenty-six years ago I contributed a paper to the Lille conference on Galen, in which I discussed the authenticity of the two treatises on theriac, concluding then that the *Ad Pamphilianum* was pseudonymous, the *Ad Pisonem* genuine.[4] While I still hold to the first conclusion, the arguments of Robert Leigh, and Véronique Boudon have forced me to reconsider my verdict on the latter.[5] One of my arguments in favour of Galen being the author of the latter was certainly ill-founded. The observation there that the general agreement of the text of Andromachus's poem on theriac in the *Ad Pisonem* with that in the genuine *De antidotis* was an indication that they had the same ultimate source is indeed true, but for a different reason than I had supposed.[6] In both works as they stand, the poem is an integral part of the tract and cannot easily be removed from its surrounding context, but the same textual agreement in both places is not proof that the author himself had copied from the same manuscript twice. Rather, it was the Renaissance editors who had used the same manuscript in two different places. Secondly, the list of anomalies, both factual and stylistic, is far longer and more significant than I had believed in 1995. If we continue to believe in the authenticity of the *Ad Pisonem*, it must be admitted there are some unusual words and considerable differences from genuine texts, not all of them easily explained by the notion of a senile Galen, no longer remembering every detail of what he had once said or written in his earlier manner. On the other hand, if the arguments for pseudonymity are accepted, then the coincidence is remarkable: the author was a doctor whose career and very many of whose views resemble those of Galen.[7] He is a Hippocratic and a Platonist, who had spent time at Alexandria, and who had served a series of emperors down at least to the first decade of the third century.[8]

Nutton, '*De virtutibus centaureae*: a Pseudo-Galenic text on pharmacology', *Galenos*, 8, 2014, pp. 149–75, is the only modern edition. The slight change in the title from the more familiar one adopted in V. Nutton, '*De virtute centaureae*: a neglected Methodist text?', in *Body, Disease and Treatment in a Changing World. Latin texts and contexts in ancient and medieval medicine*, eds D. Langslow and B. Maire, Lausanne, 2010, pp. 213–22, is the result of my collation of all the MSS.

[4] V. Nutton, 'Galen on theriac: problems of authenticity', in *Galen on Pharmacology: Philosophy, History and Medicine*, ed. A. Debru, Leiden, New York, Cologne, 1997, pp. 133–51.

[5] Leigh, *On Theriac to Piso* (n. 3 above), pp. 19–61. For the arguments of Boudon, see below, pp. 13–30 and her edition (n. 3 above), pp. lxxiv–lxxx.

[6] Galen, *De antidotis* I.6: XIV, 32–422 K.; *Ad Pisonem* 6–7, not printed in K. as too similar to the earlier citation.

[7] The possibility of a deliberate pastiche would be extremely strange for a medical book. The apparent citation by Julius Africanus also argues against this possibility.

[8] Respectively XIV, 228, 252, 281, 285; 213, 218–19; 237; 216–18 K.

He shared Galen's verbosity as well as his dismissive view of Asclepiades, and was familiar with various details of Roman history, even if the manner in which he uses his historical examples differs from that of Galen.[9] Furthermore, if Julius Africanus in his *Cestoi*, written in the 220s or slightly later, is citing this treatise rather than a passage that was their joint source, one must conclude that the treatise, and presumably also its author, had already attracted a wide readership.[10] But since relatively little is known even about elite doctors, coincidence, however implausible at first sight, must remain a strong possibility.[11]

The three texts have many similarities. All of them survived in Greek until the fourteenth century when they were translated into Latin in whole or in part by Niccolò da Reggio, but *De virtutibus* was lost in Greek after 1341. But there are also major differences. The two tracts on theriac, for example, circulated together for some time, and within the main manuscript tradition of the Greek Galen. They are both referred to by Hunayn ibn Ishaq in his *Risala* in the ninth century as genuine works of Galen.[12] Earlier still, in the early sixth century, Aetius of Amida had cited both texts together, although explicitly attributing only the *Ad Pisonem* to Galen.[13] Above all, compared with many other Pseudo-Galenic texts, these two enjoyed a long association with genuine material. By contrast, *De virtutibus* is not mentioned by Hunayn or any Arabic author, and in Latin translation it enjoyed a *fortuna* both inside and outside the main lines of transmission. Its manuscript tradition falls into two distinct families, one, the standard Galenus Latinus tradition, culminating in the 1490 edition of the *Opera omnia*, the second, and somewhat superior one, associating with other tracts on pharmacy, in both

---

[9] XI, 223–5, 250-55 K., with J. T. Vallance, *The Lost Theory of Asclepiades of Bithynia*, Cambridge, 1990, pp. 38–9; XI, 231, 235–7, 283–4 K.

[10] Unless, of course, the work was already thought to be by Galen. Africanus, *Cestoi* 3.31.1 = fr. D56 Wallraff, with Leigh, *On Theriac to Piso* (n. 3 above), pp. 22–4; Boudon-Millot, *Thériaque à Pison* (n. 3 above), p. xcvii–xcix.

[11] If the *Ad Pisonem* is not by Galen, the argument for his death sometime in the first two decades of the 3rd century is weakened, but not destroyed. The evidence of Byzantine chronographers, for instance, favours a date under Caracalla, i.e. between 212 and 217, which is certainly compatible with the Arabic date of death at age 87.

[12] G. Bergsträsser, *Hunain ibn Ishaq, Über die syrischen und arabischen Galen-Übersetzungen*, Leipzig, 1925, p. 31, nos. 82–3; idem, *Neue Materialien zu Hunain Ibn Ishaq's Galen-Bibliographie*, Leipzig 1932, p. 93, nos. 141–2. Given Hunayn's sophisticated knowledge of Galen, it is worth noting that these tracts, together with the commentary on the Hippocratic *Oath*, are unusual in being accepted by Hunayn as genuine.

[13] Aetius of Amida, XIII.86–97, including a quotation from *Ad Pamphilianum* XIV, 302.15–303.4 K., but without mentioning the name of Galen in the lemma. Cf. also Paul of Aegina, VII.10.2: CMG IX.2 pp. 293–7, citing the *Ad Pisonem* as Galenic.

manuscript and print, down to the 1530s.[14] No other Galenic text circulated so widely on its own and in the company of so much non-classical material.

What is most striking about the two tracts on theriac, and in all probability *De virtutibus*, is that they were all written by doctors active in the time of Galen. The author of the *Ad Pisonem*, if he is not Galen, refers to events in Galen's lifetime, and was probably writing around AD 204, and that of the *Ad Pamphilianum* also seems to have been active in the late second or, more likely, in the early third century.[15] If we could identify Pamphilianus, who is very likely to have had an equestrian career in Egypt, and perhaps in Crete and Rome, we might be able to be even more precise. Although there are no secure internal criteria for his date, it would also be difficult to locate the author of *De virtutibus*, outside the period from 100 to 250, and probably even closer to Galen's lifetime. Whereas many Pseudo-Galenic texts are much later, these three are roughly contemporary, and provide rare evidence for the capacities of some doctors independent of Galen's judgements on his contemporaries. They add considerably to our knowledge of second and early third century medicine.

All three texts were written by Greek doctors living and practising in Rome; two at least declare that they studied there. The author of *De virtutibus* was an immigrant to Rome, since he writes his little tract for a brother called Papias back home somewhere in the Greek world. In Rome he attached himself to a doctor, Apollonius, whom he accompanied on his rounds and whose cases he found impressive, especially his use of centaury.[16] It is not entirely clear whether it is this teacher or his teacher's teacher, who was the expert doctor whom he credits with the first widespread use of this herb. This is good evidence for the teaching of medicine by Greek doctors in Rome to fellow Greeks, and to at least one Greek who had migrated there. Indeed, if the author is to be identified with Statilius Attalus, the Methodist contemporary and rival of Galen, this is an even more unusual instance of a young man from a medical dynasty in Asia Minor receiving instruction from a Roman doctor – but that is a hypothesis that is far

---

[14] Nutton, '*De virtutibus*' (n. 3 above), pp. 150–52.

[15] Leigh, *On Theriac to Piso* (n. 3 above), pp. 11–18, cautiously accepting the argument for the Lusus Troiae of 204 as the scene of the injury to Piso's son, XIV, 213–14 K., but pointing to other possibilities. See also Boudon-Millot, *Thériaque à Pison* (n. 3 above), pp. xlix–lii. The *Ad Pamphilianum* was written sometime after the major outbreak of plague in Rome, XIV, 299 K.

[16] *De virtutibus centaureae* 1: Apollonius igitur senex unus virorum qui valde erant approbati in Roma, cuius magister fuit expertus medicus, utebatur hoc farmaco in multis adversitatibus; et per deum miratus sum de ipso in circumambulatione. Plurimum enim propter hoc circumambulabam cum eo.

from certain.[17] Of course, it need not be supposed that any of these authors arrived in Rome without any medical knowledge whatsoever: rather, once there he attached himself to one of a group of very distinguished physicians, '*valde approbati*', from whom he received instruction in practical therapy.

The author of the *Ad Pamphilianum* had come to Rome but was now no longer there if we are to deduce from the reference to his now increased leisure and to his time in Rome as having ended – he employs the aorist εἶδον – that he had returned to the Greek East.[18] The word περιοδία that he uses may also refer to his 'going the rounds' in Rome, where he had several teachers, including one by the name of Meccius (or Maecius) Aelianus.[19] Meccius, who is otherwise unknown, had told our author about a plague that at some time in the recent past had devastated Italy, killing many, and filling both doctors and leading men with fear. It was then that he came upon theriac, which alone had any effect against the plague. He cured some, although not all, who were affected by it, and claimed that it was an effective prophylaxis, not only warding off the most serious symptoms, but also even preventing those who took theriac from falling ill at all. For, as he says, if a drink of theriac can defeat a lethal poison, it can surely also resist the damaging effects of bad air.[20] The vague way in which Meccius his very old teacher (πρεσβεύτατος) describes the plague suggests that this was probably the Antonine plague, implying that our author arrived in Rome some time later. This would fit with the author's knowledge of the habits of contemporary Romans in taking a small amount of theriac on the first or fourth day of the month, something that, if we can believe Galen's comments elsewhere about the revival of theriac under the Severi, we must place around the year 200 or a little later.[21]

All three texts show how Rome was becoming a centre of medical education, almost on a level with Alexandria. The writers see nothing strange about a well-connected young doctor or medical student from the Greek East coming to Rome and attaching himself to a leading figure there, accompanying him on his rounds

[17] The name Papias, which is relatively common in Asia Minor, was that of an *archiatros*, one of a distinguished line of *archiatroi* from Heraclea Ulpia in Caria, *CIG* 3953h = E. Samama, *Les médecins dans le monde grec*, Geneva, Droz, 2003, no. 252, cf. L. and J. Robert, *La Carie*, Paris, 1954, ii, pp. 126, 167, 178–9, with Samama, nos. 245–8. The name is borne by at least two members of the family. For Attalus as a Methodist, Galen, *Meth. med.* XIII.15: X, 909–16 K.

[18] Galen, XIV, 295 K.: κατὰ τὴν περιοδίαν εἶδον ἐν Ῥώμῃ.

[19] Galen, XIV, 299 K. Compare the use of *circumambulatio* and *circumambulare* (presumably περιοδεύειν) in *De virtutibus* 1 (n. 16 above). But the word could simply refer to a period of time.

[20] Ibid.

[21] Ibid. 298 K.; cf. Galen, *De antidotis* I.13: XIV, 65 K. note his scornful comment at I.4: XIV, 24 K., about the rich following the fashion of the emperors.

and learning from him his new techniques. There is no suggestion that what was taught there was inferior, in the way that Pliny had characterized Greek doctors in Rome long before, or that obtaining information from doctors in Rome was by now anything other than normal – and respectable in Greek eyes. This was true, whatever the theoretical stance of the author. Both authors of the theriac tracts cite Hippocrates as an authority, and the author of the *Ad Pisonem* has harsh words to say about Asclepiades and the Empiricists.[22] By contrast, the opening words of *De virtutibus*, citing the precedent of Themison, *famosus magister*, 'the famous teacher', as the author of a text on a single plant, the plantain, indicate a sympathy for Methodism. All three writers came to Rome and took advantage of what was on offer there.

Although none of their patients is specifically named, it is highly likely that they included persons of wealth and status. The author of *De virtutibus* remains anonymous, but as an expert who associated with others 'highly approved' he would hardly lack for wealthy patients.[23] The two others provide clearer evidence for the circles in which they moved. The dedicatee of the *Ad Pisonem* was a wealthy individual of senatorial or equestrian rank, as was that of the *Ad Pamphilianum*. The author of the latter also implies his wide acquaintance with others from the same social class or background. At the same time, all three authors retain links with the Greek world, directly or indirectly; as we have seen *De virtutibus* is written for a brother somewhere in the Greek East, while the author of the *Ad Pamphilianum* may have retired there. In this they resemble Galen, who may have returned at least once to Pergamum after 170, and perhaps even died there.[24]

The two authors of the theriac tracts also describe themselves as being on terms of social intimacy with many leading members of the aristocracy. That of the *Ad Pisonem* describes as 'most dear', the highly respected Arria, the female philosopher who delighted in the writings of Plato, although whether Bowersock was right to connect her with the Roman consul of 164 is unclear, especially given the number of aristocratic Arrias around.[25] Antipater, the *ab epistulis Graecis* for

---

[22] For the textual problem, resolved by a collation of the MSS, see Nutton, '*De virtutibus*' (n. 3 above), pp. 155–7. The reference is to Themison's treatise on the plantain, Pliny, *Hist. nat.* XXV.39.80 = M. Tecusan, *The Fragments of the Methodists*, vol. 1, Leiden, 2003, fr. 263. Whether any of the references in the Methodist author Caelius Aurelianus to *arnoglossa/plantago* go back to Themison is a moot point.

[23] If he was Statilius Attalus or a relation, he will have been familiar with court circles.

[24] V. Boudon-Millot, *Galien de Pergame, un médecin grec à Rome*, Paris, 2012, pp. 240–1, 243.

[25] *Ad Pisonem* 2: XIV, 219–20 K. G. W. Bowersock, *Greek sophists in the Roman Empire*, Oxford, 1969, p. 84, suggests that she was the wife of M. Nonius Macrinus, consul in 154, but the name is not

a time under Severus, is praised lavishly for his morals and rhetorical skills, and for being one of a number of leading figures who took a great interest in medicine. Marcus Aurelius is held up as the model, but there is an implication that this interest in theriac is widely shared among the Roman elite, something commented on elsewhere by Galen.[26]

The *Ad Pamphilianum*, in particular, is a remarkable text for highlighting the cosmopolitan nature of Rome, as well as the ways in which the Greeks of the Antonine period had come to share in Roman values.[27] The language of its preface is that of honorific inscriptions of the period. The health of Pamphilianus is something profoundly wished for by many in Rome, the *metropolis*, because of the benefits that he has conferred on them both in private and in public. The Greek words, εὐεργετεῖν and κοσμεῖν are often used of a civic benefactor or a magistrate, the latter being particularly used to describe the grant of a building or a fountain to a city.[28] He has been active in promoting works of public benefit, κοινωφελής, as part of his πρόνοια, care, for the citizens. His political adroitness, τὸ δέξιον, and his tact, τὸ ἐπιεικές, have gained him the universal respect, if not affection, of the communities of Crete. Both in Egypt and in the royal city (a term applied to Rome but possibly also to Alexandria) his behaviour and the renown of his name have won him many friends, something that no other Cretans, and few others, have achieved.[29] This type of language is rarely found in surviving literary works, and is at least indicative of Pamphilianus's high status, a status that will reflect on the author, who has been several times asked by him to describe the way to make and prescribe theriac.

Prefaces are, even today, opportunities for showing off, for exaggerating the importance of one's project, for acknowledging help and, as this author puts it, for indicating respect and affection, σπουδή καὶ εὔνοια, towards a dedicatee, and the preface to the *Ad Pamphilianum* is no exception. But the whole treatise is also carefully composed, with artful antitheses and comparisons. It is the work of a well-trained and well-educated writer, something characteristic of all three treatises.

---

uncommon. Leigh, *On Theriac to Piso* (n. 3 above), p. 178, points out that, according to the author, she was cured by the emperors, but this rhetorical praise of the emperors' involvement with theriac does not necessarily mean that they carried out the treatment themselves.

[26] *Ad Pisonem* 2: IV, 218, 216 K.

[27] K. Buraselis, *Theia dōrea: das göttliche kaiserliche Geschenk*, Vienna, 2007, pp. 14–21, discusses the language of the *Ad Pisonem* as typifying responses to imperial benefactions.

[28] As the various indexes to the *Bulletin Epigraphique* and the *Supplementum epigraphicum graecum* easily show.

[29] *Ad Pamphilianum* XIV, 296–7 K.

De virtutibus is the least flowery of the three; it is clear, well organized, and succinct – a preface, a short description of the two types of centaury, an account of the method of preparation, and a much longer list of applications. But it also displays learning – the allusion to Themison, and the long quotation from Crateuas in chapter two – and sound sense. The *Ad Pisonem* includes interesting historical examples, Hannibal, Mithridates and Cleopatra, all presented from a Roman point of view, as well as references to Homer, Plato and Euripides' *Hecuba*.[30] The final page, XIV, 294 K, offers an elegant way of reaching a conclusion by utilising a witty comment by Piso himself. The text itself is not entirely clear, and some emendation is necessary, but it arguably refers to an occasion when Piso was attending a sophistic debate and posed a learned question for further discussion, a πρόβλημα. When the speakers contrived to find many opportunities to continue the argument, long after it might have been regarded as settled, Piso intervened with caustic criticism.[31]

> Even the gods do not make utterance between prophecies, sometimes even oracles fall silent; winter storms make the sea unsailable, rivers dry up, and flow again, while even the earth does not produce her fruits continuously. Hence the necessity, and the propriety, of stopping occasionally, and thus allowing a swift conclusion.

The author manages at one and the same time to compliment his dedicatee and to bring his whole treatise to an elegant close (Galen's usual endings, by comparison, are often abrupt and stylistically far inferior to his openings.) It is an excellent example of the cultivated prose of the second or early third century, and, like the *Ad Pamphilianum*, of the flourishing of learned Greek culture in a specifically Roman context. Although preserved only in a Latin word-for-word translation, the stylistic merits of *De virtutibus* are also clear.

But there is a further reason why historians of medicine in particular should be interested in these tracts. All three are examples of a type of text that must once have been common, but of which these are almost the only survivors, i.e. a pharmacological tract dealing with but a single plant or substance. Two are short; the *Ad Pamphiliamum* a mere sixteen pages in Kühn's edition, the *De virtutibus* little more, and only the *Ad Pisonem*, at some 84 pages, comes close to the length of an average book in Galen. One can see why, when the cost and labour of copying might be thought too great, a work dealing with only one plant, and even one

---

[30] *Ad Pisonem* respectively XIV, 231, 235–7, 283–4, 225, 213, 236 K. Leigh, *On Theriac to Piso* (n. 3 above), pp. 152–3, emends the name of the slave to Bitoitos, for the Biotokos or Bistokos of the MSS, cf. Appian, *Mithrid.* 538.1–5.

[31] Leigh, *On Theriac to Piso* (n. 3 above), p. 253, notes the difficulty, but neither text nor translation, pp. 162–3, is satisfactory. Cf. Boudon-Millot, *Thériaque à Pison* (n. 3 above), pp. 305–309.

class of drug, theriac, might be discarded in the long process of transmission in favour of similar information contained in a bigger text on pharmacology.[32]

What unites all three tracts is that they offer a panacea, a drug that can deal with just about everything. Even if the *Ad Pisonem* largely deals with poisonous animal bites, and offers both a cure and prophylaxis, its chapter 15 contains a long list of diseases and conditions for which theriac can also be used – cachexia, tetanus, gout, worms, urinary problems, and even mental conditions. Several of these treatments, for example for mental conditions, are characterized by some form of θαυμαστός or θαυμάζειν, 'amazing'. Similarly, *De virtutibus* opens with the admission that many of the healing properties of the centaury will seem amazing at first sight to brother Papias back home. It too can cure a whole range of disorders, both inside and outside the body, and can be taken internally as well as being applied externally to wounds and bites of all kinds – historians of ancient herpetology will enjoy puzzling out what Greek word lies behind the corrupted transliterated Greek. The author of the *Ad Pamphilianum* makes a similar plea, contrasting the universal benefits of theriac with the general and erroneous belief that it is of value only against bites and poisons.[33] But, of course, poisoning is not an everyday occurrence, and if kept stored at home unused like a piece of jewellery, theriac will lose its effectiveness over time, and hence it is worth knowing how it might be used as a regular tonic, or as a protection against the bad air and poor water of distant regions. Besides, even the best of doctors may accidentally prescribe some old theriac, and it is thus useful always to have some newly prepared drug to hand.

This writer's list of conditions that theriac can cure is almost as extensive as that of the *Ad Pisonem* although it does not include mental illnesses. On the other hand, he claims that theriac can on occasions give new life to those on the point of death from heart failure. But he refuses to describe this as a universal remedy for a very good reason: to provide such a list of everything, from earache and failing sight to inflamed tonsils, is both impossible and inappropriate.[34] Such claims are akin to the patter of mountebanks, and damage the reputation of the drug more than they enhance it. Besides, to use an expensive drug like theriac for conditions where there is a much cheaper or simpler one to hand, is a waste of time and money.

[32] It is worth noting how many of the Pseudo-Galenic texts do relate to practical pharmacology, not least the *Alphabetum ad Paternianum*, ed. N. Everett, *The Alphabet of Galen. Pharmacy from Antiquity to the Middle Ages*, Toronto, 2012.

[33] *Ad Pamphilianum* XIV, 297–8 K.

[34] Ibid., XIV, 305–6 K.

The reference to mountebanks, charlatans or crowd-pullers is significant. A common feature of the landscape, they were particularly famous for their ability to cure snake bite – as illustrated in the famous illuminated Dresden manuscript of Galen. They wandered the highways and byways, touring the fairs, like Lucius of Ancona, the drug seller, *pharmacopola circumforaneus*, involved, according to Cicero in his *Pro Cluentio*, in the murder of Oppianicus's aunt.[35] The reputation of these healers, like their drugs, was double-edged: they could either kill or cure. So the claim, even by a respectable doctor, to produce a cure for all or even many diseases from one single herb or drug, a typical assertion by the mountebank, was something to be viewed with caution. The boundary between magic and medicine was always fluid, and words like 'wonderful', or 'miraculous' could apply equally to both, so it was important to distinguish one's own remarkable successes from those of lesser practitioners. Galen, for example, took great pains to argue that his prognoses had nothing miraculous about them and that he was no prophet but a true follower of Hippocrates.

To counter this taint of charlatanry all three authors employ similar tactics. One is to explain how the drug works by comparing it with others, as a cholagogue for example, but the most effective arguments appeal to experience, learning, and the standing of the addressee. Pamphilianus and Piso are men of wealth, status and intelligence. Their passion for medicine, along with their commissioning of a tract on theriac, also confirms that they are good witnesses to the expertise and honesty of the author. We do not know the standing of Dr Papias in his community – he was unlikely to have been a poor man – but the fact that it is his brother who is writing a treatise on centaury to inform him of this wonder drug strengthens the writer's claim for honesty – even if, as may be the case, this was originally meant as a private missive.

The second is the appeal to expertise. All the writers mention their own experience; the author of *De virtutibus* begins by stressing that he too at first thought that what he had heard about the multiple uses of the centaury was unlikely, if not a joke – for, he says, Apollonius was a very witty man – but his experience, first as an observer, and then in actually using the drug in his practice convinced him of its widespread effectiveness. The author of the *Ad Pamphilianum* talks of what he had learned from his distinguished teachers, as well as the use made of the drug by many leading Romans, and how he had often been asked to explain the method of preparing theriac and its use.

---

[35] Cicero, *Pro Cluentio* 40.178.

The author of the *Ad Pisonem* makes similar appeals to experience, but more than either of the others it is by his appeals to learning that he wishes to establish the credentials of theriac. His own style and eloquence, the choice words, historical examples and well-moderated sentences, proclaim that he is a man of learning, whose word can be believed. He also sets himself in a line of famous writers on pharmacology reaching back to Hippocrates – Nicander, Magnus, Damocrates, Xenocrates, and of course Andromachus, whose poem is also cited in the other theriac tract, along with Menecrates, Crito and his coevals.[36] The author of *De virtutibus* is more sparing in his citations, quoting only from Crateuas.[37] All these references and allusions serve to establish the writer's credibility and dispel any hint of charlatanry, and, in the *Ad Pisonem*, also to refute Asclepiades, who had a different sort of explanation for the success of theriac.[38] The authors are men of erudition and experience, with eminent teachers or supporters who give authority to their prescriptions.

This short paper is merely one indication of the important information that can be gained by looking at Pseudo-Galenic texts. Not only do they reveal the history of Galenism as well as the ways in which, from at least the sixteenth century onwards, and sporadically earlier still, doctors attempted to distinguish between the genuine works of Galen and the rest. They provide us with a context into which to place Galen. Whether or not the *Ad Pisonem* was written by Galen, the *Ad Pamphilianum* and, to a lesser extent, *De virtutibus* are examples of Greek doctors coming to Rome, making a success of their practice, and still retaining their links with the Greek world. All three deserve to be better known by historians, of the ancient world as well as of medicine itself.

---

[36] *Ad Pisonem* respectively XIV, 239, 261, 263, 260 (if the text is correct), 233 K., XIV, 307, 306, 308 K.

[37] *De virtutibus* 2 = Crateuas, fr. 20, but with a better text than that edited by M. Wellmann, *Pedanii Dioscuridis Anazarbei De materia medica libri quinque. Volumen iii, quo continentur… Crateuae et Sextii Nigri fragmenta*, Berlin, 1914, p. 142.

[38] *Ad Pisonem* 3 and 11: XIV, 223–4, 250–55 K.

Is the *Theriac to Piso* Attributed to Galen Authentic?

Véronique Boudon-Millot*

Various opinions have been put forward about the authenticity of the treatise *De Theriaca ad Pisonem*. Galen himself does not mention it anywhere in the Galenic corpus. As early as the 6th c. AD, however, writing about Andromachus' *Theriac* in book XIII of his βιβλία ἰατρικὰ ἑκκαίδεκα, Aetius of Amida quotes several passages from the *Theriac to Piso*, a treatise which he attributes to Galen (Annex 1). Since those chapters have not yet received a critical edition, I am quoting them from the Florence manuscript *Laurentianus Plut.* 75, 7 (12th c.), f. 23v, in which the passage about theriac (chapter 87) starts with an introduction where he clearly refers to Galen:

> ἀρκτέον δὲ ἀπὸ τῆς δι᾿ ἐχιδνῶν θηριακῆς Ἀνδρομάχου, ἣν καὶ ὁ Γαληνὸς θαυμάζει περὶ ἧς τάδε γράφει· πολλῆς οὔσης διαφωνίας περὶ γραφὰς τῆς θηριακῆς ἡμεῖς τῇ Ἀνδρομάχου ὡς ἀρίστῃ χρώμεθα καὶ εἰς τὰς βασιλικὰς χρείας οὕτως σκευάζεται.

> It is necessary to begin with the theriac of Andromachus, made with vipers, since Galen himself admires it and writes the following about it: 'since theriac recipes differ greatly, we use Andromachus' as the best, and this is how it is prepared for imperial usage: (...)'[1]

This sentence is taken directly from the *De theriaca ad Pisonem* (ch. XII.23 = XIV, 262 K.; ed. B-M, p. 63):

> τοσαύτης γὰρ οὔσης τῆς περὶ τὰς γραφὰς διαφορᾶς, ἡμεῖς τῇ τοῦ Ἀνδρομάχου ὡς ἀρίστῃ χρώμεθα, καὶ εἴς γε τὰς βασιλικὰς χρείας οὕτως σκευάζομεν.

This demonstrates that in the 6th c. AD Aetius was already reading the treatise with Galen's name.[2]

---

* Following the completion of this paper, I published *Galien, Thériaque à Pison*, texte établi et traduit par Véronique Boudon-Millot, Paris, CUF, 2016 – all references are to that edition (= ed. B-M).

[1] See the Latin edition given by Cornarius in 1542, p. 713: *Ordiemur autem a theriaca Andromachi ex viperis: Cuius admiratione ductus Galenus haec de ea scribit. Quum multa discordia sit circa theriaces descriptiones, nos Andromachi descriptione ut longe optima utimur, quae etiam in regum usus apparatur.*

[2] This sentence is also cited in the anonymous treatise studied by A. Touwaide (on which see below). Another parallel passage can be found in Julius Africanus' *Cestoi*, 3.31 (a Christian Jew originating from Palestine, c.160–240 AD): the description of the δρύϊνος ὄφις which lives in the roots of the oak. There is no proof that Iulius Africanus drew on the *De theriaca ad Pisonem* (14.234 ed. Kühn) for this. Rather, it is most likely that both authors used a common source.

Another proof of this can be found slightly further down, when Aetius discusses theriac salts. Aetius indeed has drawn most of this chapter 97 (titled ἄλες θηριακοὶ ἐκ τῶν Μαρκιανοῦ οἷς συμφωνεῖ ὁ Γαληνός) from the last two chapters of *De theriaca ad Pisonem* (ch. XVIII and XIX) which he again attributes to Galen.

Paul of Aegina, at the beginning of the 7th c. AD, wherever he quotes the *De theriaca ad Pisonem*, refers to it with the name of Galen: ἐν δὲ τῷ Περὶ τῆς θηριακῆς ὁ Γαληνός φησιν τὴν τρίφυλλον τὴν τῷ ὑακίνθῳ ὁμοίαν etc. (Paulus Aegineta, VII, 3: I.L. Heiberg, CMG IX 2, 1924, p. 257, 23–28). And in the 9th c. AD, Ḥunayn ibn Isḥāq also cites the *De theriaca ad Pisonem* in the *Risāla*: 'His book *De theriaca ad Pisonem*: this book is made of a single section. Ayūb (al-Ruhawī) translated it into Syriac. I think that Yaḥyā Ibn al-Biṭrīq translated it into Arabic. I own a manuscript among my books.' *Risāla* n. 83 = G. Bergsträsser, p. 31; J. C. Lamoreaux, p. 90 § 88). The brevity of this notice, and the fact that Ḥunayn did not himself translate the treatise into Arabic seem to indicate that he may not have considered the *De theriaca ad Pisonem* as authentic.[3]

The extant Arabic translation, albeit attributed to Ḥunayn, is the work of a far less skilled translator. In the only extant Arabic manuscript (*Aya Sofya* 3590; f. 103b–130a), however, the *De theriaca ad Pisonem* is again attributed to Galen (*Kitāb Jālīnūs ilā Fīsūn fī al-tiryāq*).[4]

It is, again, under the name of Galen that the treatise is transmitted in the oldest Greek manuscript, *Laurentianus plut.* 74, 5 of the 12th c.: ΓΑΛΗΝΟΥ ΠΡΟΣ ΠΙΣΩΝΑ ΠΕΡΙ ΤΗΣ ΘΗΡΙΑΚΗΣ ΑΝΤΙΔΟΤΟΥ. The first doubts about the authenticity of the treatise arose in the Renaissance, even though successive editors at the time considered it as authentic. The Zwickau physician Janus Cornarius, in his annotations to the Aldine edition around 1530, takes good care to note about *De Theriaca ad Pamphilianum: non est genuinus Galeni libellus*. But he does not make any such comment about the *De Theriaca ad Pisonem*. The 17th c. editor René Chartier, however, adds in a note (*concisae notae*, tom. XIII, Paris, 1639, p. 1022) that some hold the treatise for inauthentic (*genuinum haud esse Galeni*

---

[3] He however translated some passages (cited by al-Majūsī in his *Kitāb al-malakī*) for his own work on Theriac (*Kitāb al-tiryāq*), now lost.

[4] The editor of the Arabic translation, L. Richter-Bernburg, *Eine arabische Version der pseudo-galenischen Schrift* De theriaca ad Pisonem, diss., Göttingen 1969, p. 42 n. 1, following J. Ilberg (on which see below n. 10), does not consider *Ad Pisonem* as authentic. For the state of the question, see my edition in the CUF, p. LII–LXXIV and also V. Boudon-Millot, 'L'apport des traducteurs arabes dans le débat sur l'authenticité des traités galéniques', in *The impact of Arabic Sciences in Europe and Asia*, Actes of the International Conference (Erlangen, 21–23 January, 2014) organised by Agostino Paravicini Bagliani et Danielle Jacquart, *Micrologus. Nature, Sciences and Medieval Societies*, 24, 2016, pp. 403–423.

foetum), or at least think that it must be a juvenile work (*aut saltem Galenum quo tempore eum conscripsit, adhuc iuuenem extitisse proferunt*). In fact, Chartier is following Mercurialis' judgment in the 1576 Juntine edition, who expresses doubts about the authenticity of the *De Theriaca ad Pisonem* without, however, going as far as to declare it inauthentic against the scholarly tradition.[5]

But ten years earlier, in the 1565 Juntine curated by Gadaldini (vol. VI, p. 89), one could read at the top of Julius Martinus Rota's translation: *Sunt qui negent hunc librum esse Galeni, nec sine causa, Aëtius tamen in capite de Sale Theriaco, citat Galeni verba ex hoc libro desumpta.*

Among the main arguments put forward by scholars, Mercurialis mentions essentially style (*loquendi rationem et stylum libri*) and some discrepancies (*quae… diverso modo citantur*) with the rest of the corpus.[6]

Those, however, as Mercurialis himself notices, are partly subjective arguments that are easily dismissed (*haec omnia argumenta scio facile posse refelli*). Thus Mercurialis concludes with caution that the *De Theriaca ad Pisonem* is probably a juvenile work.[7]

---

[5] Mercurialis (1530–1606) curated the Juntine printed in Venice in 1576–1577. See Mercurialis' judgement on the Juntine of 1576, f. 89rv accessible here: http://www.e-rara.ch/doi/10.3931/e-rara-10392; about this work, see http://www.rechercheisidore.fr/search/resource/?uri=10670/1.zke1x2.

[6] Mercurialis adds the issue of the title (*De theriaca ad Pisonem* in the Greek tradition, but *De theriaca ad Cesarem* for the Arabs), a divergence which however can be easily explained through a misreading in Arabic: see M. Steinschneider, 'Die griechischen Ärzte in arabischen Übersetzungen', in *Virchows Archiv*, 124, 1891, p. 292, nr. 55: https://archive.org/stream/diearabischenue01steigoog#page/n211/

[7] See E. Coturri, *Claudio Galeno. De theriaca ad Pisonem*, Florence, 1959, p. 15. But according to V. Nutton, who once made a case for authenticity, it should rather be a work written in his old age: V. Nutton, 'Galen on Theriac. Problems of Authenticity', in A. Debru (ed.), *Galen on Pharmacology*, Leiden, 1997, pp. 133–151 (esp. pp. 133–134 and p. 151), already Swain, *Hellenism and Empire*, Oxford, 1996, pp. 368–72. But see also V. Nutton, 'The Seeds of Disease: an Explanation of Contagion and Infection from the Greeks to the Renaissance', Medical History 27, 1983, pp. 1–34 where he notes p. 6: 'a possibly suppositious work, *On theriac, for Piso*, whose author ascribed the destructiveness of plague to the inspiration of "something deadly" in the air. But both authorship and text are too uncertain to be relied upon for an opinion of Galen, and, typical of medical authors, the passage does not give any clear idea of the way in which the bad air was actually bad, whether it was changed qualitatively or now contained extraneous matter such as seeds or poisons.' At n. 21, Nutton specifies: 'Galen, *On theriac for Piso* 16: XIV 281 K. For the date, not before AD 198, cf. the reference to joint emperors at 1: XIV 212 K. It is assumed genuine by A. v. Premerstein, 'Das Troiaspiel', *Festschrift O. Benndorf*, Vienna, 1898, pp. 261–266, but it has long been considered spurious, cf. L. Richter-Bernburg, *Eine arabische Version der pseudogalenischen Schrift De Theriaca ad Pisonem*, Diss., Göttingen, 1969, p. 42. The question deserves further investigation, for the biographical details fit a court doctor active among the Roman aristocracy'. Against authenticity, see *Claudii Galeni Chronologicum Elogium, R.P. Philippo Labbeo Scriptore, cum Iacobi Mentelii V.C. ad*

It is now time to examine what is known with certainty about this treatise, before trying to bring plausible arguments for or against its authenticity. One thing is certain: as demonstrated by Vivian Nutton, the date of the treatise lies between 204 and 211.[8] The redaction of the *De Theriaca ad Pisonem* is indeed posterior to 204, date of the *Lusus Troiae* mentioned at the beginning of the treatise, and prior to 211, date of Septimius Severus's death. An allusion at the beginning of the *De Theriaca ad Pisonem* to 'the very great current emperors' (ἐπὶ δὲ τῶν νῦν μεγίστων αὐτοκρατόρων) and to Antipater (mentioned at II, 13 – XIV, 218 K.; ed. B-M, p. 9), in fact Aelius Antipater of Hierapolis, secretary *ab epistulis graecis*, allows us to date the redaction of the treatise to the reign of Septimius Severus, in the period when he shared the Empire with his two sons Caracalla (196) and Geta (198), before his own death in 211 and Antipater's fall from grace.[9] This point is not in question. J. Ilberg himself, while locating Galen's death in 199, had already indicated in a *Rheinisches Museum* article from 1896, that the *De Theriaca ad Pisonem* had been composed under Septimius Severus, shortly after the authentic *De antidotis* ('nicht viel später als die eben besprochenen verfasst zu sein scheint'), and that for obvious chronological reasons it could not be by Galen. But Ilberg had at the same time dismissed any in depth study about the *De Theriaca ad Pisonem*.[10] Therefore, without questioning the date proposed by Nutton, it seems that it is time to explore the issue a little further.

Among the main arguments likely to put the authenticity of the treatise in doubt, I will mention briefly the excessively deferential tone of the author towards the emperors and the gods, the many anecdotes (stories of Cleopatra

eundem Epistola Galen (Paris, Claude Cramoisy, 1660, pp. 22–35 on *Theriac to Piso*). His conclusions were accepted by J.C. Gottlieb Ackermann in the *Historia literaria* printed in Kühn, vol. I, p. CLVI; see also the discussion at *Vita Galeni* pp. XXXI-XXXVIII.

[8] More precise dates, between 204 and 211, have been suggested. According to V. Nutton, 'Galen on Theriac ...', p. 150, the most accurate date could be 207: 'A date of composition for the *Ad Pisonem* of around 206–7 would seem most likely, long enough after the *Lusus Troiae* but before the downfall of Antipater, although an even later date before 211 cannot be excluded.' Identifying the games which Piso's son attended with the *Lusus Troiae* of 204, as suggested by V. Nutton, remains difficult. The date of 204 however was again favoured by R. Leigh, *On Theriac to Piso, attributed to Galen*, Leiden, 2016, p. 18 with an additional argument: Septimius Severus, he argues, did not settle in Rome until 204, and it is unlikely that such a ceremony took place in his absence. Nevertheless, the only indisputable historical landmarks are 198 (when Septimius Severus associates Caracalla to the Empire) and 211 (Septimius Severus dies, and Geta is assassinated).

[9] Antipater complained to Caracalla over Geta's assassination at the end of 211.

[10] J. Ilberg, 'Über die Schriftstellerei des Klaudios Galenos. III', *Rheinisches Museum*, 51, 1896, p. 193.

and Mithridates),[11] the excessively long catalogue of diseases that theriac cures (ch. XV), and the strange legend according to which Hippocrates had the idea of lighting fires to remove the plague.[12] All this has already been noted and dismissed as more or less conclusive.[13] In order to rest on more solid ground, as represented by style and vocabulary, I will simply mention four examples taken from four categories of words: adverbs, verbs, adjectives and nouns.

Adverbs: they appear in very high numbers; many are *hapax legomena* in the Galenic corpus or absolute *hapax legomena*, while others appear only in inauthentic works:

- Examples of *hapax legomena* in the Galenic corpus (adverbs in *Ad Pisonem* absent from the rest of the *corpus*): ἐνθέσμως (ch. II. 7 = XIV, 216 K.; ed. B-M, p. 8); παιδαριωδῶς (ch. IIIB. 6 = XIV, 224 K.; ed. B-M, p. 14); ἀπταίστως (ch. V. 3 = XIV, 230 K.; ed. B-M, p. 20); φιλοκάλως (ch. II. 12 = XIV, 218, 5 K.; ed. B-M, p. 9); ἱστορικῶς (ch. XV. 18 = XIV, 275, 8 K.; ed. B-M, p. 76); ἀπερισκέπτως (ch. XVI. 4 = XIV, 278, 15 K.; ed. B-M, p. 79); ἀτερπῶς (ch. VIII.14 = XIV, 237 K.; ed. B-M, p. 39).
- Examples of adverbs found only in inauthentic works: φιλαλήθως (2 occurrences ch. IIIB. 6 et 7 = XIV, 224 K.; ed. B-M, p. 14 + *Def. med.* XIX, 348, 2 K.); εὐπρεπῶς (ch. VIII. 11 = XIV, 236, 1 K.; ed. B-M, p. 38 + *De fasciis*, XVIIIA, 771, 14 K.)
- Example of absolute *hapax legomenon*: ἀκνίσως (ch. XIII. 14 = XIV, 266 K.; ed. B-M, p. 67) 'without odour or smoke'.[14]

The **noun** σύγκρισις is used five times in the *Theriac to Piso* with the sense of κατασκευή (itself being used only twice) to designate the body constitution, while σύγκρισις is used only eight times in the rest of the corpus with a different meaning: aggregation of atoms (in the context of the polemics with Epicurus' and Democritus' disciples).

The **verb** εὔχομαι (two occurrences in the whole corpus) is used towards the end of the treatise to ask the gods to grant health to Piso (ch. XIX. 16 = XIV, 294

---

[11] V. Boudon-Millot, 'Du nouveau sur la mort de Cléopâtre: au croisement de l'histoire des textes et de l'histoire de l'art', *REG* 128–2, 2015, pp. 331–353.

[12] J. Jouanna, *Hippocrate*, Paris, 1992, p. 53 and p. 585 n. 34 and 35. The confusion, in *Ad Pisonem*, between the Northern pestilence and that which struck Athens in 430 does not fit Galen. In fact, it is a strong argument against authenticity.

[13] V. Nutton, 'Galen on Theriac … ', p. 151.

[14] Not ἀκνίστως as in XI, 266, 13 K.: ἀκνίσως is the reading in L, ἀκνίστως a correction in the Aldine.

K.; ed. B-M, p. 95: παρὰ τῶν θεῶν εὔχομαι), a prayer of which no other example is to be found in the corpus.

The **adjective** θεῖος is used to qualify the emperor Marcus Aurelius (ch. II. 7 = XIV, 216, 14 K.; ed. B-M, p. 8: τὸν θεῖον Μάρκον); but this adjective, which is rarely used in the Galenic corpus, is only used by Galen to qualify Hippocrates (5 occurrences), Homer (1 occurrence) and Plato (2 occurrences).[15]

While it is difficult to imagine Galen, even in his old age, praying to the gods for his dedicatee's health, it is even more difficult to imagine him this gullible. Indeed the author of the *Theriac to Piso* repeatedly uses phrases such as φασι/φασιν (220, 232, 234, 235 [3 times]; 238; 240; 243; 244; 283 =; ed. B-M, p. 11, 21, 35, 37, 40, 42, 46, 84); ὡς φασιν (233; ed. B-M, p. 35); ἔτι τὸ θαυμασιώτερόν φασιν (234; ed. B-M, p. 36) and all kinds of stories: τὸ αὐτὸ ἱστορεῖσθαι λέγουσι (244; ed. B-M, p. 47); καί φησί τις ἀρχαῖος λόγος (244; ed. B-M, p. 47); ἀλλ᾽ οὗτος ὁ λόγος οὐ δοκεῖ μοι αὐτάρκης εἶναι (245; ed. B-M, p. 47). Thus he does not shy away from giving credit to the strange story according to which a female bear gives birth to a shapeless mass of flesh that she then shapes up into a bear cub with her tongue (ch. XI. 15 = XIV, 254–255 K.; ed. B-M, p. 55).

> τίνα δ᾽ οὐ πείθει λέγειν θαυμάσιόν τι χρῆμα τὴν φύσιν ὑπάρχειν ὁρῶντα τὸ ὑπὸ τῆς ἄρκτου γιγνόμενον ἔργον; ἀποτίκτει μὲν γὰρ ἡ ἄρκτος ἅπασι τοῖς γεννωμένοις ὁμοίως ζῴοις. ἔστι δὲ σὰρξ μόνη γεννωμένη ἄπλαστός τε καὶ ἀδιάρθρωτος, μορφὴν μὲν οὐδεμίαν ἔχουσα, εὐθὺς δὲ ὑπὸ τῆς γεννώσης τῇ φυσικῇ τέχνῃ διατυπουμένη. τῇ γὰρ γλώττῃ ὥσπερ χειρί τινι χρωμένη ἡ τεκοῦσα οὕτω μεμορφωμένον ζῷον τὸ τεχθὲν ἀποτελεῖ.

> For who will not concede that nature is a wonderful thing, upon seeing the miracle accomplished by the she-bear? For the she-bear gives birth just as all engendered animals do. But it is only flesh that is engendered, without any shape or articulations, and having no form, but it immediately receives an imprint from she who engendered it through the art of nature. For with her tongue, which she uses as she would a hand, the mother finishes what she engendered into a fully formed animal.

But how can we be certain that Galen did not believe this legend (also mentioned by Pliny, Ovid and Aulus Gellius)?[16] Galen, as it happens, mentions it in the *De compositione medicamentorum secundum locos* I, 2 (Kühn XII, 425–426), in order to dismiss it. The narrative occurs in a totally different context, about a prescription against premature baldness. The recipe was given to Galen by a friend of his,

---

[15] V. Boudon-Millot, 'Le divin Hippocrate de Galien', in J. Jouanna and M. Zink (eds.), *Hippocrate et les hippocratismes: médecine, religion, société*, Actes du XIVe colloque hippocratique de Paris (8–10 novembre 2012), Paris, AIBL, coll. "Colloques", 2014, pp. 253–269.

[16] Pliny, *Nat. hist.* VIII, 126 and Ovid, *Met.* XV, 379.

named Claudius, who wrote it up in in the form of a riddle (424, 2 συμβολικῶς). Galen thus sets out to find the key to the riddle. One of the ingredients is called 'fat of shapeless foetus' (423, 2 βρέφους ἀμόρφου στέατος), a phrase that Galen proposes to interpret as referring to the shapeless cub of the she-bear (425, 16–18 βρέφους δ'ἀμόρφου δοκεῖ μοι λέγειν τῆς ἄρκτου). Indeed, Galen explains, 'people say that the she-bear gives birth to a shapeless being, like a chunk of flesh, but that the mother, in licking it, gives it a shape' (425–426: αὐτὴν γὰρ φασιν ἀποκυΐσκεσθαι μὲν ἄμορφον, ὡσανεὶ σαρκῶδές τι μέρος. ἐκλειχούσης δὲ τοῦτο τῆς μητρὸς διαμορφοῦσθαι τὸ ζῷον). But while the author of *Ad Pisonem* believes this wonderful tale (using the phrase τίνα δ' οὐ πείθει), Galen in the *De compositione medicamentorum secundum locos*, using the verb φασιν, distances himself from this story which he cannot believe: βρέφους δ'ἀμόρφου δοκεῖ μοι λέγειν τῆς ἄρκτου. ταύτην γὰρ φασιν ἀποκυΐσκεσθαι μὲν ἄμορφον, ὡσανεὶ σαρκῶδές τι μέρος ἐκλειχούσης δὲ τοῦτο τῆς μητρὸς διαμορφοῦσθαι τὸ ζῷον.

Even better, the author of *Ad Pisonem* (henceforth Pseudo-Galen) mentions among various snakes the basilisk (ch. VIII. 3 = XIV, 233–234 K.; ed. B-M, p. 35), which he describes as follows:

ὁ μὲν γὰρ βασιλίσκος, ἔστι δὲ τὸ θηρίον ὑπόξανθον καὶ ἐπὶ τῇ κεφαλῇ τρεῖς ὑπεροχὰς ἔχον, ὥς φασιν, καὶ ὅτι ὁραθεὶς μόνον καὶ συρίττων ἀκουσθεὶς ἀναιρεῖ τοὺς ἀκούσαντας καὶ τοὺς ἰδόντας αὐτόν· καὶ ὅτι τῶν ἄλλων ζῴων, εἴ τι καὶ ἅψαιτο τοῦ ζῴου ἀνηρημένου, καὶ αὐτὸ τελευτᾷ εὐθέως, καὶ διὰ τοῦτο πᾶν αὐτοῦ τὸ γένος τῶν ἄλλων θηρίων ἐγγὺς εἶναι φυλάττεται.

The basilisk, for example, is a yellowish beast with three projections (horns?) on the head, they say. And also, that seeing it and hearing its hissing is enough to kill those who heard and saw it. And that if any other animal touches it when it is dead, it also dies instantly, and that, for that reason, every other type of beast keeps away from it.

The author of *Ad Pisonem* does not express any doubt about the existence of this fabulous animal described by Nicander, *Theriaca* 396ff. (ed. J.-M. Jacques, Paris, CUF, 2002, p. 32–33 and comm., p. 130–134) as the 'king of reptiles', with the power of killing those who simply saw or heard it. Things are very different with Galen, who, in *Simple drugs* X, 1 (XII, 250, 14 K.), clearly expresses his skepticism:

βασιλίσκον μὲν γὰρ τὸ θηρίον οὐδὲ εἶδον οὐδέποτε, καὶ εἰ ἀληθῆ τὰ λεγόμενα περὶ αὐτοῦ, κινδυνῶδές ἐστι καὶ τὸ πλησίον ἀφικέσθαι τῷ ζῴῳ τούτῳ.

The basilisk snake I have never seen and if what is said about it is true, it is dangerous even to come near this animal.

19

A few lines down (XII, 251, 8 K.), Galen adds that, as far as he is concerned, he will not mention any animal that he has never seen himself:

ἐγὼ τοίνυν οὔτε βασιλίσκων οὔτε ἐλεφάντων οὔθ᾽ ἵππων Νειλώων οὔτ᾽ ἄλλου τινὸς οὗ μὴ πεῖραν αὐτὸς ἔχω μνημονεύσω.

As far as I'm concerned, I will not mention basilisks, elephants, hippopotamuses ('Nile horses') or any other animal of which I have no experience.

It would thus be very curious that Galen broke his promise and, in addition, took the time to describe with such precision (colour, shape of the head, hiss) the snake he had never seen.[17]

Even more surprising, Pseudo-Galen, from ch. X (XIV, 246 K. ff.; ed. B-M, pp. 48ff.) recommends a number of 'magical' remedies (a term I am using here with quotation marks and all due precautions).[18] Some of these remedies, sounding exotic and perhaps Egyptian (made with hippopotamus, crocodile or cobra) are also mentioned by Pliny the Elder (*Hist. Nat.* XXIX), who attributes to them an eastern origin going back to the *Magi*. Pseudo-Galen mentions here remedies made from scorpions, weasels, worms, burnt flies' or kites' heads, camels, swallows or sheep's brain, ox or mouse dung, some of which Galen explicitly stigmatised.[19] But, even more puzzling, those remedies, most of which are absent from the rest of the Galenic corpus, have many parallels with the *Cyranides*, a compilation of medical treatises gathered between the 1st and 4th c. (see table 2).[20] When, by chance, Galen mentions one of those remedies, it is to dismiss

---

[17] In his *Anat. adm.* (II, 548, 16 K.), Galen again mentions the elephant and the hippopotamus as the most remote animals from man (τῶν ἐπιπλέον ἀφεστώτων ἀνθρώπου φύσεως). He also mentions several times the elephant (whose heart he would dissect at Rome). He mentions hippopotamus skin only once (ἱπποποτάμου δέρμα, XII, 409, 4 K.), in a recipe from Archigenes against alopecia. Elsewhere he states that the products from this animal are too rare and too difficult to procure to be recommended.

[18] Paul T. Keyser, 'Science and Magic in Galen's Recipes (Sympathy and Efficacy)', in A. Debru (ed.), *op. cit.*, pp. 175–198, esp. p. 195: 'if magic be defined ... as 'excluded practices depending for their efficacy on powers in the world beyond human understanding''.

[19] Those animal remedies of magical origin, for which there is no parallel in the Galenic corpus, have been cited by Maimonides in the 12th c. in his *Medical Aphorisms* (he used the Arabic translation of *Theriac, to Piso*). Some of those remedies have been in use until the 14th c. at least. See G. Bos, 'R. Moshe Narboni: Philosopher and Physician, a critical analysis of Sefer Oraḥ Ḥayyim', *Medieval Encounters* 1, 2, 1995, pp. 219–251.

[20] The *Cyranides* are a compilation of texts attributed to Hermes Trismegistus, reworked by Harpocration of Alexandria in the 4th c. 'la première rédaction, hermétique, de la *Kyranis* doit remonter au plus tard au IIIᵉ siècle de notre ère', and the second part, the *Koiranides*, could date back 'au moins à la fin du 1ᵉʳ siècle de notre ère', according to A.-J. Festugière, *La révélation d'Hermès Trismégiste*, t. I: *L'astrologie et les sciences occultes* (1944), Paris, 1981, pp. 201–210 (pp. 205 and 210).

them or specify that he himself has never used them (see table 3). Such is the case of mouse dung recommended by Pseudo-Galen against alopecia, but explicitly criticised by Galen in *Simple drugs* (XII, 307 K.), as a repulsive, ridiculous and useless remedy (Οὕτω γοῦν καὶ τὰ τῶν μυῶν ἀποπατήματα γεγράφασιν ἀλωπεκίας θεραπεύειν, ἔστι γὰρ ὄντως αἰδεθῆναι τὰ τοιαῦτα καὶ εἰς πεῖραν ἄγειν ἁπάντων καταγινωσκόντων ὡς περιέργου τε καὶ γόητος ὃς ἂν ταῦτα πράττῃ τε καὶ λέγῃ).[21] Same thing for weasel brains, recommended by Pseudo-Galen in the treatment of epilepsy (ch. IX.9 = XIV, 240 K.; ed. B-M, p. 42), but which Galen says he has never used (*Simple drugs* XI, 1 = XII, 362, 1 K.): γαλῆν δὲ οὐδέποτε ἐκαύσαμεν.

In the long catalogue of diseases cured by theriac (ch. XV), we find yet further surprises (table n. 4). There can be found almost all the diseases mentioned in the pseudo-Galenic *Introductio sive medicus* ch. XIII, 9 (ed. C. Petit, Paris, CUF, 2009, pp. 51ff.), albeit presented in a different order. Although therapeutics is a much more developed topic in the *Introductio sive medicus* than in our treatise, aetiology and symptomatology are nevertheless very similar, to the point of illuminating many aspects of our treatise that remain allusive in the *Ad Pisonem*. The authors of *Ad Pisonem* and *Introductio sive medicus* converge especially on the important role devoted to the *pneuma* in explaining diseases. The only two ailments that have no correspondence in the *Introd. s. med.* are menstrual blood (ch. XV. 14) and cachexia (XV. 21). Since the descriptions of all diseases are much more developed in the *Introd. s. med.*, and rather than assuming that the first one could be used as a model for the second, it is most likely that both draw from a common source, such as a catalogue of diseases to which doctors were used to browsing for reference.

Even more unimaginable, how could Galen write the *Ad Pisonem*, when so many passages conflict with the rest of the corpus?

The recipe of the theriac, the choice of the ingredients and how to prepare it, as they are described in *Ad Pisonem*, offer many major contradictions with those given by Galen in *De antidotis*. It would be necessary to go over each of the many steps in this complex preparation to show this in detail, but here is a summary of those remarks:

The text we read today is neither the original nor Harpocration's but a Byzantine reworking which took place between the 4th and the 8th c. See also P. Tannery, 'Les Cyranides', *Revue des études grecques*, 17, 1904, pp. 335–349.

[21] Galen devotes two long chapter to alopecia (*Comp. med. sec. locos* I, 1 et 2: XII, 379–421 K.) and cites elsewhere about ten ingredients as effective against this ailment (*Simple drugs*: XI, 879, 885, 863, 874 and XII, 217, 327, 331 K.), but he never mentions this recipe based on mouse dung. See Paul T. Keyser, *loc. cit.*, p. 193.

- The first difference concerns the order of preparation in the recipe: while Galen in the *De antidotis* gives first the recipe of viper pastilles (I, 8: Kühn XIV, 45–49), then that of squill pastilles (I, 9: K. XIV, 49–51) and finally that of *hèduchroon* (I, 10: K. XIV, 51–54), the author of *Ad Pisonem* follows the reverse order and starts with the recipe of *hèduchroon* (ch. XIII. 1–3), then of squill pastilles (4–6), and finally that of viper pastilles (7–18). The two authors differ especially about the *hèduchroon* recipe, a scented ointment of which each accepts a different version, in verse in *De antidotis*, in prose in *Ad Pisonem*, and with or without *marum*.[22]
- They also differ on the best season to hunt vipers (beginning of spring for Pseudo-Galen, beginning of summer for Galen).[23]
- They differ about the names of ingredients forming the recipe, especially the country names from which they originate. Thus Pseudo-Galen mentions nard as 'Celtic', but in *De antidotis* (ms. L), *diktamnon* and *polion* are Cretan, nard is Indian or Celtic, *phou* is from Pontus and honey from Attica.[24] Indian nard even has two different names: ναρδοστάχυος in Pseudo-Galen, and νάρδου Ἰνδικοῦ in Galen's *De antidotis*.[25]
- Pseudo-Galen follows closely Dioscorides for the description of the various ingredients included in the composition of theriac, and clearly distinguishes, just like him, cinnamon and cassia (τὸ κινάμωμον and ἡ κασσία), unlike Galen, who, in *De antidotis* I, 14 (Kühn XIV, 69–73), reunites in the same category of medicines (ταὐτοῦ γένους ἐστίν) those two ingredients, which

[22] Galen, at *Antidotes* I, 10, gives a simplified recipe for *hèduchroon* which, in terms of ingredients and dosage, differs greatly from *Ad Pisonem*. Thus Galen adds *marum*, a kind of oregano (absent from Ps.-Galen), but Ps.-Galen adds marjoram: he thus fits the category of those mentioned by Galen when he states that 'some recipes have neither marjoram nor *marum*, while others have either of them' (XIV, 53: τινὲς δ' οὐδ' ὅλως ἔχουσι τὸ ἀμάρακον καὶ τὸ μάρον, ἔνιαι δὲ τὸ ἕτερον αὐτῶν ἔχουσαι μόνον).

[23] Galen, *Simple drugs* XI, 1 (XII, 318–319 K.) states that viper pastilles must be prepared at the beginning of the summer, when their flesh is best (τούτους μὲν οὖν εἰσβάλλοντος τοῦ θέρους σκευάζομεν, ἡνίκα μάλιστα βελτίστη τῶν ἐχιδνῶν ἐστιν ἡ σάρξ).

[24] In Arabic, nard is Celtic, *phou* is Cretan, gum and acacia are Arabic, cardamom is Indian (the translator read ἰνδαῖον instead of ἰδαῖον, cf. *Th. to Piso* VII. 18: Ἰδαῖον κραδάμωμον).

[25] Two kinds of nard are mentioned (v. 146: καὶ νάρδου, Γαλάτης ἣν ἐκόμισσεν ἀνήρ), which correspond to Celtic nard (νάρδου Κελτικῆς) and Indian fragrant nard in the prose recipes (v. 133: Ἰνδήν τε βάλοις εὐώδεα νάρδον). The latter corresponds to the spike of nard, ναρδοστάχυος, a word found in Paul of Aegina and rendered in Arabic as Indian nard. Galen however, in *De antidotis*, mentions here (in MS. L) νάρδου Ἰνδικοῦ. See *Ad Glauc.* (VI, 339, 4 K.): Galen makes a clear distinction between the two kinds of nard (Indian and Celtic), and the spike of nard from which myrrh is prepared: καὶ νάρδων ἀμφοτέρων Ἰνδικῆς τε καὶ Κελτικῆς, ἔτι δὲ κρόκου καὶ οἰνάνθης καὶ μαστίχης Χίας καὶ μύρων τῶν διὰ ναρδοστάχυος σκευαζομένων.

he sees as interchangeable. Galen even considers that cinammon may come from a change in cassia (καὶ γὰρ καὶ γίνεταί ποτε κιννάμωμον ἐκ μεταβολῆς αὐτῆς) and that stems of the former may grow among those of the latter, so that they seem to be one and the same tree (ὥστε ὅλον μὲν ὁρᾶσθαι τὸ οἷον δένδρον ἀκριβὲς κασσίαν).

– In general, Pseudo-Galen is less accurate than Galen. While Pseudo-Galen is content with noting that it is sufficient to form medium-sized viper trochisks (ἀνάπλασσε συμμέτρους τροχίσκους), Galen recommends to shape tiny tablets (*De antidotis* I, 8 = XIV, 47 K.: κυκλίσκους ἀναπλάττειν λεπτούς) or small light pastilles (*Simple drugs* XI, 1 = XII, 318 K.: μικροὺς ἀρτίσκους λεπτοὺς πλάσαντες) and to use stale bread so that the trochisks may dry up faster and thus avoid putrefaction, without pouring the viper juice on top (οὐχ ὡς οἱ πρὸ ἐμοῦ σκευάζοντες τῷ Καίσαρι συνετίθεσαν, ἐμβρέχοντες αὐτὸν τῷ τῶν ἐχιδνῶν ἀφεψήματι in *De antidotis* I, 8: XIV, 47 K.). Unaware of this precaution, Pseudo-Galen recommends, on the contrary, to pour the cooking stock (παραχέας τὸ αὔταρκες τοῦ ζωμοῦ) upon the pastille and viper flesh.

– Finally, while Ps. Gal. (ch. XIII. 5) recommends preparing the squill pastilles by mixing an equal measure of the best and most recent vetch flour (μίσγοντα καὶ ὀροβίνου ἀλεύρου καλλίστου καὶ νεαρωτάτου τὸ ἴσον), Galen, *De antidotis* I, 9 (XIV, 50 K.) recommends using one and a half more squill than flour, that is to say two measures of squill for one of flour (τῷ σταθμῷ δὲ ἡμιολίαν εἶναι χρὴ τὴν σκίλλαν. λέγω δὲ ἡμιολίαν, ὡς δύο μὲν ἀλεύρου μοίρας εἶναι, τρεῖς δὲ τῆς σκίλλης). It would be easy to give many more examples of different dosage.

Finally, it is really difficult to imagine Galen forfeiting his love for his dear Asian homeland, especially his native city of Pergamon. But one of the anecdotes in *Ad Pisonem* (ch. V. 5–7) is quite harsh about one of its kings (ch. V. 5–7 = K. XIV, 231; ed. B-M, p. 20):

ἐμοὶ δὲ καὶ ἐξ ἱστορίας τις ἐμήνυσε λόγος ὡς ἄρα πολεμεῖν Ῥωμαίοις τις ἐθέλων καὶ τὸ δυνατὸν ἐκ τῆς στρατιωτικῆς τάξεως οὐκ ἔχων, ἄνθρωπος δέ, φησίν, ὁ Καρχηδόνιος οὗτος, ἐμπλήσας πολλὰς χύτρας θηρίων τῶν ἀναιρεῖν ὀξέως δυναμένων, οὕτως αὐτὰς προσέβαλε πρὸς τοὺς πολεμίους. οἱ δὲ τὸ πεμπόμενον οὐ νοοῦντες καὶ διὰ τοῦτ' ἀφύλακτοι μένοντες, οὐ γὰρ ἦν τοιαῦτα εἰθισμένα ἐν τοῖς πολεμίοις πέμπεσθαι βέλη, ταχέως πίπτοντες ἀπέθνησκον· καὶ διὰ τοῦτο πολλάκις ὁ ἄνθρωπος οὗτος τῇ τοιαύτῃ πρὸς τὸ πολεμεῖν πανουργίᾳ, ὥσπερ τι καὶ αὐτὸς θηρίον ὑπάρχων, διέφυγε τῶν ἐναντίων τὰς χεῖρας.

A historical narrative revealed to me that a man, who wanted to fight against the Romans but did not have the power to do so from his military resources, this man, they say, a Carthaginian, had many jars filled with beasts capable of killing fast, and threw them at his enemies. As they were unaware of what was directed at them, and for that reason failing to protect themselves (for it was not a common kind of missile directed during hostilities), they fell rapidly and died. And thus this man escaped the hands of his enemies many times through the same trick, as though he were himself a beast.

The Carthaginian is Hannibal (247–183), son of Hamilcar, who beat Eumenes II of Pergamon (an ally of Rome) in a naval battle in 184 sometimes referred to as 'the first biological war', by throwing at his enemies terracotta jars filled with deadly snakes.[26] But it is more than unlikely that Galen, who was so in love with his homeland, should record such a painful memory of his compatriot Eumenes.

Even more surprising, and I will conclude with this example, how could we imagine that Galen, so proud of his technique and so convinced of his superiority, could concede having caused, even by force, the death of a child through a higher dose of theriac? (ch. XVII. 7–9 = K. XIV, 286–287; ed. B-M, pp. 86–87)

ἐγὼ γοῦν ἱστόρησα διαλυθέν ποτε παιδίον ὑπὸ τῆς ἀκαίρου τῆς ἀντιδότου χρήσεως. τὸ μὲν γὰρ ἐπύρεττε χρονίως καὶ ἦν ἰσχνὸν αὐτῷ πάνυ τὸ σῶμα καὶ τὴν δύναμιν ἀσθενές, μόλις δὲ καὶ διὰ πολλῆς ἐπιμελείας διαζῆν δυνάμενον, ἅπερ ἐγὼ μὲν συνορῶν ἐκ τοῦ ἰατρικοῦ λογισμοῦ καὶ πάνυ διεκώλυον αὐτῷ δίδοσθαι τοῦ φαρμάκου. κηδόμενος γάρ τις αὐτοῦ καὶ πατὴρ εἶναι δῆθεν λέγων καὶ τυραννικὴν ἐξουσίαν τοῦ κελεύειν ἔχων μᾶλλον ἤπερ τὴν ἐκ τοῦ λόγου συμβουλίαν ἀκούων ἀλόγως καὶ μετὰ πολλῆς ἀνάγκης ἐξηνάγκασέ με τοῦ φαρμάκου διδόναι τῷ παιδίῳ. τὸ δὲ ληφθὲν μὲν οὐκ ἠδυνήθη πεφθῆναι· κρεῖττον γὰρ ἦν τῆς ἰσχύος τοῦ λαμβάνοντος· διέλυσε γὰρ αὐτοῦ τὴν σύμπασαν ἕξιν καὶ τὴν γαστέρα ῥεῖν ἐποίησε, καὶ οὕτω διὰ τὴν ἄλογον τοῦ φαρμάκου χρῆσιν νύκτωρ ἀπώλετο τὸ παιδίον.

And indeed I once experienced a child whose body relaxed over an inappropriate use of the medicine: he suffered from chronic fever, had a very thin and weak body, and was just able to remain alive through abundant care. When I saw that, judging from my medical reasoning, I prevented the medicine being given to him. But someone who cared for him and claiming he was his father, but who displayed a tyrannical authority for giving orders rather than listening to sound advice, against all reason and with much insistence forced me to give the medicine to the child. But the medicine could not be concocted, for it was stronger than the patient's strength. Indeed, it relaxed his entire bodily state and caused an intestinal flow. And this is how, because of the irrational use of the medicine, the child died during the night.

---

[26] See Cornelius Nepos (c. 100–29), *Vit. Hann.* (c. X–XI) in Cornelius Nepos, *Vitae cum fragmentis*, edidit Peter K. Marshall, Münich and Leipzig, 2001, pp. 84–85.

It would be really astonishing that Galen, who boasts of never having experienced a death among the gladiators under his care in his second term, should concede here that he had been responsible for the death of a child.[27] The Arabic translator was obviously disturbed by this narrative, which he modified and translated as follows: 'the father forced the child to take the poison'. Similarly, Niccolò da Reggio (to whom the older Latin translation is attributed) absolves the author of the treatise, and blames instead the other physicians: *unde ego quidem prohibens dare pueri eius, medici dantes ei de ipso farmaco interfecerunt eum.*[28]

It is time to conclude. What can we say about the authorship of *Ad Pisonem* and the date around which it entered the Galenic corpus? The author who speaks about the Romans in the second or third person (284; ed. B-M, p. 84 ὁπότε γὰρ πολεμῶν πρὸς τοὺς Ῥωμαίους et 232; ed. B-M, p. 20 ὑμῖν τοῖς ὑπερέχουσι καὶ τοῖς τῶν στρατοπέδων ἄρχουσιν) is most likely a Greek. He is also probably an *archiatros*, who locates himself in a lineage of such *archiatroi* who are named (ch. XII. 18–23; ed. B-M, pp. 61–63 Andromachos, Damocrates, Magnos and Demetrios) and prepares theriac for the emperors (εἴς γε τὰς βασιλικὰς χρείας οὕτως σκευάζομεν). He has also stayed at Alexandria, where he has witnessed convicts condemned to death killed by snakes (ch. VIII.15 = XIV, 237 K.; ed. B-M, pp. 39–40). He shares the same Hippocratic background as Galen, to whom he is chronologically very close, as we have seen (early 3rd c. AD). But when he happens to quote the same Hippocratic passages as Galen, he adopts different readings, which may show that he used a different text, for which he even provides a different interpretation than that offered by the Pergamene in his commentaries.[29]

Thus, if, as I think, Galen is not the author of *Ad Pisonem*, it becomes easier to understand why the long verse recipe of Andromachos' theriac is found twice in the Galenic corpus, once in *De antidotis*, once in *Ad Pisonem*. The existence of a specific literature on theriac, highly developed at that time, invites us, in turn, to reconsider Galen's importance in the field, since he was not the only one to have written on this topic.

[27] See Galen, *Opt. med. cogn.* 4 (CMG *Suppl. Orient.* IV, pp. 103–105).

[28] V. Boudon-Millot, 'La traduction latine de la *Thériaque à Pison* attribuée à Nicolas de Reggio', *Medicina nei Secoli*, Nuova serie Vol. 25–N° 3, 2013, pp. 979–1010. I called F MS. Cesena, *Malat.* S.XXVII.4, (14th c.), which is much superior to MS. *Malat.* S. V. 4, 14th c. (= C); MS. *Malat.* S.XXVI.4 (15th c.) (= E) and MS. *Vaticanus Pal. lat.* 1211, 14th c. (= V).

[29] V. Boudon-Millot, 'Dialogues between Galen and Ps.-Galen (*Epidémies* 2, 3, 2 et *Aphorismes* 4, 5)', in P. Pormann (ed.), *The Hippocratic Corpus and its Commentators: East and West*, Proceedings of the 15th Hippocratic Colloquium (Manchester, 28 to 30 October 2015), forthcoming.

One last question remains to be solved. When did the treatise *Ad Pisonem* become part of the Galenic corpus? This must have happened between the end of the 3rd c. AD and the beginning of the 6th c. AD, when Aetius of Amida quotes *Ad Pisonem* as Galen's, which probably explains why the medical tradition widely accepted Galen as the author of this work. In any case, the fact that this treatise entered the Galenic corpus at such an early stage determined its fortune, since it was translated into Syriac, and then, in the 9th c., into Arabic, and then again into Latin by Niccolò da Reggio in the 14th c. Widely quoted as early as the Byzantine period, it was also read by Rhazes in the 9th c., Maimonides in the 12th c., and is still quoted and used by the Jewish physician Moses ben Joshua in the 14th c.

To sum up, the author of *Ad Pisonem*, probably an archiatros of the early 3rd c. AD, used among his sources a compilation of magical medicine close to the extant *Cyranides*, and a catalogue of diseases similar to that once used by the author of the *Introd. S. med.* But more importantly, the author of *Ad Pisonem* differs radically from Galen in his medical and pharmacological practice, when preparing the theriac, selecting ingredients, or defining doses, not to speak of the strange anecdotes among which he does not shy away from showing his homeland in a bad light (Hannibal's stories) or himself (death of a young child). For all those reasons, it seems very difficult to me to consider the *De theriaca ad Pisonem* as authentic.

Annexes

1. Passages of Aetius taken from *De theriaca ad Pisonem*

Aetius, Book XIII in *Laurentianus plut.* 75, 7 (*uersio latina* in Cornarius, 1542, pp. 713–722)	*De theriaca ad Pisonem* (ed. V. Boudon-Millot, Paris, 2016, CUF, p. 63ff.)
ch. 87 (f. 23v) Introduction (f. 23v) ἀρκτέον δὲ ἀπὸ τῆς δι' ἐχιδνῶν θηριακῆς Ἀνδρομάχου, ἣν καὶ ὁ Γαληνὸς θαυμάζει περὶ ἧς τάδε γράφει. πολλῆς οὔσης διαφωνίας περὶ γραφὰς τῆς θηριακῆς ἡμεῖς τῇ Ἀνδρομάχου ὡς ἀρίστῃ χρώμεθα καὶ εἰς τὰς βασιλικὰς χρείας οὕτως σκευάζεται.	ch. XII. 23 (Kühn XIV, 262; ed. B-M, p. 63): τοσαύτης γὰρ οὔσης τῆς περὶ τὰς γραφὰς διαφορᾶς, ἡμεῖς τῇ τοῦ Ἀνδρομάχου ὡς ἀρίστῃ χρώμεθα, καὶ εἴς γε τὰς βασιλικὰς χρείας οὕτως σκευάζομεν.
ch. 88 Preparation of the breads of squill (f. 23v)	ch. XIII. 4–6
ch. 89 Preparation of heduchroon (f. 24r)	ch. XIII. 1–3
ch. 90 Preparation of the breads of viper (f. 24r)	ch. XIII. 7–18
ch. 91 Other ingredients added in the theriac and Andromachus' recipe (f. 25v)	ch. XII. 12–17
ch. 92 Preparation of the antidote (f. 26r)	ch. XIV. 1–4
ch. 93 From when can you use the theriac (f. 27r)	ch. XIV. 5
ch. 94 For how long is theriac effective (f. 27r)	ch. XIV. 6
ch. 95 How to check theriac is still efective (f. 27v)	ch. XIV. 7
ch. 96 Which theriac dose is to be used, in what form and against which diseases and the story of Mithridates (f. 27v)	ch. XIV. 8 (doses) and 9 (against which diseases) + ch. XV and XVI (the story of Mithridates)
ch. 97 Theriac salts from Marcianus and Galen (f. 30r) ἅλες θηριακοὶ ἐκ τῶν Μαρκιανοῦ οἷς συμφωνεῖ ὁ Γαληνός	ch. XVIII and XIX

2. Magical remedies offering parallels with the *Cyranides*

Ps.-Galen in *De theriaca ad Pisonem* (ed. V. Boudon-Millot, Paris, CUF, 2016)	*Cyranides* (ed. D. Kaimakis, *Die Kyraniden*, Meisenheim am Glan, 1976)
ch. IX. 8 (K. XIV, 240; ed. B-M, p. 42): ἐνίοις γοῦν βοηθοῦσιν αἱ κεφαλαὶ τῶν μυιῶν, καυθεῖσαι γὰρ καὶ μετὰ μέλιτος χριόμεναι, τὰς ἀλωπεκίας ἰᾶσθαι δύνανται.	III, 28, 2 (p. 214): [Περὶ μυιῶν] Μυιῶν κεφαλαὶ λεῖαι σὺν στέατι χοιρείῳ τριβόμεναι, ἀλωπεκίας θεραπεύουσιν.
ibid.: καὶ τοῦ ἰκτίνου τὴν κεφαλήν, φασίν, ὁμοίως τοὺς ποδαγριῶντας ὠφελεῖν, εἴ τις αὐτῆς ξηρανθείσης ἄνευ τῶν πτερῶν ὅσον τοῖς τρισὶ δακτύλοις ἐπιπάσας ὕδατι πίνειν ἐθέλοι.	III, 19, 2 (p. 209): [Περὶ ἰκτίνου] Ἰκτῖνος πτηνόν ἐστιν ἱερόν. τούτου ἡ κεφαλὴ ξηρανθεῖσα ἄνευ τῶν πτερῶν καὶ λειωθεῖσα καὶ πινομένη σὺν ὕδατι ὅσον οὐγ. α΄ ποδαγρικοὺς ὠφελεῖ καὶ χειραγρικούς.
ch. IX. 9 (K. XIV, 240; ed. B-M, p. 42): ὁ δὲ τῆς χελιδόνος (sc. ἐγκέφαλος) μετὰ μέλιτος πρὸς ὑποχύσεις ποιεῖ.	III, 50, 20 (p. 237): [Περὶ χελιδόνος] ὁ δὲ ἐγκέφαλος αὐτῶν μετὰ μέλιτος, πρὸς ὑπόχυσιν ποιεῖ.
ch. IX.14 (K. XIV, 241; ed. B-M, p. 44): τὸ δὲ τοῦ χηνὸς στέαρ τὰς φλεγμονὰς μετὰ ῥοδίνου ἰᾶται·	III, 51, 10 (p. 238): [Περὶ χηνός] σὺν ῥοδίνῳ δὲ καὶ στέατι καὶ ὀπτοῖς λεκίθοις ὠῶν λειωθεὶς πρὸς φλεγμονὴν μήτρας ποιεῖ.
ch. IX.17 (K. XIV, 242; ed. B-M, p. 45): καρκίνος γοῦν ὁ ἀπὸ τῶν ποταμῶν λειωθεὶς καὶ καταπλασθεὶς ἀναβάλλει τοὺς σκόλοπας καὶ τὰς ἀκίδας	IV, 28, 7 (p. 264): [Περὶ καρκίνου] Καρκίνοι ποτάμιοι... λεῖοι δὲ ἐπιτεθέντες βελοτρώτοις ἐξάγουσι τὰς ἀκίδας τῶν βελῶν, καὶ σκόλοπας καὶ ἀκάνθας καὶ ὅσα τοιαῦτα ἀποβάλλει.
ibid.: ὁ δὲ σκορπίος σὺν ἄρτῳ ἐσθιόμενος ὀπτὸς θρύπτει τοὺς ἐν τῇ κύστει λίθους.	I, 24, 46 (p. 107): Ὀπτὸς δὲ ὁ κοινὸς σκορπίος ἐσθιόμενος ὑπὸ λιθιώντων ποιεῖ αὐτοὺς ἐξουρεῖν τὸν λίθον ἀβασανίστως.
ch. IX.19 (K. XIV, 243; ed. B-M, p. 46): ὁ δὲ ἱέραξ ἑψηθεὶς μετὰ μύρου σουσίνου ἀμβλυωπίας ἰᾶται.	III, 18, 5 (p. 208): [Περὶ ἱέρακος] ἡ δὲ χολὴ αὐτοῦ σὺν γλυκεῖ καὶ κρόκῳ λυτῇ μιγνυμένη καὶ ἐπιχριομένη, πᾶσαν ἀχλὺν καὶ ἀμβλυωπίαν ἰᾶται. ζῶν δὲ μαδισθεὶς καὶ συνεψηθεὶς σὺν ἐλαίῳ σουσίνῳ ἄχρι τακῇ καὶ διηθουμένου τοῦ ἐλαίου, ὅντινα χρίσεις ἐξ αὐτοῦ πᾶσαν ἀχλὺν καὶ ἀμβλυωπίαν ἰάσει.
ibid.: ὁ δὲ κορυδαλὸς ὀπτὸς τρωγόμενος θαυμασίως τοὺς κωλικοὺς πολλάκις ὠφέλησεν.	III, 20, 2 (p. 209): [Περὶ κορυδάλου] Κορύδαλος στρουθίον ἐστὶ πᾶσι γνωστόν, λόφον ἔχον ἐν τῇ κεφαλῇ. οὗτος ἑψηθεὶς καὶ ἐσθιόμενος συνεχῶς σὺν τῷ ζωμῷ, κοιλιακοὺς ὠφελεῖ καὶ δυσεντερικούς.

3. Magical remedies retained by the author of *Ad Pisonem* but excluded by Galen

Ps.-Galen in *De theriaca ad Pisonem*	Galen
ch. IX. 13 (K. XIV, 241; ed. B-M, p. 44): **καὶ ἡ τῶν μυῶν ἄφοδος** λεία μετ' ὄξους ἀλωπεκίας θεραπεύει· ἐν ποτῷ δὲ λαμβανομένη τοὺς ἐν κύστει θρύπτει λίθους·	*On simples* (Kühn XII, 307): Περὶ μυῶν κόπρου. **ἔστι γὰρ ὄντως αἰ-δεθῆναι τὰ τοιαῦτα** καὶ εἰς πεῖραν ἄγειν ἁπάντων καταγινωσκόντων ὡς περιέργου τε καὶ γόητος ὅς ἂν ταῦτα πράττῃ τε καὶ λέγῃ.
ch. IX.9 (K. XIV, 240; ed. B-M, p. 42): μετ' ὄξους πινόμενος ἐπιληπτικοὺς ἰᾶται καὶ **ὁ τῆς γαλῆς** (sc. ἐγκέφα-λος) ὁμοίως.	*On simples* XI, 1 (Kühn XII, 321, 15): **Γαλῆν δὲ οὐδέποτε ἐκαύσαμεν,** ἐφ' ἧς γεγράφασι τὴν τέφραν κατα-χριομένην μετ' ὄξους ὠφελεῖν ποδα-γρικούς τε καὶ ἀρθριτικούς, ὡς ἱκα-νῶς διαφορεῖν πεφυκυῖαν, σκελετευ-θεῖσαν δὲ πινομένην ἐπιλήπτους

4. List of diseases cured by theriac in *Ad Pisonem* ch. XV = Ps.-Galen, *Introductio siue Medicus* ch. XIII. 9ff. (ed. C. Petit, Paris, CUF, 2009, p. 51ff.)

De theriaca ad Pisonem	*Introductio sive medicus*
κεφαλαίας (XV. 1)	ch. XIII. 21 κεφαλαία
σκοτώματα (XV. 1)	ch. XIII. 23 τὰ δὲ σκοτώματα
τῶν φρενιτικῶν παρακοπὰς (XV. 2)	ch. XIII. 9 φρενῖτις
ταῖς ἐπιληψίαις (XV. 3)	ch. XIII. 22 ἐπιληψία
τοῖς δυσπνοοῦσιν (XV. 4)	ch. XIII. 13 ἡ δὲ περιπνευμονία
τοὺς αἷμα δὲ ἀνάγοντας πάνυ (XV. 5)	ch. XIII. 27 αἰτίαι δὲ αἵματος ἀναγωγῆς τρεῖς
ἐλμίνθων τοῖς ἐντέροις ἐγκειμένων (XV. 7)	ch. XIII. 41 ἕλμινθες δὲ πάθος ἐντέρων
τὰς ἡπατικὰς δὲ διαθέσεις (XV. 8)	ch. XIII. 30 αἱ δὲ περὶ τὸ ἧπαρ... φλεγμοναὶ
τὸν ἴκτερον (XV. 8)	ch. XIII. 15 ἴκτερος δέ
καὶ τοὺς σπλῆνας τοὺς ἐσκιρρωμένους (XV. 9)	ch. XIII. 30 αἱ δὲ περὶ... σπλῆνα φλεγμοναὶ... καὶ σκιρρώδεις καχεξίας ἐπιφέρουσαι τῷ σώματι

De theriaca ad Pisonem	Introductio sive medicus
τοὺς ἐν νεφροῖς λίθους ... καὶ τὰς τῆς κύστεως δυσουρίας (XV. 10)	ch. XIII. 32 πάθη δὲ συνίστανται περὶ νεφροὺς ταῦτα... 34 περὶ δὲ κύστιν ταῦτα συνίσταται τὰ πάθη ...
τὰς περὶ τὴν κοιλίαν δυσπεψίας τε καὶ ἀτονίας (XV. 11)	ch. XIII. 36 ἡ δὲ περὶ κοιλίαν καὶ ἔντερα ἀρχὴ
τὰς δυσεντερίας αὐτὰς καὶ τὰς λειεντερίας (XV. 11)	ch. XIII. 38 δυσεντερία δέ ἐστι πάθος περὶ τὰ ἔντερα 39 λειεντερία δὲ γίνεται μὲν ἀπὸ τῆς δυσεντερίας
τοὺς εἰλεωδῶς τὰ ἔντερα διατιθεμένους (XV. 12)	ch. XIII. 17 εἰλεὸς δὲ
τοῖς χολεριῶσι (XV. 12)	ch. XIII. 16 ἡ δὲ χολέρα
ἐπὶ τῶν καρδιακῶν (XV. 13)	ch. XIII. 14 ἡ δὲ καρδιακὴ διάθεσις
ἐπὶ τῶν καταμηνίων αἱμάτων ἀγωγὸς (XV. 14)	
καὶ τοὺς ποδαγριῶντας (XV. 16–19)	ch. XIII. 42 καὶ ποδάγρα
καὶ τοὺς ὑδεριῶντας (XV. 20)	ch. XIII. 31 ὑδρώπων δὲ
τῆς καχεξίας λεγομένης (XV. 21)	
τοῖς ἐλεφαντιῶσι (XV. 22)	ch. XIII. 43 ἡ δὲ ἐλεφαντίασις τὸ πάθος
τοὺς δὲ τετανικῶς σπωμένους (XV. 23)	ch. XIII. 19 τέτανος δὲ
τὰς παραλύσεις τῶν μερῶν (XV. 24)	cf. ch. XV. 3 πρὸς παραλύσεις ποιοῦντα

Easy Remedies – Difficult Texts: the Pseudo-Galenic *Euporista*[1]

Laurence Totelin

In the last twenty years, there has been a revival of interest in ancient pharmacology in general, and in Galenic pharmacology in particular.[2] There is, however, one area which has been neglected, and where much work remains to be done: the *Euporista* genre, which was very successful in antiquity. *Euporista* are collections of remedies that were – at least allegedly – easy to procure and prepare; they devote very little space to theoretical aspects of pharmacology. Among the *Euporista* treatises written in antiquity, we can mention those of Apollonius Mys (first century BC), constituted of at least two books, of which several fragments are preserved in the works of Galen and other medical authors;[3] those attributed to Dioscorides and dedicated to a certain Andromachus (first–second century CE);[4] the Latin *Euporiston* of Theodorus Priscianus, in three books (fourth century CE);[5] and Oribasius's work which he dedicated to Eunapius (fourth century CE). Here I will focus on the three books of *Euporista* (*De remediis parabilibus*) transmitted under the name of Galen, two books of which are almost certainly Pseudo-Galenic.

[1] Unless stated otherwise, all translations from the Greek and Latin are mine.

[2] For an overview of the topic, and bibliography, see L. M. V. Totelin, 'Technologies of Knowledge: Pharmacology, Botany, and Medical Recipes', *Oxford Handbooks Online* (10.1093/oxfordhb/9780199935390.013.94), 2016. On Galenic pharmacy, see in particular *Galen on Pharmacology, Philosophy, History and Medicine*, ed. A. Debru, Leiden, 1997; S. Vogt, 'Drugs and Pharmacology', in *The Cambridge Companion to Galen*, ed. R. J. Hankinson, Cambridge, 2008, pp. 304–22; C. Petit, 'Galen, Pharmacology and the Boundaries of Medicine: A Reassessment', in *Collecting Recipes: Byzantine and Jewish Pharmacology in Dialogue*, eds L. Lehmhaus and M. Martelli, Berlin, 2017, pp. 51–79.

[3] Fragments in Galen, *De simpl. med. temp. et fac.* 6, proemium, XI, 795 K.; 11.1.49, XII, 367 K.; *De comp. med. sec. loc.* 1.8., XII, 475 K.; 2.1, XII, 502 K.; 2.2, XII, 582 K.; 3.1, XII, 612, 616, 646, 651 K.; 3.3, XII, 686 K.; 5.1, XII, 814 K.; 5.5, XII, 858, 864, 865 K.; 6.8, XII, 979 K.; 6.9, XII, 995 K.; Oribasius, *Eun.* Praef. 1.5.4; Philumenus, *De venetatis animalibus eorumque remediis* 5.5; 17.10; 19.1; 20.3; 23.3; 32.3; 33.5; 35.4; Alexander, *Therapeutica* 1.599. See C. Fabricius, *Galens Exzerpte aus älteren Pharmakologen*, Berlin/New York, 1972, pp. 182–3; *Herophilus: the Art of Medicine in Early Alexandria. Edition, Translation and Essays*, ed. H. von Staden, Cambridge, 1989, p. 543.

[4] Edition: *Pedanii Dioscuridis Anazarbei De materia medica libri quinque. Edidit M. Wellmann. Volumen III quo continentur liber V, Crateuae et Sextii Nigri fragmenta, Dioscuridis libri De simplicibus*, ed. M. Wellmann, Berlin, 1914, pp. 151–317.

[5] Edition: *Theodori Prisciani Euporiston libri iii: cum physicorum fragmento et additamentis pseudo-Theodoreis*, ed. V. Rose, Leipzig, 1894.

They span 270 pages in the fourteenth volume of Kühn's edition (1827), which is known to be unreliable.[6]

From Galen's *Euporista* to Kühn's Text

Galen himself composed a book of *Euporista*, to which he referred on several occasions in his other treatises. In his treatise *On the Powers of Simple Medicines*, he mentioned it several times in the future tense:

εἰρήσεται δὲ καὶ ἡμῖν ἐπιπλέον ὑπὲρ αὐτῶν ἐν τῇ περὶ συνθέσεως φαρμάκων πραγματείᾳ καὶ τῇ τῶν εὐπορίστων

We will discuss these substances thoroughly in our treatise on the composition of remedies and in that on remedies easily procured.[7]

εἰρήσεται δὲ κἀν τοῖς εὐπορίστοις

This will also be discussed with the remedies easily procured.[8]

ῥηθήσεται γὰρ ἐπιπλέον ἔν τε τοῖς περὶ συνθέσεως φαρμάκων κἀν τοῖς περὶ τῶν εὐπορίστων

This will be discussed thoroughly in [the treatises] on the composition of remedies as well as in those on remedies easily procured.[9]

περὶ ὧν ἐν τοῖς εὐπορίστοις ἐπιπλέον εἰρήσεται

These will be discussed thoroughly in [the treatises] on remedies easily procured.[10]

In the same treatise *On the Powers of Simple Medicines*, Galen alluded once to his *Euporista* in the present tense: ἐν τοῖς εὐπορίστοις γράφεται φαρμάκοις (this is written in [the treatises] on remedies easily procured).[11] A final reference to remedies easily procured is found in *On the Powers of Simple Medicines*, this time in the past tense: εὐπόριστα γὰρ ἁλιεῖς ὅλως ἐδίδασκον φάρμακα (I have given thorough instruction on the remedies from the sea that are easily procured).[12]

In two other treatises, *On the Properties of Foodstuffs* and *On the Therapeutic Method*, Galen mentioned his *Euporista* in the past tense:

---

[6] Book I goes from page 311 to page 389; book II goes from page 390 to page 491; book III goes from page 492 to page 581.

[7] *De simpl. med. temp. et fac.* 6.1.1, XI, 799 K.

[8] *De simpl. med. temp. et fac.* 6.2.2, XI, 846 K.

[9] *De simpl. med. temp. et fac.* 9.1.4, XII, 183 K.

[10] *De simpl. med. temp. et fac.* 10.2.24, XII, 302 K.

[11] *De simpl. med. temp. et fac.* 6.1.1, XI, 801 K. Note that this reference is to the same chapter as that in n. 7.

[12] *De simpl. med. temp. et fac.* 9.3.9, XII, 217 K.

περὶ ἀνδράχνης. ὡς ἔδεσμα μὲν ὀλίγην τε τροφὴν ἔχει καὶ ταύτην ὑγρὰν καὶ ψυχρὰν καὶ γλίσχραν, ὡς φάρμακον δ᾽ αἱμωδίαν ἰᾶται διὰ τὴν ἄδηκτον γλισχρότητα, περὶ ἧς ἐπὶ πλέον ἐν τῇ τῶν Εὐπορίστων φαρμάκων πραγματείᾳ λέλεκται.

Concerning purslane: when eaten, it contains very little nourishment, and is wet, cold, and sticky; as a drug, it treats teeth ailments through its non-pungent stickiness, on which topic much has been said in my treatise on remedies easily procured.[13]

καὶ σὺ τοίνυν ὅσα μὲν ἐκ Μεθόδου θεραπευτικῆς ἐντεῦθεν μάνθανε, τὰ δ᾽ ἐκ μόνης τῆς πείρας ἐγνωσμένα κατὰ τὰς περὶ τῶν φαρμάκων πραγματείας ἔχεις ἠθροισμένα, μίαν μὲν τὴν περὶ τῆς δυνάμεως αὐτῶν, ἑτέραν δὲ τὴν περὶ τῆς συνθέσεως, καὶ τρίτην τὴν περὶ τῶν εὐπορίστων ὀνομαζομένων, ἐν αἷς ἐπιδέδεικταί μοι τίνα μὲν ἐκ μόνης τῆς πείρας εὕρηται φάρμακα, τίνα δὲ ἐκ μόνου τοῦ λόγου, τίνα δ᾽ ἐξ ἀμφοτέρων.

Accordingly, also among those things that you must learn here from the Method of Medicine are those known from experience alone, collected together for you in the writings on medications: the first on their potency, the second on the composition, and the third on what is called their ease of procurement.[14]

The dating of Galen's writings is complex, as he wrote some of his treatises over a long period of time (this is the case of *On the Powers of Simple Medicines*), and the tense in which cross-references are cast is not always the best indicator of the order in which works were composed.[15] Nevertheless, one could suggest that Galen wrote his pharmacological books in the order he gave in the passage of *On the Therapeutic Method* XIII (itself written after 193 CE): *On the Powers of Simple Medicines*; *On the Composition of Drugs according to Types* and *On the Composition of Drugs according to Places*; and *Euporista*. A date in the early years of Septimius Severus's reign seems plausible.

By the fourth century, unfortunately, the work of Galen on *Euporista* appears not to have been widely available. Oribasius could not use it to compose his own collection of remedies easily procured, as he explained in the preface to his *Books to Eunapius*:

εἰ μὲν οὖν ἐσῴζετο τὰ τῷ θαυμασίῳ Γαληνῷ γραφέντα περὶ τῶν εὐπορίστων φαρμάκων, εἶχες ἂν τὸ σπουδαζόμενον ἐξ αὐτῶν· ἐπεὶ δ᾽ οὔτε ταῦτα ἦλθεν εἰς ἡμᾶς, τά τε γραφέντα Διοσκορίδῃ καὶ Ἀπολλωνίῳ καὶ τοῖς ἄλλοις ἅπασιν εὐπόριστα παντελῶς εἰσιν ἀδιόριστα καὶ οὔτε ἀσφαλῶς οὔτε ἱκανῶς ἔχειν μοι δοκεῖ, διὰ τοῦτο ἑτοίμως ὑπήκουσά σου τῇ βουλήσει.

---

[13] *De alim. fac.* 2.46, VI, 634 K.

[14] *Meth. med.* 13.6, X, 896 K. Translation: I. Johnston and G. H. R. Horsley, *Galen. Method of Medicine*, Volume III: Books 10–14, Cambridge, MA, 2011: p. 351, slightly modified.

[15] For a list of possible dates for Galen's writings, see Boudon-Millot, 2012, pp. 345–74.

If the books on remedies easily procured written by the amazing Galen were preserved, you would have the most important material from these. However, since they have not reached us, and considering that the *Euporista* written by Dioscorides, Apollonius and all the others are entirely disorganized and seem to me to be neither reliable nor sufficient, I readily yield to your request [Eunapius].[16]

Several centuries later, however, Hunayn ibn Ishaq (late ninth century CE–tenth century CE), seems to have had access to the Galenic *Euporista*. When discussing stomach ailments, Hunayn gave two recipes which he had apparently found in Galen's works on remedies easily procured.[17] In another treatise, however, Hunayn admitted that he had never seen a Greek copy of Galen's *Euporista*:

This treatise [Galen's *Euporista*] is in two books: its purpose is apparent from the title. I have never come across any Greek manuscripts of this treatise, nor have I heard of anybody who owned a copy, although I sought very carefully to find one. Sergius [of Resaina] translated it [into Syriac]: at present, the Syriac copies are corrupt and bad. One book, dealing with the same subject, was added to it, and was attributed to Galen, although it is not by Galen, it is by Philagrius. I have seen this book; indeed I translated it, with other books also by Philagrius, into Syriac for Bukhtīshū. Commentators on treatises did not merely add this book [to Galen's *De remediis parabilibus*], they also interpolated much irrational material, extraordinary and strange receipts, and drugs which Galen would never have seen or even heard of. I came across a statement by Oribasius that he had not found any copies of this treatise in his time. Some of my friends asked me to read the Syriac version and to correct it in any way which I thought would agree with Galen's opinion. This I did.[18]

Thus, according to Hunayn, Galen's *Euporista* was a treatise in two books. It had

---

[16] Oribasius, *Libri at Eunapium* Proemium 5, ed. J. Raeder, *Oribasii Synopsis ad Eustathium, Libri ad Eunapium*, CMG VI.3, Leipzig/Berlin, 1926, pp. 317–18.

[17] *Fī awjāʿ al-maʿida*, MS Madrid, Escorial Library, 852, III, fol. 67b, lines 5–11: 'Prescriptions mentioned by Galen in his book *On Drugs that are easily obtained*. For stomach ailments: receipt of a drug useful for the weak stomach; place anise and caltrops inside a wet linen cloth, then soak in hot water; give this infusion to the patient to drink. Another drug, for the weak stomach, [which also relieves] distress: three or four branches of mentha are to be infused in sweet pomegranate juice; boil and give to the patient to sip little by little.' Translation: A. Z. Iskandar, *A Descriptive List of Arabic Manuscripts on Medicine and Science at the University of California*, Leiden, 1984, p. 10.

[18] Hunayn, *Fi'l-adwiya allatī yashul wujūduhā*. Translation: Iskandar, *A Descriptive List* (n. 17 above), p. 10 n. 21, slightly modified. The square brackets are in Iskandar's translation. I substituted 'book' for 'treatise' and vice versa, in line with the common use among classicists: a treatise is composed of several books. See also G. Bergsträsser, *Hunain ibn Ishaq über die syrischen und arabischen Galen-Übersetzungen, zum ersten Mal herausgegeben und übersetzt von G. Bergsträsser*, Leipzig, 1925, p. 31; F. Sezgin, *Geschichte des arabischen Schrifttums. Band III. Medizin – Pharmazie – Zoologie – Tierheilkunde bis ca. 430*, Leiden, 1970, pp. 120–21; M. Ullmann, *Die Medizin im Islam*, Leiden, 1970, p. 49 no. 54.

been translated into Syriac by Sergius (sixth century CE), but the Syriac translation was corrupt by Hunayn's time. To the two books of Galen's *Euporista* had been added a third, which Hunayn believed to be by Philagrius (fourth century CE), with further interpolations which mentioned drugs that were not available during Galen's time. As we will see, the third book of *Euporista* in Kühn's edition does indeed include recipes with ingredients that Galen would never have encountered, but it may well have a core that dates to the fourth century CE or earlier. The editor of Philagrius, Rita Masullo, however, argued that she could not discover anything in *Euporista* III that could be attributed to Philagrius.[19]

The earliest Greek manuscript that contains a *Euporista* treatise attributed to Galen is MS Vaticano, Biblioteca Apostolica Vaticana, Urbinas gr. 67 (fols 268ʳ–275ᵛ), which dates to the thirteenth century. The text corresponds to *Euporista* I in Kühn's edition. In fact, only one preserved Greek manuscript includes all three books of *Euporista* attributed to Galen (see Table 1): MS Vaticano, Biblioteca Apostolica Vaticana, Barberinus gr. 147 (fols 48–161), which dates to the fifteenth or sixteenth century.

The situation is similar with the Latin translations of the Galenic *Euporista*: each of the three books was translated separately, and the translations did not always circulate together.[20] The earliest Latin translation was that of book II by Niccolò da Reggio in 1336 (see below for some of the other translations).[21] Translations by Ioannes Guinterius (book I), Hubertus Barlandus (book I), Sebastianus Scrofa (book I), Iunius Paulus Crassus (books II and III), and Ioannes Baptista Rasarius (books II and III) followed in the sixteenth century.

In the classic Juntine edition of 1565, the Latin translations of the three Galenic books of *Euporista* are transmitted together.[22] While book I is clearly attributed to Galen, books II and III are presented in a more ambivalent manner; doubt is cast on their authenticity:

---

[19] *Filagrio frammenti: testo edito per la prima volta, con introduzione, apparato critico, traduzione e note*, ed. R. Masullo, Naples, 1999, p. 23.

[20] See R. J. Durling, 'A Chronological Census of Renaissance Editions and Translations of Galen', *Journal of the Warburg and Courtauld Institutes*, 24, 1961, pp. 230–305 (no. 98); the online Catalogo delle traduzioni Latine, *De remediis facile parabilibus* (http://www.galenolatino.com/index.php?id=10&L=&uid=91, accessed February 2021).

[21] See Catalogo delle traduzioni Latine, De remediis facile parabilibus II *tradotto da Niccolò da Reggio: De facile acquisibilibus* (http://www.galenolatino.com/index.php?id=11&L=&uid=366, accessed February 2021).

[22] Vol. 8, *classis* 7: book I starts on fol. 153ʳ and ends on fol. 160ᵛ; book II on fol. 169ᵛ; book III ends on fol. 177ᵛ

Book I: *Galeni de remediis paratu facilibus libellus ab Huberto Barlando philiatro latino sermoni traditus.* (Galen's treatise *On Remedies Easily Prepared*, translated into Latin by Hubertus Barlandus, philosopher–physician).

Book II: *Galeno ascriptus liber de medicinis facile parabilibus ad Solonem medicorum principem Iunio Paulo Crasso Patavino interprete. Censura: Liber, cuiuscumque is fuerit, non omnino inutilis* (Book *On Remedies Easily Prepared* ascribed to Galen, dedicated to Solon, most distinguished among physicians. Translated by Iunius Paulus Crassus of Padua. Judgement: This book, whoever composed it, is not entirely useless).

Book III: *Liber tertius de medicamentis quae ad manum sunt, Galeno ascriptus, Iunio Paulo Crasso Patavino interprete. Censura: Liber ordine ac iudicio vacans* (Third book on drugs which are at hand, ascribed to Galen. Translated by Iunius Paulus Crassus of Padua. Judgement: this book lacks organization and discernment).

The Greek text of the Galenic *Euporista* was first published in 1679, as part of the tenth volume of René Chartier's *Operum Hippocratis Coi et Galeni Pergameni Archiatron*.[23] In this edition, again, book I is presented as authentic (*Galeni De remediis parabilibus liber primus*, p. 574), but books II and III are considered spurious (*Galeno ascriptus liber II. De remediis parabilibus ad Claudianum Solonem Medicorum principem*, p. 602; *Galeni De remediis parabilibus liber III. Ascriptitius*, p. 638).[24] Chartier most probably used manuscripts held in Paris to establish his text.

In volume XIV of his monumental (if often unreliable) edition, Karl Gottlob Kühn simply reproduced the text from Chartier's edition, but removed the subtitle of book II, therefore making it look as if he considered it authentic and a continuation of book I (*Galeni De remediis parabilibus liber secundus*, p. 390).[25] However, Johan Christian Gottlieb Ackermann, in his *Historia litteraria Claudii Galeni*, which Kühn included in volume I of his *Claudii Galeni Opera*, expressed strong doubts over the authenticity of books II and III of the *Euporista*. Ackermann, in turn, had lifted those words from Albrecht von Haller's *Biblioteca botanica*:

These three books were not composed by a single author. The first book is dedicated to Glaucon; it cites *The Method of Healing to Glaucon*, and it is the oldest [of the three]. It is composed mostly in the spirit of Galen. It contains many medicaments from Archigenes, whose books Galen used often in other pharmacological works... The

---

[23] This edition was published posthumously by Chartier's son-in-law, A. Pralard. As a result, the *Euporista* in the Chartier edition are not accompanied by the short notes that the editor usually gave on his sources and where he shared his thoughts on the authenticity of treatises.

[24] Book I starts on p. 574 of vol. 10; book II on p. 602; and book III on p. 638.

[25] The subtitle of Book III is identical in Chartier and Kühn: *Galeni De remediis parabilbus liber tertius adscriptitius.*

second book of remedies easily procured is dedicated to the archiatros Claud. Solon, whom Galen does not mention anywhere else ... Many superstitious and absurd ideas are put forth there, which clearly are inconsistent with the spirit of Galen. The third book is the worst. Galen himself is cited within it. It is full of ignorance and superstition. It was written by a Christian, who ascribes powers to a candle kindled in the sanctuary of Paul the Apostle, and talks about the Anargyroi saints [Cosmas and Damian]. Von Haller correctly tells us that this book belongs to the times of the Emperors of Constantinople.[26]

While the Renaissance Latin editors, von Haller, Chartier and Ackermann were justified in classifying books II and III of the Galenic *Euporista* as spurious, it is important to move beyond negative prejudices, and study these texts for what they are. They may be impossible to date, but they represent a form of pharmacology which is interesting in and of itself. In the second half of this paper, I will ask basic questions about these texts: How are they organized? What do their proemia tell us? What types of recipes do they contain? Which authorities do they mention? What do the Pseudo-Galenic *Euporista* have in common with other similar texts? Such questions will open the way for further studies of the *Euporista* genre in antiquity.

Euporista Book I

Book I starts with a rather long proemium, in which the author claimed to be writing for people who lived outside of towns and travelled to deserted and wild places:

δίκαιον ᾠήθην κατ᾽ ἐμὴν δύναμιν εἰσενέγκασθαι ἐπικουρίαν τοῖς ἐν ὁδοῖς, μάλιστα καὶ κατ᾽ ἀγροὺς καὶ κατά τινας ἐρήμους τόπους διατρίβουσιν, ἐφ᾽ ὧν τὰ μὲν πάθη ῥᾳδίαν καὶ ἀπροσδόκητον ἔχει τὴν κατὰ τῶν σωμάτων φορὰν καὶ δύναμιν.

---

[26] J. C. G. Ackermann ap. Kühn, 1821, pp. cliv-clv: *Neque hi libri tres ab uno auctore compositi sunt. Primus ad Glaucon., in quo etiam de methodo medendi ad Glaucon. librum citat, et antiquior, et ad Galeni ingenium magis compositus. Multa continet medicamenta ex Archigene, cujus libris Galenus in aliis libris de medicamentis crebro usus est ... Alter de medicamentis paratu facilibus liber, ad Claud. Solonem, achiatrum, scriptus, cujus Galenus alias non meminit ... multa etiam superstitiosa et absurda in eo proponuntur, quae ab ingenio Galeni plane abhorrent. Tertius liber pessimus est. Galenus ipse in eo passim citatur. Est plenus ignorantiae et superstitionum, et scriptus a Christiano, qui vires adeo adscripserit candelae ad ignem in sacello Pauli Apostoli accensae, atque de sanctis anargyris loquitur. Incidere hunc librum in tempora imperatorum Constantinopolitanorum, Haller ... recte monet.* Ackermann's text is summarised from H. von Haller, *Bibliotheca botanica qua scripta ad rem herbariam facientia a rerum initiis recensentur. Tomus 1. Tempora ante Tournefortium*, Zurich, 1771, pp. 150–51.

I thought it good to offer help, according to my power, to those who travel, and particularly those who spend time in the wild and in deserted places, on whom diseases have easy and unexpected effect and power.[27]

The author then stated that he would not use expensive remedies, but rather those that are easily found and cheap; he would not fill his treatise with theory, but rather make it accessible to laypeople (*idiōtai*). He further went on to explain the way in which he ordered his material, the head-to-toe order. To him, starting with the head made sense because:

αὕτη γὰρ καθάπερ τις ἀκρόπολίς ἐστι τοῦ σώματος καὶ τῶν τιμιωτάτων καὶ ἀναγ-καιοτάτων ἀνθρώποις αἰσθήσεων οἰκητήριον, διὸ καὶ τὴν ἀρχὴν τῶν βοηθημάτων ἀπ' αὐτῆς ποιησόμεθα.

In some ways, [the head] is the acropolis of the body and the dwelling place of the noblest and most necessary human feelings, and for that reason, we start with the remedies for it.[28]

The remedies are then divided into seventeen chapters, organized from head to toe, beginning with headaches and ending with diseases that affect the extremities (gout and arthritis), followed by a final chapter on the bites of poisonous animals.[29] No space is given to gynaecological ailments. In many ways, *Euporista* I is a very traditional collection of recipes, with little of great note.

Archigenes, a famous late-first century CE pharmacologist, is mentioned on two occasions in *Euporista* I: in relation to headaches caused by wine and rheumy eyes.[30] The author commented that Archigenes had made use of amulets in the treatment of headaches:

ἐπεὶ δὲ τὰ περίαπτα ἔγραψεν ὁ Ἀρχιγένης τοῖς κεφαλαλγοῦσιν, οὐκ ἄτοπον ᾠήθην καὶ ταῦτα ἀναγράψαι πρὸς τὰς ἐκ μέθης καὶ ἐγκαύσεως κεφαλαλγίας.

Since Archigenes wrote recipes of amulets against headaches, we did not think it out of place to record those against headaches caused by drunkenness and heat-stroke.

---

[27] *De rem. para.* 1, proemium, XIV, 312 K.

[28] *De rem. para.* 1, proemium, XIV, 314 K.

[29] Topics of chapters: 1) afflictions inside the head (headaches); 2) afflictions on the outside of the head (alopecia); 3) ears; 4) nose; 5) eyes; 6) afflictions of the face; 7) teeth; 8) mouth, throat; 9) organ of sound; 10) mouth of the cavity; 11) liver; 12) spleen; 13) epigastrion; 14) backside; 15) kidneys and bladder; 16) gout, arthritis; 17) poisonous drugs.

[30] *De rem. para.* 1.1, XIV, 321 K. and 1.5, XIV, 343 K. On Archigenes, see A. Touwaide, 'Arkhigenes of Apameia', in *The Encyclopedia of Ancient Natural Scientists: The Greek Tradition and its Many Heirs*, eds P. T. Keyser and G. L. Irby-Massie, London, pp. 160–61.

Galen gave a similar, but longer, justification for including Archigenes' amulet recipes in his *On the Composition of Drugs according to Places*.[31] The amulet recipes attributed to Archigenes, for their part, are very similar in *Euporista* II and in *On the Composition of Drugs according to Places*. In particular, they both include an interesting statement on the name of chicory in Latin: ἤ κιχώριον, τὸ Ῥωμαϊστὶ καλούμενον ἴντυβον λάχανον (chicory, the vegetable which is called *intubum* in Latin).[32]

Towards the end of *Euporista* I, in the chapter on gout, we find a reference to *Therapeutics to Glaucon*, written in the first person, as if the author of our treatise was indeed Galen:

εἴρηται δὲ ἡμῖν περὶ τούτων ἐπὶ πλεῖστον ἐν τοῖς ἐμοῦ πρὸς Γλαύκωνα θεραπευτικοῖς γεγραμμένοις δυσὶ βιβλίοις, καὶ ἐν ἄλλοις πλείοσι, διὸ βραδύνειν οὐ χρὴ ὡς ἐν εὐπορίστοις περὶ τούτων λέγοντα.

We have said much about these matters in the two therapeutic books to Glaucon, and in many other places, and for this reason it is not necessary to dwell on these in the *Euporista*.[33]

Similarly, the treatise ends with an address to Glaucon, the recipient of *Therapeutics*:

ὁ μὲν οὖν τέταρτός μοι λόγος, ὦ Γλαῦκων, ἐνθάδε πέρας ἐχέτω· εἰ δέ σοι χρεία γένηται καὶ τοῦ πρὸς Σαλομῶντα τὸν ἀρχίητρον γεγραμμένου ἡμῖν συντάγματος, δηλώσας ἑτοίμως λήψῃ, θαυμάσεις δὲ πάνυ δεξάμενος.

Let this be the end of my fourth treatise, Glaucon. If you need more, consult the treatise that we have written for the Archiatros Solomon – you will find much to admire there.[34]

The reference to a 'fourth treatise' is a little puzzling (Kühn did not translate τέταρτος into Latin). Perhaps 'fourth' refers to the fact that Galen wrote three main pharmacological treatises before the *Euporista*: *On the Powers of Simple Medicines*; *On the Composition of Drugs according to Places*; and *On the Composition of Drugs according to Types*. I would suggest that this concluding statement is an interpolation, a very clumsy attempt at linking *Euporista* I to *Euporista* II. Indeed, *Euporista* II is dedicated to a certain Solon, who may well be the same person as

---

[31] *De comp. med. sec. loc.* 2.2, XII, 574 K.

[32] Galen made the same linguistic observation at *De alim. fac.* 2.41, VI, 628 K. On the plant name *intubus* (or *intubum*), see J. André, *Les noms des plantes dans la Rome antique*, 2nd ed, Paris, 2010, 131–32.

[33] *De rem. para.* 1.16, XIV, 384 K.

[34] *De rem. para.* 1.17, XIV, 389 K.

the Solomon of the *explicit* to book one. According to Caroline Petit, Σαλομῶντα (found in Barberinus gr. 147 and Chartier's edition) is a late mistake for Σωλόμονα (as found in Urbinas gr. 67). It would be tempting to correct it to Σόλωνα.[35]

Euporista Book II

Euporista II starts with a short proemium, in which the book is presented to Solon:

> προοίμιον. ἐπειδὴ μὲν ἠξίωσας ὡς περὶ εὐπορίστων σοι γράφειν, ὦ Σόλων τιμιώτατε, χαρίζεσθαί σοι νενόμικα τά μοι διὰ τῆς πείρας ἐγνωσμένα γράφειν τε καί σοι ἐπιστέλλειν, ἀπὸ τῶν τριχῶν πρὸς τὰς πόδας προβαίνων, ὅπως ἄνθρωπος ῥαδίως αὐτὰ προσλαμβάνειν δύνηται. ἀρχόμεθα μὲν οὖν πρῶτον ἀπὸ τῶν τριχῶν.

> Since I have deemed worthy to write to you about remedies that are easily procured, most honourable Solon, I will tell you the usages that I have learnt through practice and recommend them to you, starting with the hair, and proceeding towards the feet, in a way that people can easily grasp. We start first with the hair.[36]

The identity of the dedicatee is uncertain. In some manuscripts, including Barberinus gr. 147 (fol. 75ᵛ), the dedicatee is named as Claudianus Solon. Galen mentioned both a Claudianus and a Solon in his *On the Composition of Drugs according to Places*. Claudianus is introduced as a companion (*hetairos*) of Galen, while Solon is presented as a dietician to whom a recipe for an earache is attributed.[37] It is not possible to determine whether Claudianus and Solon are one and the same person; and if they are the same person, whether they can be identified with the dedicatee of *Euporista* II.

Euporista II then contains 28 chapters, organized in the head-to-toe order, starting with remedies that are unashamedly cosmetic in nature (when Galen had expressed reluctance towards including cosmetics in his *On the Composition of Drugs According to Places*), and ending with aphrodisiacs and antidotes against venomous bites.[38] *Euporista* II is noteworthy in several respects. Firstly, it names

---

[35] Caroline Petit, personal communication, 2017.

[36] *De rem. para.* 2, proemium, XIV, 390 K.

[37] Claudianus: *De comp. med. sec. loc.* 1.2, XII, 423–24 K.: τοῦτο τὸ φάρμακον οὕτω γεγραμμένον εὗρε Κλαυδιανὸς ὁ ἑταῖρος ἡμῶν ἐκ πυκτίδι διφθέρᾳ (Claudianus our companion found this remedy thus written in a parchment notebook). Solon: *De comp. med. sec. loc.* 3.1, XII, 630 K. Nutton suggests that Galen alluded to Claudianus, without naming him, at *De indolentia* 33: V. Nutton, 'Avoiding Distress', in *Galen: Psychological Writings*, ed. P. Singer, Cambridge, 2013, pp. 43–106 (88 n. 67).

[38] Topics of chapters: 1) hair; 2) diseases of the head; 3) ears; 4) eyes; 5) nostrils; 6) face (cosmetics); 7) mouth; 8) teeth (with some cosmetics); 9) gums; 10) uvula; 11) throat; 12) bronchi and pharynx; 13) thorax and lungs; 14) pleurisy; 15) breasts; 16) remedies against smelly armpits; 17) 'stomach'

several authorities, some of whom are otherwise unknown: Hippion 'of the Centaurs' (ὁ Κενταύριος), otherwise unknown, is the creator of a remedy for those who spit blood;[39] Herophilus, perhaps the famous Hellenistic physician, is cited in relation to a remedy against phthisis, which is not recorded anywhere else;[40] Marcellus, perhaps the first-century pharmacologist, is mentioned in relation to a remedy for the spleen;[41] and a certain Priscus of Samos, otherwise unknown, is cited in relation to a remedy against the stone.[42] *Euporista* II also contains a couple of authorial interventions, one of which points to an author based in Asia: τούτῳ ἔσωσα ἡγεμόνα κατὰ τὴν ἡμετέραν Ἀσίαν (this saved a leader in our Asia).[43] The historical Galen regularly referred to his native Asia, in the pharmacological treatises in particular.[44]

Another characteristic is the presence of some remedies that may be called magical, as von Haller and Ackermann had noted. For instance, we can point to the following test to determine whether someone is epileptic:

> ἐπιθυμίαμα τῷ γνῶναι εἰ ἔστιν ἐπιληπτικός. λίθον ἐπιθυμίασον τὸν γαγάτην, αὐτῷ συμπεριβαλὼν, ὡς μὴ διασκίδνασθαι τὴν ὀσμὴν καὶ καταπεσεῖται εἴπερ ἑάλω τῷ πάθει.

> Fumigation to know whether someone is epileptic. Fumigate lignite, fully covering it lest the smell be overwhelming, and the patient will drop if the disease has seized.[45]

However, neither von Haller nor Ackermann singled out this recipe. Instead, they focused on the presence of ingredients such as deer horn in the second book of *Euporista*, an ingredient which was in fact rather common in ancient pharmacology.

---

remedies; 18) vomiting and diarrhoea; 19) liver; 20) jaundice and kidneys; 21) spleen; 22) dropsy; 23) prolapse of the navel; 24) belly; 25) stones; 26) gynaecological diseases; 27) aphrodisiacs; 28) bites of animals. On Galen's attitudes to cosmetics, see *De comp. med. sec. loc.* 1.2, XII, 434–35 K.

[39] *De rem. para.* 2.13, XIV, 442–43 K.

[40] *De rem. para.* 2.13, XIV, 444 K. = Herophilus, *Art of Medicine* (n. 3 above), fr. 256.

[41] *De rem. para.* 2.21, XIV, 459 K. On Marcellus, see P. T. Keyser, 'Marcellus', in *The Encyclopedia of Ancient Natural Scientists: The Greek Tradition and its Many Heirs*, eds P. T. Keyser and G. L. Irby-Massie, London, 2008, p. 527.

[42] *De rem. para.* 2.25, XIV, 474 K.

[43] *De rem. para.* 2.019, XIV, 453 K. The pronoun ἐγώ appears at *De rem. para.* 2.20, XIV, 455 K. and 2.24, XIV, 470 K.

[44] Galen used the phrase παρ'ἡμῖν to refer to Asia twenty times in his pharmacological treatises. See L. M. V. Totelin, 'And to end on a poetic note: Galen's authorial strategies in the pharmacological books', *Studies in History and Philosophy of Science Part A*, 43, 2, 2012, pp. 307–15 (309).

[45] *De rem. para.* 2.2, XIV, 402 K.

A final noteworthy characteristic of *Euporista* II is the emphasis it puts on cosmetics and gynaecology, two topics that often went hand in hand in ancient pharmacological treatises. The treatise opens with recipes for hair dyes, and it displays an interest in beautifying the body throughout. Thus, chapter 16 contains remedies against smelly armpits;[46] the chapter on teeth includes recipes to whiten them;[47] and the chapter on breasts includes recipes to preserve their beauty and pertness.[48] Gynaecology is represented in chapter 15, which deals with breast diseases and medicaments promoting and checking lactation, and in the very long chapter 26, which contains 38 sections.[49]

As I have argued more fully elsewhere, *Euporista* II presents strong parallels with the gynaecological *Metrodora* compilation, preserved in a single Florence manuscript (MS Florence, Biblioteca Medicea Laurenziana, Plut. 75.3).[50] The *Metrodora* compilation also mixes gynaecology with cosmetics. There are even cases of parallel recipes between *Euporista* II and the *Metrodora* compilation, such as the case of a recipe to straighten drooping breasts.[51] Both collections also include recipes to restore virginity, which, while different from each other, testify to a concern that is not found in Galen's pharmacological treatises.[52] The similarities between *Euporista* II and *Metrodora* are particularly pronounced, but other ancient *Euporista* treatises displayed an interest in gynaecology. This is the case for the third book of Theodorus Priscianus's *Euporiston* and the fourth book of Oribasius's *Books to Eunapius*. *Euporista* II ends without a conclusion and without any link to *Euporista* III.

---

[46] *De rem. para.* 2.16, XIV, 449 K.

[47] *De rem. para.* 2.8, XIV, 426–27 K.

[48] *De rem. para.* 2.15, XIV, 447 and 449 K.

[49] Chapter 15: XIV, 446–49 K.; chapter 26: XIV, 475–486 K.

[50] See L. Totelin, 'The Third Way: Galen, Pseudo-Galen, Metrodora, Cleopatra and the Gynaecological Pharmacology of Byzantium', in *Collecting Recipes: Byzantine and Jewish Pharmacology in Dialogue*, eds L. Lemhaus and M. Martelli, Berlin, 2017, pp. 103–22. For editions of the Metrodora compilation, see A. P. Kousis, "Metrodora's Work 'On the Feminine Diseases of the Womb' according the Greek Codex 75,3 of the Laurentian Library', *Praktika ēs Akadēmias Athēnōn*, 20, 1945, pp. 49–60; G. Del Guerra, *Metrodora: medicina e cosmesi ad uso delle donne: la antica sapienza femminile e la cura di sé*, Milan, 1953.

[51] *De rem. para.* 2.15.1, XIV, 446 K. cf. Metrodora 49, MS Florence, Biblioteca Medicea Laurenziana, Plut. 75.3, fol. 17ᵛ.

[52] *De rem. para.* 2.26.12, XIV, 478 K. cf. Metrodora 32, MS Florence, Biblioteca Medicea Laurenziana, Plut. 75.3, fol. 15ʳ. See A. E. Hanson, 'The Hippocratic *Parthenos* in Sickness and Health', in *Virginity Revisited: Configurations of the Unpossessed Body*, eds B. MacLachlan and J. Fletcher, Toronto, 2007, pp. 40–65.

Euporista Book III

Euporista III is clearly different from the two other books we have examined so far. It starts *in medias res*, with recipes for a swollen uvula; it has no chapter divisions and does not follow the head-to-toe order. It appears to be constituted of several recipe clusters, composed in different periods. Some of the recipes would not be out of place in an authentic Galenic treatise, but others are clearly much later. Several include Christian elements. Thus, a recipe against pains in the womb is attributed to the *Anargyroi* saints, that is, Cosmas and Damian.[53] Another recipe is attributed to a monk called Barlama (Barlaam).[54] An interesting remedy to preserve the health of cows involves a candle – presumably a liturgical candle.[55] Finally, one remedy claims to chase away demons.[56]

Several recipes in *Euporista* III are written in late Byzantine Greek. That is the case for recipes clustering over two pages of Kühn's edition (XIV, 562–63 K.), in which we find the words γούλα to refer to the throat of a cock; μοὺρ given as a synonym for σμύρνα, myrrh; and ζουφάς to refer to hyssop.[57] Most remarkable, however, is a long recipe for garum attributed to a certain Ioachos of Martyropolis (near Amida), which contains among many other ingredients sugar (σάκχαρ), and ambergris (ἄμβαρ), and uses the word τζιαρίκη (probably of Ottoman origin) to refer to a measure, as well as the late word τράμια for the drachm.[58] Also noteworthy is a recipe which gives the name of an ointment 'in the Saracen language', that is, in Arabic.[59] A large cluster of recipes, then, appear to date to the late Byzantine period.

[53] *De rem. para.* 3, XIV, 536 K.: πρὸς πόνον μήτρας τῶν ἁγίων ἀναργύρων. λαβὼν ἄσαρον μετὰ γλήχωνος δὸς πιεῖν (Against pains in the womb, recipe of the Anargyroi saints, take hazelwort with pennyroyal; give to drink).

[54] *De rem. para.* 3, XIV, 548 K.: περὶ κεφαλαλγίας Βαρλαμὰ μοναχοῦ.

[55] *De rem. para.* 3, XIV, 525–26 K.: εἰς τὸ μὴ νοσεῖν βόας. ἐλάφου κέρας θὲς ἐπάνω πανίου καὶ ἐπάνω ἄψον κανδήλαν καὶ μὴ ἐπιλάθου τὴν ἡμέραν καὶ κατὰ χρόνον ἐπικαλοῦ τὸν ἅγιον Δημούσαριν καὶ Ἄρσον, φυλάξοντας τὰ κτήνη καὶ τὸν βίον σοῦ (To prevent cows from being ill: place a deer horn above a bobbin, and above this attach a candle, and do not forget it [?] for a day. During that time pray to the holy Demousaris [?] and Arsus [?] that they might preserve your beasts and your own life).

[56] *De rem. para.* 3, XIV, 561 K.: πρὸς φαρμακείας. καρίδιον καὶ πλατυκύμινον καὶ ζωχίου ῥίζαν ἀποτριτώσας δὸς πιεῖν μετ' οἴνου παλαιοῦ καὶ φορείτω καὶ γλανέων ὀστᾶ, καὶ γὰρ καπνιζόμενα δαίμονας διώκει (Against charms: small crab, broad cumin, root of thistle; boil down to a third; give to drink with old wine, and let the patient bear [?] a fumigation of sheat-fish bones, for they chase away demons).

[57] All three words are recorded in the Lexikon zur byzantinischen Gräzität.

[58] *De rem. para.* 3, XIV, 547–48 K.

[59] *De rem. para.* 3, XIV, 557 K.: ἄλειμμα δόκιμον ... λεγομένου Σαρακινιστὶ τλεν (Excellent unguent ... called *tlen* in the Saracen language).

As noted by von Haller and Ackermann, Galen himself is cited as a source in *Euporista* III. He is presented as the author of two long recipes: one for squill vinegar and one for squill wine.[60] The recipe for squill vinegar is prefaced with an anecdote about the philosopher Pythagoras who managed to live to the age of 107 thanks to the power of this preparation. The philosopher Pythagoras generously shared his knowledge with the world, thus benefitting numerous emperors. 'Galen' then switches to the first person, asserting that he will expound the infallible power of the medicament.[61]

Conclusion

The three Pseudo-Galenic *Euporista* are a heteroclite collection. Book I is quite similar to the Galenic *On the Composition of Drugs according to Places*, and even shares some recipes with it. However, in the spirit of the *Euporiston* genre, Book I contains only short recipes, with ingredients that are – for the most part – common or easily substituted. This book may be authentically Galenic.

Book II is particularly interesting in that it openly offers cosmetic recipes, which Galen frowned upon. It also has a strong emphasis on gynaecology, and in particular on breast ailments, for which Galen had very little interest. In many ways, *Euporista* II complements *Euporista* I very well. The compilator's attempt at linking the two books together may be very awkward, but it does make good practical sense.

Book III is much more varied and may have evolved over a long period of time, perhaps only gaining its final form in the fifteenth century, to which belongs our earliest preserved manuscript. It was probably attached to the two other books of *Euporista* because it contained remedies allegedly by Galen.

[60] Squill vinegar: XIV, 567–69 K.; squill wine: XIV, 569–70 K.
[61] *De rem. para.* 3, XIV, 567–69 K.

Table One: Greek Manuscripts, in Approximate Chronological Order[62]

Manuscript	Century	book I	book II	book III
Rome, Biblioteca Apostolica Vaticana, Urbinas gr. 67	13th	✓		
Milan, Biblioteca Ambrosiana B 126 sup	14th		✓	
London, Wellcome Library, MS 60	15th	✓		
Milan, Biblioteca Ambriosiana, Q 94	15th–16th		✓	
Vaticano, Biblioteca Apostolica Vaticana, Barberinus gr. 147	15th–16th	✓ (without prologue)	✓ (up to XIV, 462 K.)	✓ (last words differ)
Bibliothèque nationale de France, suppl. gr. 684	15th-18th			(a similar, but different text)
Paris, Bibliothèque nationale de France, suppl. gr. 636	16th	✓ (up to XIV, 364 K.)		
Moscow, Gosudarstvennyj, Sinod. gr. 508	16th-17th		✓	

[62] Table compiled by Caroline Petit and Laurence Totelin, based on Caroline Petit's direct inspection of the Vatican Library manuscripts and the information found on the Pinakes website (http://pinakes.irht.cnrs.fr/notices/oeuvre/3784/, accessed February 2021) and Diels's list of manuscripts, 1905, pp. 99–100. The MS Bibliothèque Nationale de France, Suppl. grec 764, which preserves a fragment of the text at ff. 37–44, could not be consulted.

Les manuscrits grecs des *Definitiones medicae* pseudo-galéniques

Marie Cronier

Les *Definitiones medicae* (ὅροι ἰατρικοί) figurent parmi les plus célèbres ouvrages dont l'attribution à Galien, attestée unanimement dans les manuscrits, a été rejetée de longue date.

Tradition manuscrite

La tradition manuscrite des *Definitiones medicae* a été étudiée en détail par Jutta Kollesch, dont on regrette que l'édition annoncée ne soit pas encore parue à ce jour.[1] Ce travail fondamental a bien montré les difficultés de reconstitution de la forme originelle qu'a pu prendre le traité. La présente contribution se situe dans le prolongement des travaux de Jutta Kollesch, en tirant parti de l'analyse matérielle et historique des manuscrits.

Voici un liste des témoins manuscrits :[2]

- Athos, Μονὴ Κουτλουμουσίου, 248 (Lampros 3321), 17e s., fols 197–221.[3]
- Berlin, Staatsbibliothek (Preussischer Kulturbesitz), Phillipps 1526 (gr. 122), 16e s., fols 38v–62v, texte complet, sans titre.[4]
- Bologna, Biblioteca Universitaria, 3632, milieu du 15e s., fols 129r–131v, version abrégée (seulement une sélection de définitions à l'intérieur de l'œuvre).[5]

[1] J. Kollesch, *Untersuchungen zu den pseudogalenischen Definitiones*, Berlin, 1973.

[2] À l'exception du Marc. gr. IV.10, tous ces manuscrits. ont été signalés par Kollesch, *Untersuchungen* (n. 1 ci-dessus), pp. 47–8, qui corrige et complète la liste de H. Diels, 'Die Handschriften der antiken Ärzte. I. Teil. Hippokrates und Galenos', *Abhandlungen der Königlichen Preußischen Akademie der Wissenschaften zu Berlin 1905*, Berlin, 1905, p. 111, et H. Diels, 'Bericht über den Stand des interakademischen Corpus medicorum antiquorum und Erster Nachtrag zu den in den Abhandlungen 1905 und 1906 veröffentlichten Katalogen : Die Handschriften der antiken Ärzte, I. und II. Teil', *Abhandlungen der Königlichen Preußischen Akademie der Wissenschaften zu Berlin 1907*, Berlin, 1908, p. 36.

[3] S. Lampros, *Catalogue of the Greek Manuscripts on Mount Athos*, t. I, Cambridge, 1895, p. 305.

[4] W. Studemund and L. Cohn, *Verzeichnisse der Königlichen Bibliothek zu Berlin*, t. I : *Codices ex bibliotheca Meermanniana Phillippici graeci nunc Berolinenses*, Berlin, 1890, pp. 49–50.

[5] A. Olivieri and N. Festa, 'Indice dei codici greci delle biblioteche Universitaria e Comunale di Bologna', *Studi italiani di filologia classica*, 3, 1895, pp. 385–495 (446). Pour la datation au milieu

- Firenze, Biblioteca Medicea Laurenziana, Plut. 74.14, fin du 15ᵉ s., fols 1ʳ–26ʳ, texte complet.[6]
- København, Det Kongelige Bibliotek, GKS 1648 4°, fin du 15ᵉ s., fols 1ʳ–8ᵛ. Fragment : début du texte jusqu'à ὥστε κουφίζεσθαι τὸ ἡγούμενον τῆς ψυχῆς (μέρος) (XIX, 365.9 K.: déf. 71).[7]
- Leipzig, Universitätsbibliothek, gr. 52, 16ᵉ s., fols 40ʳ–56ᵛ, texte complet.[8]
- London, British Library, Addit. 11888, fin du 15ᵉ ou début du 16ᵉ s., fols 1ʳ–24ʳ, texte complet.[9]
- London, Wellcome Library, MS. 289, 16ᵉ s., fols 1ʳ–30ʳ, texte complet.[10]
- Milano, Biblioteca Ambrosiana, B 90 sup. (gr. 115), début du 16ᵉ s. fols 1ʳ–42ᵛ, texte complet.[11]
- Milano, BA, T 19 sup. (gr. 742), fin du 15ᵉ s., fols 122ʳ–178ʳ, texte complet.[12]
- Modena, Biblioteca Estense e Universitaria, α.V.6.12 (gr. 210), début du 16ᵉ s., fols 387ʳ–414ᵛ, texte complet.[13]
- Moskva, Gosudarstvennyj Istoričeskij Musej (Государственный Исторический музей / Musée historique d'État), Synod. gr. 51 (Vladimir 464), milieu du 14ᵉ s., fols 328ᵛ–340ʳ, texte complet.[14]

du 15ᵉ siècle et l'identification du scribe comme Démétrios Angélos, voir B. Mondrain, 'Démétrios Angélos et la médecine : contribution nouvelle au dossier', in *Storia della tradizione e edizione dei medici greci. Atti del VI Colloquio internazionale, Paris 12–14 aprile 2008*, eds V. Boudon-Millot, A. Garzya, J. Jouanna and A. Roselli, Napoli, 2010, pp. 293-322 (300–313).

[6] A. M. Bandini, *Catalogus codicum manuscriptorum Bibliothecae Mediceae Laurentianae ...*, t. I–III, Florence, 1764–70, réimpr. Leipzig, 1961, t. III, col. 115–6.

[7] B. Schartau, *Codices graeci Haunienses. Ein deskriptiver Katalog des griechischen Handschriftenbestandes der Königlichen Bibliothek Kopenhagen*, Copenhagen, 1994, pp. 138–9.

[8] V. Gardthausen, *Katalog der griechischen Handschriften der Universitäts-Bibliothek zu Leipzig*, Leipzig, 1898, pp. 72–3. Dans l'attente de la parution du catalogue des manuscrits de Leipzig réalisé par Friederike Berger, on consultera la très bonne notice descriptive qu'elle a établie pour ce manuscrit sur le site Manuscripta mediaevalia (http://www.manuscripta-mediaevalia.de/dokumente/html/obj31584930).

[9] Une reproduction du manuscrit est disponible sur le site internet de la British Library, accompagnée d'une notice descriptive (http://www.bl.uk/manuscripts/).

[10] P. Bouras-Vallianatos, 'Greek Manuscripts at the Wellcome Library in London : A Descriptive Catalogue', *Medical History*, 59, 2015, pp. 275–326 (316–7).

[11] E. Martini and D. Bassi, *Catalogus codicum graecorum Bibliothecae Ambrosianae*, Milan, 1906, p. 126.

[12] *Ibidem*, p. 854.

[13] V. Puntoni, 'Indice dei codici greci della Biblioteca Estense di Modena', *Studi italiani di filologia classica*, 4, 1896, pp. 379–536 (508) ; voir aussi la description de G. De Gregorio sur le site internet *Commentaria in Aristotelem Graeca et Byzantina* (https://cagb-db.bbaw.de), en particulier pour une datation dans les années 1510-30 et l'identification des copistes.

[14] Archim. Vladimir (Filantropov), Систематическое описание рукописей Московской Сино-

– München, Bayerische Staatsbibliothek, cod. gr. 109, 1re moitié du 16e s., fols 1^r–21^v, texte complet.[15]

– München, BSB, gr. 469, fin du 13e ou début du 14e s., fols 78–82^v,[16] début du texte seulement.[17]

– Oxford, Bodleian Library, D'Orville 3 (Auct. X.1.1.3), fin du 15e s., fols 191^r–213^v, texte complet.[18]

– Paris, Bibliothèque nationale de France, gr. 2153, 1re moitié ou milieu du 15e s., fols 29^r–36^v, texte complet.[19]

– Paris, BNF, gr. 2167, 16e s., fols 269^v–281^v, texte complet.[20]

– Paris, BNF, gr. 2175, 16e s., fols 50^r–81^v, texte complet.[21]

– Paris, BNF, gr. 2282, 2nde moitié du 15e s., fols 53^v–99^v, texte complet.[22]

– Paris, BNF, suppl. gr. 35, fin du 15e s., fols 1^r–23^v, texte complet.[23]

– Paris, BNF, suppl. gr. 446, début du 10e s., fols 70^r–91^r, texte mutilé au début (manque 1 folio).[24]

дальной (Патриаршей) библиотеки/Sistematičeskoe opisanie rukopisej Moskovskoj Sinodal'noj (Patriaršej) biblioteki Moscou, 1894, pp. 701–3 (n° 464). Pour une datation au milieu du 14e siècle, voir B. Mondrain, 'Les écritures dans les manuscrits byzantins du xive siècle. Quelques problématiques', *Rivista di Studi Bizantini e Neoellenici*, 44, 2007, pp. 157–96 (181 et 183), qui renvoie aux travaux de B. Fonkič pour l'identification d'un des scribes comme Constantin Sophos. Selon B. Mondrain, le *Mosquensis* serait le résultat d'une volonté de rassembler les œuvres complètes de Galien. Le même scribe a également rassemblé 'tout Hippocrate' dans un autre volume, le *Vaticanus gr. 277*. Il faut cependant remarquer que dans le *Mosquensis* les *Definitiones medicae* ont été ajoutées à la fin, par un autre scribe, sur un papier différent (communication personnelle de B. Mondrain, que je remercie).

[15] M. Molin Pradel, *Katalog der griechischen Handschriften der Bayerischen Staatsbibliothek München*, t. II : *Codices graeci Monacenses 56–109*, Wiesbaden, 2013, pp. 325–6.

[16] On utilise la numérotation de l'angle supérieur externe.

[17] I. Hardt, *Catalogus codicum manuscriptorum graecorum Bibliothecae Regiae Bauaricae*, t. IV, Munich, 1810, pp. 451–4.

[18] F. Madan, *A Summary Catalogue of Western Manuscripts in the Bodleian Library at Oxford*, t. IV, Oxford, 1897, p. 38.

[19] Le texte n'est pas recensé dans l'inventaire d'H. Omont (voir note suivante) ni dans le répertoire de Diels, 'Die Handschriften' (n. 2 ci-dessus). Sa présence est signalée par Kollesch, *Untersuchungen* (n. 1 ci-dessus), p. 47 n. 2.

[20] H. Omont, *Inventaire sommaire des manuscrits grecs de la Bibliothèque nationale et des autres bibliothèques de Paris et des Départements*, t. II, Paris, 1888, pp. 208–9.

[21] Omont, *Inventaire* (n. 20 ci-dessus), p. 209.

[22] Omont, *Inventaire* (n. 20 ci-dessus), p. 229.

[23] C. Astruc, M.-L. Concasty, C. Bellon and C. Förstel, *Catalogue des manuscrits grecs. Supplément grec numéros 1 à 150*, Paris, 2003, pp. 94–6.

[24] H. Omont, *Inventaire sommaire des manuscrits grecs de la Bibliothèque nationale et des autres bibliothèques de Paris et des Départements*, t. III, Paris, 1888, p. 262. Voir aussi la description du contenu dans M. Cronier, 'Un témoin problématique de Théophile : le *Parisinus suppl. gr. 446*', in

- Paris, BNF, suppl. gr. 1328, 16ᵉ s., fols 1ʳ–87ʳ, texte complet.[25]
- Vaticano, Biblioteca Apostolica Vaticana, Ottob. gr. 311: 15ᵉ s. pour cette partie, fols 112ᵛ–117ʳ [26] (longs extraits).[27]
- Vaticano, BAV, Palat. gr. 199, début du 14ᵉ s.,[28] fols 192ʳ–193ʳ, 194ᵛ–195ʳ, 198ᵛ, 272ʳ, extraits.[29]
- Vaticano, BAV, Palat. gr. 297, début du 14ᵉ s. pour cette partie, fols 3ʳ–16ᵛ, 19ʳ–39ʳ, longs extraits avec une présentation en deux livres.[30]
- Vaticano, BAV, Vat. gr. 1614, fin du 15ᵉ s., fols 125ʳ–156, texte complet.[31]
- Venezia, Biblioteca Nazionale Marciana, gr. IV.10 (coll. 833), début du 16ᵉ s., fols 11ᵛ–141ʳ.[32]

Un corpus médical problématique. Les traités attribués à Théophile Protospathaire (VIIᵉ–IXᵉ s.) et la relecture chrétienne des enseignements hippocratiques et galéniques (Paris, 27–28 novembre 2014), eds A. Guardasole and C. Magdelaine, Paris (à paraître).

[25] C. Astruc and M.-L. Concasty, *Bibliothèque nationale. Catalogue des manuscrits grecs. Troisième partie : Le Supplément grec, Tome III : Numéros 901–1371*, Paris, 1960, p. 628.

[26] E. Féron and F. Battaglini, *Bibliothecae Apostolicae Vaticanae... Codices manuscripti graeci Ottoboniani*, Rome, 1893, p. 166.

[27] Après le prologue, on trouve une sélection de définitions. La dernière correspond à la *Def.* 220 de Kühn : Τί ἐστι ῥυθμός; κίνησις ἐν χρόνοις ... ἐν οἷς συστέλονται (XIX, 409.7 K.).

[28] H. Stevenson, *Bibliothecae Apostolicae Vaticanae... Codices Palatini graeci*, Roma, 1885, pp. 99–101. Pour la datation au tout début du 14ᵉ siècle, voir B. Mondrain, 'Nicolas Myrepse et une collection de manuscrits médicaux dans la première moitié du xivᵉ siècle. À propos d'une miniature célèbre du *Parisinus gr. 2243*', in *I testi medici greci. Tradizione e ecdotica. Atti del III Convegno Internazionale, Napoli 15-18 ottobre 1997*, eds A. Garzya and J. Jouanna, Naples, 1999, pp. 403–18 (408–11).

[29] Le texte des *Definitiones medicae* n'est pas copié en tant que tel mais beaucoup de définitions ont été insérées d'une part à l'intérieur d'un traité anonyme *De pulsibus*, d'autre part dans les livres V et VI d'Aétios. La liste exhaustive des extraits est donnée par A. Mavroudis, 'Τὸ ψευδο-γαληνικό ἔργο Ὅροι ιατρικοί και ο κώδικας Vaticanus Palat. gr. 199', *Ἑλληνικά*, 44, 1994, pp. 319–40 ; voir aussi A. Mavroudis, 'Τὸ ανώνυμο έργο Περί σφυγμού στον κώδικα Vaticanus Palat. gr. 199 και το Περί της του ανθρώπου κατασκευής του Μελετίου', *Ἑλληνικά*, 41, 1990, pp. 235–65.

[30] Stevenson, *Codices Palatini Graeci* (n. 28 ci-dessus), pp. 166–7. La première partie du manuscrit (fols 3ʳ–42ᵛ ; les fols 1–2 sont d'anciennes gardes de papier) est due au même copiste que le *Pal. gr.* 199 et peut donc être datée, comme lui, au tout début du 14ᵉ s. (voir Mondrain, 'Nicolas Myrepse' (n. 28 ci-dessus), pp. 411–12). L'ordre des folios doit être reconstitué de la manière suivante (d'après une précédente numérotation du 16ᵉ s., indiquant qu'il manque au début 18 folios) : fols 17–22, 41, 3–16, 24, 25, 23, 26–40. Le fol. 42, qui contient un fragment du livre VI d'Aétius (chap. 29–36), se trouvait plus loin dans le manuscrit original. Le fol. 17 contient le début du livre IV de Paul d'Égine. Le fol. 18 est illisible, le fol. 19 contient des recettes attribuées à Archigène, Rufus et Logadios.

[31] C. Giannelli, *Bibliothecae Apostolicae Vaticanae... Codices Vaticani Graeci. Codices 1485–1683*, Città del Vaticano, 1950, pp. 278–9.

[32] E. Mioni, *Bibliothecae Divi Marci Venetiarum codices graeci manuscripti. Volumen I, Pars altera : Classis II, Codd. 121–198 – Classes III, IV, V. Indices*, Rome, 1972, p. 204.

– Venezia, BNM, gr. V.9 (coll. 1017), 1re moitié ou milieu du 15e s., fols 500^r–507^v (longs extraits, entre les *def.* 50 [XIX, 360.10 K.] et 381 [XIX, 441.9 K.]).[33]

– Venezia, BNM, gr. Z. 521 (coll. 316), milieu ou 2nde moitié du 13e s., fol. 100^{r-v}[34] (fragment : fin du traité).[35]

– Wien, Österreichische Nationalbibliothek, med. gr. 16, fin du 13e s. pour cette partie, fols 287^r–309^r, texte complet.[36]

On laissera ici de côté les très nombreux manuscrits ne contenant qu'un petit nombre d'extraits.

Les éditions imprimées

Le traité a été édité pour la première fois en grec dans la monumentale édition aldine de Galien (1525) puis de nouveau dans l'édition basiléenne de 1538.[37] Ainsi que l'a indiqué Jutta Kollesch dans ses travaux désormais classiques, le texte de ces deux éditions a été établi à partir de la famille A (voir *infra*) :[38] cela n'est guère surprenant puisque c'est à cette branche qu'appartiennent quasiment tous les témoins qui se trouvaient en Europe occidentale dans la première moitié du 16e siècle.[39]

Un changement majeur dans la constitution du texte des *Definitiones medicae* apparaît avec l'édition de René Chartier, parue en 1638.[40] Comme l'a très bien montré J. Kollesch, Chartier part de la basiléenne mais remanie considérablement le texte, en faisant appel à un manuscrit de la Bibliothèque royale de France qui peut être identifié avec l'actuel *Par. gr.* 2153, lequel contient un texte beaucoup

---

[33] Mioni, *Bibliothecae Divi Marci* (n. 32 ci-dessus), pp. 265–70.

[34] E. Mioni, *Bibliothecae Divi Marci Venetiarum codices graeci manuscripti. Volumen II : Thesaurus Antiquus. Codices 300–625*, Rome, 1985, pp. 390–93.

[35] On trouve les définitions suivantes : 86 fin (XIX, 368.5 K.), 448, 437–47, 449–62, 465–86 (cet ordre est bien celui de tous les manuscrits de la famille A de Kollesch, voir *infra*).

[36] H. Hunger and O. Kresten, *Katalog der griechischen Handschriften der Österreichischen Nationalbibliothek, II. Codices Juridici et Medici*, Vienne, 1969, pp. 60–62.

[37] Édition aldine : *Galeni Opera omnia*, Venise, 1525, t. IV, 3e partie, fols 11^r–17^r; édition basiléenne : *Galeni Pergameni… opera omnia*, Basel, 1538, t. IV, p. 390–403.

[38] Kollesch, *Untersuchungen* (n. 1 ci-dessus), p. 48, n. 4.

[39] La seule exception, à ma connaissance, est constituée par le *Par. gr.* 2153, qui se trouvait à la fin du 15e siècle dans la collection de Gioacchino Turriano (1416–1500), lequel léga de son vivant sa bibliothèque au monastère vénitien dei Santi Giovanni e Paolo, où le volume a dû rester jusqu'à son achat dans les années 1560 par Jean Hurault de Boistaillé.

[40] *Operum Hippocratis Coi et Claudii Galeni Pergameni medicorum omnium principum Tomus II. Τὰ εἰσαγωγικὰ quae in artem medicam introducunt*, Paris, 1638, pp. 232–81.

plus développé que celui de la famille textuelle utilisée pour les éditions aldine et basiléenne (famille A). Les interventions de Chartier vont d'ailleurs beaucoup plus loin, puisqu'il ajoute un nombre important de passages totalement étrangers au texte transmis dans les manuscrits (mais qui proviennent en fait d'autres médecins grecs) et opère de nombreux remaniements dans l'organisation de l'ouvrage. Ce travail a été très bien analysé par J. Kollesch et ne demande pas davantage de développements.[41]

Quant à l'édition de Kühn, on sait également depuis les travaux de J. Kollesch que pour les *Definitiones medicae* elle reprend mot pour mot celle de Chartier. Il s'avère ainsi que le texte de l'édition de Kühn n'est absolument pas représentatif de celui que nous transmettent les manuscrits, en-dehors même des divergences que ces derniers présentent entre eux. En conséquence, toute analyse de ce traité, de son organisation, de son contenu, évitera absolument de s'appuyer sur l'édition de Kühn mais devra, idéalement, remonter aux manuscrits.[42] À défaut, on pourra prendre pour référence le texte des éditions de la Renaissance (aldine et basiléenne), qui reflètent au moins un état textuel bien attesté dans les manuscrits et remontant au plus tard à la seconde moitié du 13e siècle (époque où l'on peut situer la réalisation de son plus ancien témoin, le *Marc. gr.* 521).

Les familles textuelles

À l'intérieur de la tradition manuscrite des *Definitiones medicae*, Jutta Kollesch distingue deux familles : la famille A, comportant 19 manuscrits, et la famille B, avec 10 manuscrits.[43] À mon sens, la notion de famille dans un sens philologique n'est valable que pour A, dont Jutta Kollesch a montré que les témoins présentent une réelle unité de texte. La famille B, en revanche, est totalement hétéroclite et ne mérite pas le nom de 'famille'.

---

[41] Voir en particulier : J. Kollesch, 'René Chartier Herausgeber und Fälscher der Werke Galens', *Klio*, 48, 1967, pp. 183–98; J. Kollesch, 'René Chartier als Herausbeger der Werke Galens', in *Antiquitas Graeco-Romana ac tempora nostra. Acta Congressus Internationalis habiti Brunae diebus 12–16 mensis Aprilis MXMLXVI*, eds J. Burian and L. Vidman, Praha, 1968, pp. 525–30; en dernier lieu : C. Petit, 'René Chartier (1572-1654) et l'authenticité des traités galéniques', in *René Chartier (1572–1654) éditeur et traducteur d'Hippocrate et Galien. Actes du colloque international de Paris (7 et 8 octobre 2010)*, eds V. Boudon-Millot, G. Cobolet and J. Jouanna, Paris, 2012, pp. 289–91.

[42] Par exemple, comme l'a très bien montré J. Kollesch, Max Wellmann avait remarqué la présence d'un extrait d'Arétée de Cappadoce dans le texte des *Definitiones medicae* et en avait déduit que l'auteur des *Definitiones medicae* utilisait ce traité. En fait, c'est Chartier qui l'utilisait ! Voir Kollesch, 'René Chartier Herausgeber' (n. 41 ci-dessus), pp. 186-7.

[43] Kollesch, *Untersuchungen* (n. 1 ci-dessus), p. 48.

La famille A

Jutta Kollesch réunit dans la famille A les manuscrits suivants : *Ath. Koutloum.* 248 ; *Berol. Phill.* 1526 ; *Flor. Laur.* 74.14 ; *Haun.* GKS 1648 4° ; *Lips. gr.* 52 ; *Lond. Add.* 11888 ; *Lond. Wellc.* 289 ; *Mediol. Ambros.* B 90 sup. et T 19 sup. ; *Mut.* α.V.6.12 ; *Monac. gr.* 109 ; *Oxon. Bodl. D'Orv.* 3 ; *Par. gr.* 2167, 2175 et 2282 ; *Par. suppl. gr.* 35 et 1328 ; *Vat. gr.* 1614 ; *Venet. Marc. gr.* 521.

L'unité philologique très bien mise en évidence par J. Kollesch peut être renforcée, me semble-t-il, par une unité chronologique et même géographique. En effet, tous les manuscrits de cette famille A sont 'récents' (c'est-à-dire qu'ils ne sont pas antérieurs à la fin du 15e siècle) et ont été produits en Occident.[44] Voici les éléments qui permettent de l'établir pour chaque manuscrit :

- *Berol. Phill.* 1526. Il fait partie du petit nombre de manuscrits de Guillaume Pellicier (1490–1567) que ce dernier n'a pas fait exécuter sur commande pendant son séjour à Venise (1539–1542) mais s'est procurés d'une autre manière : en effet, il daterait plutôt du début du 16e siècle.[45] Il formait originellement un unique livre avec l'actuel *Berol. Phill.* 1529,[46] qui porte une note d'appartenance au chanoine Simon Charpentier. Charpentier, qui a donc possédé le *Phill.* 1526, est connu par ailleurs comme possesseur du *Leidensis Voss. gr.* F. 53.[47] Les deux manuscrits (*Phill.* 1526 + 1529 et *Voss. gr.* F. 53) ont un format très proche[48] et contiennent des ouvrages de médecine : peut-être ont-ils été réalisés dans le même atelier,[49] pour un même commanditaire ? Ce commanditaire serait peut-être Guillaume Cop (Wilhelm Kopp, † 1532), médecin du roi François Ier et connu comme

---

[44] Il y a cependant deux exceptions : l'*Athous Koutl.* 248 et le *Marc. gr.* 521, dont il sera bientôt question.

[45] Voir A. Cataldi Palau, 'Les copistes de Guillaume Pellicier, évêque de Maguelonne (1490-1567)', *Scrittura e civiltà*, 10, 1986, pp. 199–237 (199 n. 1).

[46] A. Cataldi Palau, 'Les vicissitudes de la collection de manuscrits grecs de Guillaume Pellicier', *Scriptorium*, 40, 1986, pp. 32–53 (44). Le *Phill.* 1529 contient le *De compositione medicamentorum per genera* de Galien et quelques opuscules médicaux.

[47] Le *Voss. gr.* F. 53 (première moitié du 16e s.) contient l'*Ad Glauconem* puis le *De locis affectis* de Galien. Par la suite, il a appartenu à Paul Petau (1568–1614) et à son fils Alexandre Petau (1610–72), puis à la reine Christine de Suède (1626–89). Son appartenance à Simon Charpentier n'est pas attestée par une note de possession mais est signalée dans le registre de la bibliothèque de Leyde. Voir K. A. De Meyïer, *Bibliotheca Universitatis Leidensis. Codices manuscripti. VI. Codices Vossiani graeci et Miscellanei*, Leiden, 1955, p. 61.

[48] *Voss. gr.* F. 53 : 305 × 215 mm ; *Phill.* 1526 : 300 × 200 mm ; *Phill.* 1529 : 310 × 220 mm.

[49] Cela pourrait être montré par une analyse paléographique et codicologique, que je n'ai pas encore effectuée.

traducteur de Paul d'Égine et d'Hippocrate. Cop aurait en effet possédé au moins le *Voss. gr.* F. 53.[50]

– *Laur.* 74.14. Datable dans la seconde moitié 15ᵉ s., il a été réalisé par un copiste anonyme mais qui était très vraisemblablement un Occidental, comme l'indiquent, me semble-t-il, certaines caractéristiques graphiques ainsi que la présence de réclames verticales et de remarques en latin de sa propre main.

– *Lips. gr.* 52. Le manuscrit aurait été réalisé en France, sans doute à Paris, vers 1517, par un copiste anonyme à qui on doit aussi les *Lips. gr.* 50 + 51 (Galien).[51] Pour le *Lips. gr.* 50, notre scribe a utilisé comme modèle le *Leid. Voss. gr.* F. 53,[52] qui appartenait alors à Guillaume Cop (voir *supra*). Il est donc possible que pour le *Lips. gr.* 52, il ait pris pour modèle le *Phill.* 1529, possédé par le même propriétaire.

– *Lond. Addit.* 11888. Sa souscription indique qu'il a été copié par un certain Nicolas. Ce dernier est attesté à la fin du 15ᵉ siècle et au début du 16ᵉ à Venise et Padoue, notamment comme collaborateur de Zacharias Calliergis.[53]

– *Lond. Wellc.* 289. Selon P. Bouras-Vallianatos, le manuscrit aurait été copié en Italie aux environs de 1535.[54]

– *Ambros.* B 90 sup. Datable au début du 16ᵉ siècle, il porte une note d'acquisition auprès d'un certain Pinatellus en 1525. On trouve en marge de nombreuses variantes textuelles, qui constituent sans doute un travail préparatoire à une édition. Il a ensuite appartenu à Girolamo Mercuriale (1530-1606).

– *Ambros.* T 19 sup. Son copiste peut être identifié comme Démétrios Damilas,[55] actif à Florence, Milan et Rome notamment, à la fin du 15ᵉ siècle. Il s'agit d'un manuscrit de luxe, copié sur du parchemin très fin,

---

[50] Selon l'indication du registre de la bibliothèque de Leyde ; voir De Meyïer, *Bibliotheca* (n. 47 ci-dessus), p. 61.

[51] Voir la description de F. Berger sur *Manuscripta mediaevalia* (n. 7 ci-dessus).

[52] Voir F. Gärtner, *Galeni De locis affectis I–II* (CMG V 6, 1, 1), Berlin, 2015, p. 62.

[53] Voir E. Gamillscheg and D. Harlfinger, *Repertorium der griechischen Kopisten 800–1600*, I : *Handschriften aus Bibliotheken Grossbritanniens*, Vienne, 1981, nº 330 et II : *Handschriften aus Bibliotheken Frankreichs und Nachträge zu den Bibliotheken Grossbritanniens*, Vienne, 1989, nº 447.

[54] Voir Bouras-Vallianatos, 'Greek Manuscripts' (n. 10 ci-dessus).

[55] Voir S. Martinelli Tempesta, 'Per un repertorio dei copisti greci in Ambrosiana', in *Miscellanea Graecolatina. I*, ed. F. Gallo, Milano/Roma, 2013, pp. 101–53 (137). Sur Démétrios Damilas, voir en dernier lieu D. Speranzi, 'Prima di Aldo. Demetrio Damilas disegnatore di caratteri', in *Manuciana Tergestina et Veronensia* (Graeca Tergestina 4), eds F. Donadi et al., Trieste, 2015, pp. 143–61, avec la bibliographie antérieure.

manifestement pour un commanditaire occidental (non identifié).

– *Mutin.* α.V.6.12 (gr. 210). Datable dans les années 1510–30 d'après les filigranes, le manuscrit a été copié notamment par Aristobule Apostolis et Jean Sévère de Lacédémone, vraisemblablement pour le prince Alberto Pio de Carpi (1475–1531) qui en est, en tout cas, le premier possesseur attesté.[56]

– *Monac. gr.* 109. De la première moitié du 16e siècle, il est dû au même copiste que les *Monac. gr.* 16 (fols 459r–474v) et 170 (pp. 1–84) et, comme eux, il a appartenu au médecin florentin Pietro Vettori (1499–1585), qui en est sans doute le commanditaire ou du moins l'un des premiers possesseurs.[57]

– *Bodl. D'Orv.* 3 (Auct. X.1.1.3). De la fin du 15e siècle, il est sans doute rattachable au milieu des collaborateurs d'Alde Manuce.[58]

– *Par. gr.* 2167. C'est un volume composé de divers fragments reliés ensemble et remontant au 16e siècle. Il serait pour partie une copie d'impression de l'Aldine.[59] Par la suite, il appartenu à John Clement († 1572), puis à Claude Joly (en 1666), avant d'être finalement acquis par Jean-Baptiste Colbert en 1677.

– *Par. gr.* 2175. Copié par une main occidentale de la fin du 15e siècle ou début du 16e s. (mais qui utilise une foliotation en lettres grecques), il porte (f. Ir) un *ex-libris* du médecin Jean Ruel († 1537) connu comme traducteur de Dioscoride, au-dessous d'une devise en français qui doit indiquer un autre possesseur (non identifié) : 'Dieu faict tout pour le mieulx'. Le manuscrit a ensuite appartenu à Jacques-Auguste de Thou (1553–1617).

– *Par. gr.* 2282. Datable dans la 2nde moitié du 15e siècle, il est dû à un unique scribe, anonyme, dont la main rappelle un peu celle de Jean Moschos. Le manuscrit a appartenu à Janus Lascaris (1445–1534) avant d'arriver, comme bon nombre de ses livres, dans la bibliothèque du Cardinal Ridolfi (1501–50). Selon Caroline Petit, il aurait été utilisé dans le cercle d'Alde Manuce :[60]

---

[56] Voir la description de G. De Gregorio sur le site internet du CAGB (n. 13 ci-dessus).

[57] Voir Molin Pradel, *Katalog* (n. 15 ci-dessus), pp. 325–6.

[58] Voir Petit, *Galien. Le médecin* (n. 53 ci-dessus), p. cxx et n. 178.

[59] Voir : C. De Stefani, 'Contributi della versione araba all'edizione del testo greco del "De differentiis febrium" di Galeno', in *Ecdotica e ricezione dei testi medici greci. Atti del V Convegno Internazionale, Napoli 1-2 ottobre 2004*, eds V. Boudon-Millot, A. Garzya, J. Jouanna and A. Roselli, Naples, 2006, pp. 111–16 (111 n. 1) (pour le *De differentiis febrium*) ; C. Petit, 'La tradition manuscrite du traité des Simples de Galien. Editio princeps et traduction annotée des chapitres 1 à 3 du livre I', in *Storia della tradizione e edizione dei medici greci. Atti del VI Colloquio internazionale, Paris 12–14 aprile 2008*, eds V. Boudon-Millot, A. Garzya, J. Jouanna and A. Roselli, Naples, 2010, pp. 143–65 (pour le *De simplicibus* de Galien).

[60] Voir Petit, *Galien, Le médecin* (n. 53 ci-dessus), p. cxx et n. 178.

ce n'est guère surprenant car on sait que Lascaris mit beaucoup de ses manuscrits à la disposition de cet éditeur.

– *Par. suppl. gr.* 35. Ses filigranes indiquent une datation à la fin du 15e siècle. Pour la seconde partie (fols 60–242), il a été copié par l'*Anonymus Harvardianus* (fols 61ʳ–120ʳ, 129ʳ–242ʳ) et Paul le Relieur (fols 121ʳ–126ʳ, les fols 126ᵛ–128ᵛ étant blancs),[61] dans l'entourage d'Alde Manuce, sans doute pour le médecin de Ferrare Niccolò Leoniceno (1428–1524), à qui en tout cas il a appartenu.[62] Quant à la première partie (fols 1ʳ–54ᵛ, les fols 55ʳ–59ᵛ étant blancs), où se trouvent le *Definitiones medicae*, elle peut être attribuée à Andronic Éparque selon Brigitte Mondrain[63] et doit être située à une époque un peu antérieure (2e moitié du 15e siècle).

– *Par. suppl. gr.* 1328. Son attribution au 16e siècle en fait encore un *recentior*. La suite de son histoire le situe en France : une note indique qu'il se trouvait au château de Malesherbes et il porte un *ex-libris* de Louis-Michel Le Peletier de Saint-Fargeau (1760–93).[64]

– *Vat. gr.* 1614. Il s'agit d'un livre de luxe, copié sur parchemin, produit vraisemblablement à Florence pour les Médicis. On le trouve en tout cas dans l'inventaire de la bibliothèque de Pierre de Médicis en 1495. C'est matériellement un jumeau du *Laur.* 6.6, copié par le même scribe (Laurent Kyathos),[65] sur une page de mêmes dimensions avec le même nombre de lignes. Comme ce dernier, il porte (fol. 7ʳ) une miniature peinte par Actavantius de Actavantiis.[66]

– *Haun.* GKS 1648 4°. Il s'agit du premier cahier (quaternion) d'un manuscrit qui devait contenir à l'origine l'ensemble du texte. La présence d'une réclame dénote une production occidentale : sur une base paléographique, le

---

[61] Voir P. Hoffmann, 'Un mystérieux collaborateur d'Alde Manuce : l'*Anonymus Harvardianus*', *Mélanges de l'École française de Rome. Moyen Âge, Temps modernes*, 97, 1985, pp. 45–143 (116–17).

[62] S. Fortuna, 'Nicolò Leoniceno e le edizioni aldine dei medici greci (con un'appendice sulle sue traduzioni latine)', in *Ecdotica e ricezione dei testi medici greci. Atti del V Convegno Internazionale, Napoli 1–2 ottobre 2004*, eds V. Boudon-Millot, A. Garzya, J. Jouanna and A. Roselli, Naples, 2006, pp. 443–64 (452).

[63] B. Mondrain, 'La lecture et la copie de textes scientifiques à Byzance pendant l'époque paléologue', in *La produzione scritta tecnica e scientifica nel medioevo : Libro e documento tra scuole e professioni. Atti del Convegno internazionale di studio dell'Associazione italiana dei Paleografi e Diplomatisti Fisciano – Salerno (28–30 settembre 2009)*, eds G. De Gregorio and M. Galante, Spoleto, 2012, pp. 607–32 (620).

[64] C. Astruc and M.-L. Concasty, *Le Supplément grec* (n. 25 ci-dessus), p. 628.

[65] Traducteur de Lucien, il est connu comme copiste d'un manuscrit daté de 1498 à Florence (*Par. gr.* 2844).

[66] Giannelli, *Codices Vaticani Graeci* (n. 31), pp. 278–9.

manuscrit a été attribué à la dernière période d'activité de Jean Scoutariotes, soit dans les années 1490.[67] Il a ensuite appartenu au cardinal Domenico Grimani (1461–1523).[68]

– *Marc. gr.* IV.10. Quoiqu'il ne soit pas mentionné par Jutta Kollesch, c'est sans doute également dans cette famille qu'il faut le ranger. Il s'agit d'un manuscrit de luxe, sur parchemin, copié à la fin du 15e siècle par César Stratégos probablement pour Gioacchino Turriano (1416–1500)

L'*Athous Koutloumous* 248 (Lampros 3321), du 17e siècle, est en revanche très susceptible d'avoir été produit dans l'Orient méditerranéen. Il n'est pas impossible qu'il descende d'une édition imprimée, comme cela arrive souvent pour les manuscrits grecs produits à cette époque dans l'empire Ottoman.

Mis à part le cas particulier de l'*Athous*, tous les manuscrits de la famille A de Kollesch sont donc des productions occidentales, dont aucune ne semble antérieure à la fin du 15e siècle. Le plus vraisemblable est que la multiplication des copies à cette période résulte de l'arrivée en Occident d'un unique manuscrit, dont tous ces *recentiores* descendraient, directement ou non. Je n'ai pas encore déterminé quel était ce manuscrit mais pour l'heure j'aurais tendance à vouloir orienter les investigations en direction du *Par. suppl. gr.* 35 où, comme on l'a vu, le texte des *Definitiones medicae* a été copié par le médecin Andronic Éparque. Originaire de Constantinople où il avait suivi l'enseignement de médecine de Jean Argyropoulos, Andronic s'exila après la chute de la ville (1453) pour finalement s'établir à Corfou dans la seconde moitié du 15e siècle. Il possédait une importante bibliothèque de textes médicaux, largement mise à profit par son fils Georges, son petit-fils Antoine et son entourage.[69] Même si ses filigranes semblent indiquer une datation dans la seconde moitié du 15e siècle, le *Par. suppl. gr.* 35 est donc peut-être susceptible de nous aider à remonter la piste.

De fait, dans cette famille A, le seul manuscrit quelque peu ancien est le *Marc. gr.* 521, de la seconde moitié du 13e siècle, malheureusement très mutilé : on ne conserve plus qu'un folio, avec la fin du texte. Pour ce passage, le texte du

---

[67] S. Martinelli Tempesta, 'Il codice Milano, Biblioteca Ambrosiana, B 75 sup. (gr. 104) e l'evoluzione della scrittura di Giovanni Scutariota', in *The Legacy of Bernard de Montfaucon : Three Hundred Years of Studies on Greek Handwriting. Proceedings of the Seventh International Colloquium of Greek Palaeography (Madrid-Salamanca, 15–20 September 2008)*, eds A. Bravo García and I. Pérez Martín, Turnhout, 2010, pp. 171–86 (174 n. 10).

[68] Voir D. Jackson, 'A List of Greek Mss of Domenico Grimani', *Scriptorium*, 62, 2008, pp. 164–9 (165).

[69] Sur ce personnage voir B. Mondrain, 'Janus Lascaris copiste et ses livres', in *I manoscritti greci tra riflessione e dibattito : Atti del 5 Colloquio internazionale di paleografia greca, Cremona, 4–10 ottobre 1998*, ed. G. Prato, Firenze, 2000, pp. 417–26 (424–5).

Marc. gr. 521 est très proche de celui des autres manuscrits de cette famille mais ne peut en être le modèle (notamment en raison de plusieurs omissions dans le *Marc. gr.* 521, par exemple la dernière définition). Le *Marc. gr.* 521 nous permet cependant de souligner que la forme transmise par la famille A n'est pas une création occidentale récente mais remonte à la période byzantine et était déjà attestée dans la seconde moitié du 13ᵉ siècle. Elle mérite donc d'être comparée aux autres manuscrits anciens pour une analyse de la structure du texte.

On soulignera en passant que, dans cette famille A, les *Definitiones medicae* sont presque toujours copiées avec l'*Introductio siue medicus* pseudo-galénique, ce qui n'arrive jamais dans les manuscrits anciens mais témoigne de l'intérêt particulier des Occidentaux pour ces textes à l'usage des débutants.[70]

La famille B

La famille B de Jutta Kollesch comprend les manuscrits suivants : pour le texte complet, les *Mosq. synod. gr.* 51 (Vlad. 464), *Par. gr.* 2153, *Par. suppl. gr.* 446 et *Vind. med. gr.* 16 ; pour des versions incomplètes ou abrégées, les *Bonon.* 3632, *Monac. gr.* 469, *Vat. Pal. gr.* 199 et 297, *Ott. gr.* 311 et *Marc. gr.* V.9.

Il me semble important de souligner que, contrairement à la famille A, ce qui est désigné comme 'famille B' est un groupe qui ne présente pas d'unité philologique : de fait, la famille B réunit tous les témoins qui ne font pas partie de la famille A mais ceux-ci ne comportent pas entre eux de parentés particulières. Bien au contraire, comme le fait remarquer déjà Jutta Kollesch, ces manuscrits se caractérisent chacun par des ajouts et des omissions qu'on ne trouve nulle part ailleurs. Ainsi, le *Par. gr.* 2153 présente une forme extrêmement 'augmentée' (qui se retrouve aussi, nous le verrons dans le *Mosquensis*); mais le *Par. suppl. gr.* 446 comporte aussi beaucoup d'ajouts qui lui sont propres (par exemple la séquence finale consacrée à l'ostéologie) ainsi que bon nombre d'omissions et de transpositions de définitions; c'est le cas également du *Vind. med. gr.* 16, pour ne parler que des témoins qui conservent la forme complète du texte. En revanche, je n'ai pas pour l'instant réussi à mettre en évidence de fautes communes qui permettraient de faire remonter ces témoins à un chef de file d'une famille quelconque.

La seule exception est constituée par le *Mosq. syn. gr.* 51 et le *Par. gr.* 2153 : tous deux sont étroitement apparentés, notamment en ce qu'ils présentent un ordre des

---

[70] Petit, 'René Chartier' (n. 41 ci-dessus), p. 289, recense neuf manuscrits présentant les deux textes.

questions extrêmement perturbé, exactement le même dans les deux cas.[71] Cette perturbation provient probablement d'un problème matériel sur un ancêtre, où des cahiers avaient été reliés dans le désordre. Le copiste du *Mosquensis*, conscient du problème, laisse régulièrement des lignes blanches au niveaux des jonctions problématiques. En revanche, ce n'est que très rarement le cas dans le *Par. gr.* 2153. Ce dernier, datable vers le milieu du 15ᵉ siècle, a toute chance d'être un descendant du *Mosquensis*, qui remonte au milieu du 14ᵉ siècle,[72] et il me semble qu'il pourrait donc être omis, en tant que *descriptus*, dans l'analyse de la famille B.

À mon sens donc, en dehors de la famille A et du *Par. gr.* 2153, chacun des manuscrits des *Definitiones medicae* représente une forme particulière de ce traité et il ne semble pas y avoir à l'époque byzantine de 'famille' textuelle pour ce texte à vocation didactique et pratique qui est, par nature, voué à être complété ou écourté, au gré des intérêts et des visées des copistes et des lecteurs. La seule 'famille' qui peut être individualisée, la famille A, doit son existence au fait qu'à la Renaissance, en Occident, on a recopié ce texte sans intervenir sur lui, ce qui ne devait certainement jamais se produire à l'époque byzantine ni même antérieurement.

Un texte aux formes variables

Une fois cette mise au point faite, il ne reste, en fin de compte, plus beaucoup de témoins sur lesquels s'appuyer pour analyser le traité et les formes qu'il a pu prendre. Parmi les manuscrits conservant ou ayant conservé le texte 'complet', nous n'avons en somme que quatre témoins ou groupes de témoins : (1) le *Par. suppl. gr.* 446 ; (2) le *Vind. med. gr.* 16 ; (3) le *Mosq. syn. gr.* 51 ; (4) la famille A.

Les autres témoins, en effet, nous conservent seulement une forme réélaborée et partielle :

- *Monac. gr.* 469 (fin du 13ᵉ-début du 14ᵉ siècle). Après un début mutilé (et donc sans titre), sont copiées les questions 8–111 (avec quelques déplacements ou omissions de définitions). Juste à la suite (au bas du fol. 82ᵛ), sous le

---

[71] Dans le *Mosq.* 51, cette perturbation est encore augmentée aujourd'hui par plusieurs interversions de l'ordre des folios. Il faut restituer la séquence originelle suivante : fols 328–332, 337, 338, 336, 333–335, 339–340. Une fois ce rétablissement effectué, l'ordre des questions est dans le *Mosq.* 51 strictement identique à celui du *Par. gr.* 2153.

[72] Cette solution me semble plus économique que celle de J. Kollesch, qui proposait que tous deux descendent d'un même modèle (Kollesch, 'René Chartier Herausgeber' (n. 41 ci-dessus), p. 184 n. 4). D'après mes sondages (qui devront naturellement être complétés par une analyse exhaustive), le *Par. gr.* 2153 ne conserve jamais une leçon meilleure que le *Mosq. syn. gr.* 51, sauf par conjecture aisée.

titre Γαληνοῦ περὶ τῶν ἐτησίων καιρῶν ὧν δεῖ διαιτᾶσθαι, on trouve la fin de l'*Epistula ad Ptolemaeum regem de hominis fabrica*, souvent attribuée à Hippocrate.[73]

– *Pal. gr.* 297 (début du 14ᵉ s.). Ce manuscrit, auquel il faut vraisemblablement rattacher d'un point de vue philologique les extraits conservés dans le *Pal. gr.* 199,[74] constitue un remaniement assez fort. Il présente un découpage en deux livres.[75] Le traité comporte de nombreux ajouts de définitions et se présente entremêlé d'extraits d'autres auteurs, sans séparation ni indication aucune.[76] La fin n'est pas bien marquée : la dernière question qui concorde avec l'édition de Kühn se lit au fol. 38ʳ (cf. *Def.* 183, XIX, 398.1–2 K.). Arrivent alors (fol. 38ʳ⁻ᵛ) sans séparation des extraits du livre V d'Aétius (chap. 3-6 au fol. 38ʳ⁻ᵛ et chap. 12 au fol. 39ʳ) puis, toujours sans séparation ni titre, un extrait des *Problemata* d'Alexandre d'Aphrodise (*Probl.* 83, fol. 39ʳ). Le bas du fol. 39ʳ et les fol. 39ʳ-40ʳ sont occupés par des *diaireseis* accompagnées de questions-réponses, sur les fièvres et sur le pouls, et d'un extrait du commentaire de Stéphanos au *Pronostic* d'Hippocrate (sans titre), puis (fol. 40ᵛ) le début du traité *De febribus* attribué dans les manuscrits à Théophile ou Stéphanos, parfois à Palladios,[77] mais avec ici l'indication d'une origine galénique (ἐκ τῶν Γαληνοῦ). En somme, il s'agit donc bien moins du texte des *Definitiones medicae* que d'un traité formé en prenant pour base cet ouvrage. La combinaison de plusieurs sources pour composer un nouveau texte semble bien une caractéristique de ce manuscrit, et peut-être même du copiste. Aimilios Mavroudis a ainsi montré que le traité *De pulsibus* contenu dans le *Pal. gr.* 199, dû au même copiste, provient de Paul d'Égine mais comporte aussi des extraits du *De natura hominis* de Mélétios, ainsi que des *Definitiones medicae*.[78] Dans ce dernier manuscrit, comme l'a bien mis en évidence Aimilios Mavroudis, les *Definitiones medicae* sont à

---

[73] *Anecdota medica Graeca*, ed. F. Z. Ermerins, Leiden, 1840, pp. 279–97 (293, 14–297, 12).

[74] Le *Pal. gr.* 199 ne contient que des extraits (voir *supra*). Je n'ai pas encore achevé son analyse philologique mais j'aurais tendance à le croire apparenté d'un point de vue textuel au *Pal. gr.* 297 du fait que tous deux ont été copiés par un même scribe.

[75] Le livre II s'ouvre (fol. 36ʳ) sur une définition des différentes parties de la médecine qui mentionne Hippocrate, Galien et Magnos (cf. *Def.* 10 de l'éd. XIX, 351.8 K.).

[76] On trouve par exemple à la fin du livre I, fol. 35, le chapitre I, 61 de Paul d'Égine (sans nom d'auteur) puis une série de questions sur les bains tirées d'Aetius, qui est en revanche explicitement cité.

[77] Édition sous le nom de Palladios : J. Ideler, *Physici et medici Graeci minores*, t. I, Berlin, 1841, pp. 107–20.

[78] Mavroudis, 'Το ανώνυμο έργο' (n. 29 ci-dessus).

leur tour intégrées dans différents ouvrages, dont celui d'Aetius d'Amide.

- *Marc.* V.9 (milieu du 15ᵉ siècle). Ne conservant que quelques extraits, il n'est mentionné ici que parce qu'il est copié par le même scribe que le *Par. gr.* 2153, à savoir le médecin bibliophile Démétrios Angelos.[79] Cela conduit à soupçonner une parenté entre les deux : un premier sondage laisserait effectivement penser que le *Marc. gr.* V.9 descend pour cette partie du *Par. gr.* 2153. Mais, en l'absence d'une analyse exhaustive, il reste possible que Démétrios Angelos, qui avait accès à un grand nombre de manuscrits et qui s'intéressait de près au texte de Galien, ait fait appel à un autre témoin. On sait par exemple qu'il a annoté un autre manuscrit qui contient une version abrégée des *Definitiones medicae*, le *Bonon.* 3632.[80]
- *Ott. gr.* 311 (15ᵉ s.). On ne lit qu'un peu moins de la première moitié du texte (jusqu'à la *Def.* 220), avec d'importantes lacunes qui semblent indiquer un ancêtre défectueux. Le manuscrit a appartenu à Constantin Lascaris (1434/1435–1501), qui a ajouté des textes au début et à la fin.

Quant aux manuscrits qui conservent la forme complète, on est forcé de constater qu'ils présentent un texte en somme assez variable. Le *Mosq. syn. gr.* 51, par exemple, comporte beaucoup plus de définitions non seulement que la famille A mais aussi que tous les autres témoins. Cependant, la nature de ces ajouts ferait parfois penser qu'il s'agirait non pas de compléments mais d'omissions dans le reste de la tradition (par endroits, on a l'impression de *saut du même au même* chez les autres lorsque le texte est plus long). À son tour, le *Vind. med. gr.* 16 donne en beaucoup d'endroits des définitions inconnues par ailleurs. C'est le cas également du *Par. suppl. gr.* 446 qui, à côté de ses nombreuses omissions, présente lui aussi beaucoup d'ajouts, à commencer la section d'ostéologie sur laquelle s'achève chez lui le traité.[81] En somme, chacun des témoins, à sa manière, comporte des compléments ou des omissions qui lui sont propres. Et il semble que nous touchons à la principale caractéristique du texte, qui est la variation : l'ajout et l'omission à volonté. De ce fait, toute tentative de reconstitution d'une hypothétique forme d'origine semble particulièrement ardue, et presque d'emblée vouée à l'échec.

---

[79] Sur ce personnage, voir Mondrain, 'Démétrios Angélos' (n. 5 ci-dessus).

[80] Voir Mondrain, 'Démétrios Angélos' (n. 5 ci-dessus), pp. 310–13. Démétrios Angélos n'a cependant pas annoté dans le *Bonon.* 3632 le texte des *Definitiones medicae*.

[81] Voir le développement très détaillé de Kollesch, *Untersuchungen* (n. 1 ci-dessus), pp. 41–2.

Les traductions en latin et en arabe

Jusqu'à présent, il n'a pas été possible d'identifier de traduction latine ancienne qui aurait été conservée jusqu'à nous avant la Renaissance.[82] Cependant, quelques brefs extraits d'une traduction latine de nos *Definitiones medicae* ont été repérés dans une branche de la tradition manuscrite des *Quaestiones medicinales* du pseudo-Soranus : d'un point de vue linguistique cette traduction doit remonter à la fin de l'antiquité.[83] Même si les deux manuscrits qui conservent ces extraits ne sont pas antérieur au début du 12ᵉ siècle, et même s'il ne s'agit que de quelques définitions, nous avons ici une trace très ancienne de l'existence de notre traité et de sa circulation.

L'arabe présente un cas similaire au latin : aucune traduction arabe des *Definitiones medicae* n'a été identifiée jusqu'à présent, mais nous avons des traces de ce qu'il en a au moins existé une. Elle est citée par Hunain Ibn Ishaq, et on en conserverait quelques extraits chez Razi (mort en 925) et al-Baladi (mort en 990).[84] Après les bribes d'une traduction latine tardo-antique, ces attestations indirectes en arabe, dont la première (Hunain) remonterait au milieu du 9ᵉ siècle et serait donc antérieure au plus ancien manuscrit grec conservé (*Par. suppl. gr.* 446, du début du 10ᵉ s.), constitueraient la seconde plus ancienne trace de l'existence de ce traité.

---

[82] Diels, 'Die Handschriften' (n. 2 ci-dessus), suivi par Stefania Fortuna dans son catalogue en ligne (*Galeno. Catalogo delle traduzioni latine*, www.galenolatino.com), ne signale que la traduction conservée dans le *Laur.* 73,9 (16ᵉ s.) et due à Euphrosynus Boninus (Frosino Bonini, † 1525). Élève d'Ange Politien, 'artium et medicinae doctor et physicus Florentinus', Bonini est attesté comme correcteur dans l'officine des Junte. Outre les *Definitiones medicae*, on connaît de lui plusieurs traductions du grec au latin : l'*Introductio* pseudo-galénique (conservée avec la traduction des *Definitiones* dans le *Vat. lat.* 4423 ; voir à son sujet Petit, *Galien. Le médecin* (n. 53 ci-dessus), pp. cxv-cxvi), Paul d'Égine ou encore le commentaire de Jean Philopon aux *Analytica posteriora* d'Aristote. Quatre autres traductions latines de la Renaissance sont signalées dans R. J. Durling, 'A Chronological Census of Renaissance Editions and Translations of Galen', *Journal of the Warburg and Courtauld Institutes*, 24.3–4, 1961, pp. 230–305 (285 nº 48).

[83] Voir J. Kollesch, 'Zum Fortleben der pseudogalenischen Definitiones medicae in der Medizin des lateinischen Mittelalters', *Beiträge zur Geschichte der Universität Erfurt*, 14, 1968–9, pp. 55–9 ; en dernier lieu, la synthèse de K.-D. Fischer, 'Die vorsalernitanischen lateinischen Galenübersetzungen', *Medicina nei secoli. Arte e scienza*, 25.3, 2013, pp. 673–714 (683-4).

[84] Voir M. Ullmann, *Die Medizin im Islam*, Leiden/Köln, 1970, p. 38, nº 3.

Structure et organisation

À l'issue d'un prologue adressé à Teuthras, connu par ailleurs comme destinataire de traités authentiques de Galien,[85] où est clairement marquée la visée pédagogique de l'entreprise, le texte se présente comme une série de 'définitions' exprimées sous forme de questions et de réponses. C'est une caractéristique des textes à vocation pédagogique mais aussi pratique : elle permet d'une part l'enseignement et la mémorisation ; d'autre part le repérage aisé et rapide dans l'exercice de la pratique médicale.[86]

Dans les manuscrits, contrairement à ce qui apparaît dans l'édition de Kühn (et déjà dans celle de Chartier), les questions ne sont jamais numérotées. En revanche, on trouve presque systématiquement la question exprimée au style direct avant la réponse (parfois même avec les mentions ἐρώτησις/ἀπόκρισις) : ces questions, très largement attestées par la tradition manuscrite, sont bien présentes dans l'édition de Chartier mais ont été supprimées dans cette de Kühn. Il faut cependant noter d'importantes variations entre les manuscrits dans la formulation des questions. Quant à la réponse, elle commence généralement en reprenant les termes de la question. Dans quelques manuscrits (par exemple le *Vind. med. gr.* 16) cette reprise est omise, sans doute pour éviter les lourdeurs de la répétition, ou pour économiser l'espace sur la page.

Visant à embrasser l'ensemble de la médecine, le texte présente une importante étendue : on peut prendre comme point de repère les 487 définitions de l'édition de Chartier puis Kühn, même si ce dénombrement peut varier considérablement selon la manière de compter. Bien souvent, par exemple, ce sont plusieurs définitions qui sont données pour une même notion ; et, à l'intérieur d'une définition, on peut trouver de nouvelles définitions (portant sur des termes utilisés pour la première définition) qui ne sont pas toujours individualisées dans les manuscrits ni les éditions.

Les définitions se succèdent les unes aux autres de manière brute, sans mise en valeur d'une quelconque logique organisationnelle. À la lecture, il apparaît

---

[85] Galien dédie à son ami Teuthras deux traités, le *Glossarium hippocraticum* et le *De pulsibus ad tirones*. Dans le *De indolentia*, il relate sa rencontre avec ce personnage ainsi que sa mort (voir *Galien. Ne pas se chagriner*, texte établi et traduit par V. Boudon-Millot et J. Jouanna, avec la collaboration d'A. Pietrobelli, Paris, 2010, p. 12 § 34 et le commentaire pp. 105-6 et pp. 108–9). On peut remarquer que le *De pulsibus ad tirones* fut largement lu et commenté à Alexandrie.

[86] À propos de la structuration des traités d'initiation sous forme de questions-réponses, voir Kollesch, *Untersuchungen* (n. 1 ci-dessus), pp. 35–46 ('II. Der Frage- und Antwortdialog als medizinisches Lehrbuch') ; plus particulièrement pour la médecine, A. M. Ieraci Bio, 'L'ἐρωταπόκρισις nella letteratura medica', in *Esegesi, Parafrasi, Compilatori in età tardoantica. Atti del III Convegno Nazionale dell'Associazione di Studi Tardoantici (Pisa, 7–9 ottobre 1993)*, ed. C. Moreschini, Naples, 1995, pp. 187–207.

cependant qu'elles sont regroupées en séquences thématiques. L'édition de Chartier (suivie par Kühn), qui a opéré des regroupements arbitraires, n'aide pas le lecteur moderne à s'en apercevoir. Logiquement, l'ouvrage s'ouvre sur la définition de ce qu'est une définition puis sur d'autres notions apparentées ; on définit ensuite la médecine, ses parties, les différentes écoles médicales, le médecin, etc. Vient enfin ce qui concerne le corps humain et ses différents constituants, de la tête aux pieds. Sont ensuite passées en revue toutes les affections, de manière plus ou moins développées.[87]

Origine

L'attribution des *Definitiones medicae* à Galien est générale dans tous les manuscrits qui conservent le début de l'œuvre (on ne peut rien dire du plus ancien témoin, le *Par. suppl. gr.* 446, dans lequel le commencement du traité est mutilé) : de fait, la première remise en cause de son authenticité se trouve seulement dans l'Aldine de 1525, où l'ouvrage apparaît, au tome IV, dans la liste des traités jugés apocryphes. Néanmoins, si son inauthenticité ne fait guère de doute, la question de son origine et de sa datation est loin d'être tranchée : on présentera ici quelques éléments permettant d'orienter les recherches.

La présentation sous forme de questions et de réponses ne nous apporte pas d'indice décisif pour une datation. On l'a vu, c'est une pratique attestée dès Platon et Aristote puis à l'époque hellénistique ; encore en vogue à la fin de l'Antiquité, elle jouit toujours d'un grand succès pendant la période byzantine. Tout ce qu'on peut en dire est qu'elle est typique d'un contexte d'enseignement.

Comme on l'a vu, la première trace assez solide de l'ancienneté des *Definitiones medicae* se trouve dans les quelques bribes d'une traduction latine ancienne qui, d'après ses caractéristiques linguistiques et stylistiques, remonterait à la fin de l'Antiquité. L'arabe, nous venons de l'évoquer, confirme également que l'ouvrage était connu au moins au milieu du 9e siècle.

Au niveau de la tradition indirecte, un point qui mérite d'être souligné est la présence de nombreuses citations des *Definitiones medicae* dans l'*Apotherapeutike* de Théophile, vaste compilation médicale byzantine qu'Anna Maria Ieraci Bio situe au plus tôt au 10e siècle. Outre notre traité, l'*Apotherapeutike* fait appel à de multiples sources dont Hippocrate, Galien et les encyclopédistes tels que

---

[87] Sur l'organisation du traité, voir la très bonne présentation de Kollesch, *Untersuchungen* (n. 1 ci-dessus), pp. 47–57.

Paul d'Égine, Aetius d'Amide et Alexandre de Tralles.[88] Un élément intéressant pour notre propos me semble le fait, relevé par Anna Maria Ieraci Bio, que l'*Apotherapeutike* témoigne de l'utilisation de matériel issu de l'école médicale d'Alexandrie, en particulier des *diaireseis* exégétiques.[89]

De fait, et en dehors même de toute analyse du contenu des *Definitiones medicae*, quelques indices externes invitent à explorer la piste alexandrine dès lors que l'on cherche à remonter dans l'histoire de leur transmission. Il faut tout d'abord remarquer que ce traité est transmis dans au moins trois manuscrits qui semblent conserver des restes de l'enseignement médical d'Alexandrie :

- le *Par. suppl. gr.* 446: il contient des ouvrages à destination des débutants (*Ad Glauconem, Ad Antonium de pulsibus*), qui faisaient partie du canon galénique en vigueur à Alexandrie, mais aussi le traité *De febribus* attribué à Stéphane d'Alexandrie, parfois à Théophile ou Palladios, lequel semble issu d'un commentaire non conservé à l'ouvrage galénique *De differentiis febrium*.[90]
- le *Vind. med. gr.* 16: l'unité codicologique contenant les *Definitiones medicae* (fols 284–359, sur papier oriental) conserve aussi le *De febribus* de Stéphane/Théophile/Palladios (fols 325^v–326^v, 310^r–v, 327^r–328^v) mais elle est surtout célèbre pour ses *diaireseis* exégétiques (fols 329^r–359^v), dont c'est la seule attestation. L'origine alexandrine de ces schémas n'est plus à discuter.[91]
- le *Pal. gr.* 297: dans sa partie ancienne (fols 3–42), on trouve des *diaireseis* juste à la suite des *Definitiones medicae* (fols 39^v–40^r), accompagnées d'un extrait du commentaire de Stéphane au *Pronostic* d'Hippocrate. Sur le verso suivant (fol. 40^v) se lit le début du *De febribus* de Théophile/Stéphane/Palladios.

---

[88] A. M. Ieraci Bio, 'Sur une Ἀποθεραπευτική attribuée à Théophile', in *Storia e ecdotica dei testi medici greci. Atti del II Convegno Internazionale. Parigi 24–26 maggio 1994*, ed. A. Garzya, Naples, 1996, pp. 191–205, en particulier p. 194 pour une liste des sources identifiées, parmi lesquelles les *Definitiones medicae* figurent à plusieurs reprises.

[89] Voir A. M. Ieraci Bio, '*Disiecta membra* della scuola iatrosofistica alessandrina', in *Galenismo e medicina tardoantica. Fonti greche, latine e arabe. Atti del Seminario Internazionale di Siena (Certosa di Pontignano, 9–10 settembre 2002)*, ed. I. Garofalo, Naples, 2003, pp. 9–51 (28-9) : six *diaireseis* mises en évidence et analysées.

[90] Voir C. Schiano, 'Il trattato inedito "Sulle febbri" attribuito a Giovanni Filopono : contenuto, modelli e struttura testuale', in *Galenismo e medicina tardoantica. Fonti greche, latine e arabe. Atti del Seminario Internazionale di Siena, Certosa di Pontignano, 9 e 10 settembre 2002*, eds I. Garofalo and A. Roselli, Naples, 2003, pp. 75–100, en particulier p. 94 ; Cronier, 'Un témoin problématique' (n. 24 ci-dessus).

[91] Voir Ieraci Bio, '*Disiecta membra*' (n. 90 ci-dessus), pp. 15–17.

Ces trois manuscrits contiennent les *Definitiones medicae* dans des formes relativement différentes et ont des origines géographiques variées : une région indéterminée, mais provinciale, de l'empire byzantin pour le *Par. suppl. gr.* 446 (l'Italie méridionale ?) ; peut-être la Morée franque pour le *Pal. gr.* 297 ; Constantinople pour le *Vind. med. gr.* 16.[92] On ne peut donc pas envisager l'idée qu'ils auraient été produits immédiatement dans le même milieu. Au contraire, ils semblent davantage refléter la diffusion en différents endroits et à différentes époques d'un enseignement originel.

Mais ces trois témoins importants des *Definitiones medicae* se caractérisent aussi par le fait qu'ils conservent des textes très rares, dont ils sont quasiment les attestations uniques et sur l'origine desquels on ne sait à peu près rien :

- La *Synopsis artis medicae* de Léon le médecin ou le philosophe, que l'on lit dans le *Paris. suppl. gr.* 446 (fols 146[r]–168[r]) et ses descendants[93] mais aussi de manière anonyme et partielle dans le *Vind. med. gr.* 16 (fols 311–318[v] : livres I–IV).[94]
- Les *Eclogae medicamentorum* du pseudo-Oribase, connues essentiellement par le même *Par. suppl. gr.* 446 (fols 168[r]–261[v]) mais dont un passage est cité dans le *Pal. gr.* 297 (fol. 17[v]), au niveau du chap. 1.3 du livre IV de Paul d'Égine : il s'agit du chap. 76, 11–19.[95]

D'un manuscrit à l'autre, pour ces deux traités, on observe une fois encore de grandes variations textuelles, si bien qu'il est impossible non seulement que l'un descende de l'autre, mais aussi qu'ils remontent immédiatement à un même milieu. Au contraire, les parentés sont réelles mais lointaines.

[92] Pour le *Par. suppl. gr.* 446, voir Cronier, 'Un témoin problématique' (n. 24 ci-dessus) ; pour le *Pal. gr.* 297, voir Mondrain, 'Nicolas Myrepse' (n. 28 ci-dessus), p. 412 ; l'origine géographique des fols 284-359 du *Vind. med. gr.* 16 n'est pas établie avec certitude mais mes recherches sur la tradition du *De materia medica* de Dioscoride m'ont permis de montrer que d'autres parties du manuscrit ont été réalisées à Constantinople au 14e siècle et que le volume a été constitué dans son état actuel dans cette ville au cours du 15e siècle (c'est là d'ailleurs qu'il sera acquis par l'ambassadeur d'Autriche Ogier Ghislain de Busbecq au début des années 1560).

[93] Voir B. Zipser, 'Überlegungen zum Text der *Synopsis Iatrikes* des Leo medicus', in *Studia Humanitatis ac Litterarum Trifolio Heidelbergensi dedicata. Festschrift für Eckhard Christmann, Wilfried Edelmaier und Rudolf Kettemann*, eds A. Hornung, C. Jäkel, W. Schubert, Francfurt/Berlin/Bern, 2004, pp. 393–9 ; la *Synopsis* contient sept livres dans le *Par. suppl. gr.* 446.

[94] Voir Cronier, 'Un témoin problématique' (n. 24 ci-dessus).

[95] *Oribasii Collectionum medicarum reliquiae, libri XLIX–L, libri incerti, eclogae medicamentorum* (CMG VI, 2.2), ed. I. Raeder, Berlin, 1933, p. 247, l. 23–248, l. 34. Dans son contenu, ce passage est proche de celui de Paul d'Égine (IV, 1.4) mais les variantes l'apparentent davantage à l'extrait des *Eclogae*.

Dans le même sens, on peut aussi évoquer le très énigmatique *De pulsibus* de Marcellinus, qui est conservé dans la partie ancienne du *Vind. med. gr.* 16 (fols 319^r–325^v) mais aussi dans le *Bonon.* 3632 (fols 65^r–67^v), lequel contient par ailleurs une version abrégée des *Definitiones medicae*.[96]

Conclusion

Au bout du compte, les *Definitiones medicae* nous sont transmises dans des manuscrits de l'époque byzantine sous des formes fluctuantes, ce qui s'accorde bien avec la nature du texte. À partir du 14e siècle, on en conserve des attestations assez nombreuses, qu'une analyse philologique approfondie, laquelle n'a pas pu être menée dans le cadre de ce travail, devrait permettre de classer. Auparavant, en revanche, le traité ne semble avoir été conservé que dans des manuscrits très isolés les uns des autres qui, chacun à sa façon, ont manifestement sauvé du naufrage quelques restes d'un enseignement médical ancien pour lequel nous ne disposons par ailleurs de quasiment aucune trace.

Trois manuscrits importants en particulier, le *Par. suppl. gr.* 446 et, pour leur partie ancienne, le *Pal. gr.* 297 et le *Vind. med. gr.* 16, auquel il faut peut-être adjoindre le *Bonon.* 3632, paraissent refléter de manière lointaine un héritage commun, peut-être celui de l'école d'Alexandrie, qui aurait été transmis de manière indépendante dans différentes régions, en donnant lieu à des développements divers.

Il faut néanmoins rappeler que les *Definitiones medicae* sont également transmises par des manuscrits qui n'offrent *a priori* pas de relations particulières avec Alexandrie. À cet égard, la version 'augmentée' donnée par le *Mosq. syn. gr.* 51 (et, à sa suite, par le *Par. gr.* 2153) mériterait une analyse philologique approfondie : il est en effet possible qu'elle ne soit pas tant une version 'augmentée' qu'une version non-réduite. Alexandrie – si cette hypothèse est vérifiée – ne serait donc peut-être que l'un des relais par lesquels l'ouvrage nous est parvenu.

La multiplicité des formes sous lesquelles nous a été transmis le traité atteste la vitalité de sa circulation. C'est, pour notre connaissance de cet ouvrage, une chance dont ne bénéficie pas la grande majorité des traités du corpus galénique.

---

[96] Voir H. von Staden, 'Les manuscrits du *De pulsibus* de Marcellinus', in *Storia e ecdotica dei testi medici greci. Atti del II Convegno Internazionale. Parigi 24–26 maggio 1994*, ed. A. Garzya, Napoli 1996, pp. 407–25: selon H. von Staden, le *Vind. med. gr.* 16 est le meilleur témoin ; quant au *Bonon.* 3632, il offre des passages inconnus par ailleurs et apparaît très isolé d'un point de vue philologique.

Four Works on Prognostic Attributed to Galen (Kühn vol. 19): New Hypotheses on Their Authorship, Transmission, and Intellectual Milieu[1]

Caroline Petit

In 1830 was published one of the last volumes of what is still the standard reference edition of Galen's works in Greek: tome XIX of the famously unreliable Kühn edition (1821–1833). While the many problems of this edition have often been pointed out, in terms of language, punctuation, and more importantly its reliance on the seventeenth-century edition made by René Chartier, the depths of Kühn's manipulations have not been entirely revealed. Most volumes are thematically arranged, but with volume XIX, Kühn assembled a number of very different works that simply did not fit in other volumes. Among them, several crucial Galenic works have rightly attracted abundant attention, like the two bio-bibliographical treatises *De libris propriis* and *De ordine librorum suorum*, and the *Glossary*.[2] The majority of the works in volume XIX however, are of disputed authenticity or plain forgeries: some, like the *An animal sit quod in utero est* or the *Definitiones medicae* have benefited from relatively in-depth study,[3] while others are still waiting for their Karl Kalbfleisch. This paper aims at shedding light on the history of a group of such works, united by the theme of prognostic: the *Prognostica de decubitu infirmorum ex mathematica scientia*, *De urinis*, *De urinis compendium*, and *Ad Antonium de pulsibus*.[4] An enquiry into the textual transmission of those works, albeit incomplete, demonstrates the fallacies of the Kühn edition and its dangers for the novice reader of Galen. Ultimately, Kühn's shortcomings illustrate serious issues with the seventeenth-century Chartier edition, based on

[1] I am grateful to the Wellcome Trust for supporting my research on *Medical Prognostic in Late Antiquity* through a Wellcome University Award (2013–2018), of which this chapter is an offshoot. I was able to finalise this work as an invited fellow at the Institute of Advanced Study, University of Durham (2020). I wish to thank the IAS and the research community at Durham for their help and support. I am also grateful to Laurent Pernot for discussing this paper with me.

[2] See the new edition of the *Glossary* by Lorenzo Perilli (*Galeni Vocum Hippocratis Glossarium / Galeno, Interpretazione Delle Parole Difficili Di Ippocrate: Testo, Traduzione E Note Di Commento*, CMG V, 13, 1, Berlin, 2017).

[3] For example, *An animal sit quod in utero est* (K. XIX, 158–181) was edited in 1914 by Hermann Wagner ('Galeni qui fertur libellus εἰ ζῷον τὸ κατὰ γαστρός', Diss. phil. Marburg 1914); see the many studies on the *Definitiones medicae* by Jutta Kollesch, and Marie Cronier's contribution in this volume. See also the studies cited in the introduction, p. xiii.

[4] I am preparing the first critical edition of these texts.

Renaissance scholarship and a handful of randomly selected Greek manuscripts. Centuries of reliance over outdated scholarship has not only made some 'Galenic' material unusable for the modern scholar, but also erased the traces of several late antique medical texts and professors who once enjoyed a fame worthy of Galen's: Magnus of Emesa and, as I tentatively suggest, John of Alexandria.

Prognostica de decubitu infirmorum ex mathematica scientia (K. XIX, 529–573)

A rare example of a iatro-magical text in the Galenic corpus, the *Prognostica* connects health, the body and the planets in a manner that is reminiscent of Hermetic works. The work remained popular well into early modern times: in the Middle Ages, the text took different forms in Latin, under various titles, and it was attributed either to Galen or to Hippocrates.[5] The first Renaissance translation was made by the Polish physician Josephus Struthius and published in 1535. John Dee owned a copy of this translation, a reprint from 1550, which he annotated dutifully.[6] The famous polymath was clearly interested in what a Galenic text could bring to scholars of his time about astrology. Later still, a French translation by a certain Juste L'Aigneau was published in 1650, as an addition to the third edition of David L'Aigneau's *Traité pour la conservation de la santé et sur la saignée de ce temps. Augmenté d'un traité de Galien, de l'alictement des malades, etc.* L'Aigneau, a physician trained in Montpellier, is known as an adept of alchemy; in this work, he and his son clearly seem to consider the *Prognostica* as a relevant work, and a genuine Galenic piece.[7] Although this piece of information has not been much exploited, it clearly puts this pseudo-Galenic work among key sources used by physicians and alchemists of the period, following in the steps of John Dee.

René Chartier, who published the work in volume VIII of his complete works of Galen and Hippocrates, also argues in favour of its authenticity, finding it very

---

[5] P. Kibre, '*Astronomia* or *Astrologia Hippocratis*' in *Science and History: Essays in Honor of Edward Rosen. Studia Copernicana 16*, Cracow, 1977, 133–156.

[6] *Claudii Galeni Pergameni Mathematices scientiae prognostica de decubitu infirmorum, Iosepho Struthio interprete cum paraphrasi Claudii Fabri, medici surregiensis, novissime juncta*, Lyons, 1550. On Dee's ownership see my blog https://www.medicineancientandmodern.com/2016/08/07/a-tale-of-two-libraries-john-dee-1527-1609-and-galen/.

[7] About David L'Aigneau (whose name is spelled in various ways), see S. Matton, « Vie et œuvre de David Laigneau, alchimiste et médecin du roi », préface à la rééd. de : David L'Agneau, *Harmonie mystique* (1636), Paris: Gutenberg Reprints, 1986, pp. 7–38. His son Juste L'Aigneau, author of the translation of the pseudo-Galenic *Prognostica*, became a famous physician as well.

faithful to Galenic doctrines expressed in works of indisputable authenticity, such as the *De crisibus* and *De diebus decretoriis*. He defends the opuscule as follows:

Magnae experientiae liber, a plerisque tamen neglectus, quod plerique sint divinae Astrologiae ignari, quorum quidam quod ignorant, id deprimunt.[8]

It is a book of vast experience, yet neglected by the very many, because very many people are ignorant of divine Astrology, among whom some dismiss the things they do not know.

Both L'Aigneau and Chartier's attitudes reflect theoretical and practical preoccupations of their time (around the mid-seventeenth century), when the debate over the role of astrology in medicine was rife. Both are firm believers in the validity of astrology in medicine, as several fellow disciples of L'Aigneau in Montpellier in the late sixteenth century turned out to be.[9] They thus promote this text as an authentically Galenic work. Kühn himself gives no indication of doubt about this text, seemingly appropriating Chartier's inclusive approach. But the evidence to corroborate its authenticity is very thin. As Weinstock[10] pointed out in a brief article published in 1948, the work crept into the Galenic corpus as the result of a basic scribal error in a twelfth-century manuscript, the *Laurentianus Plut.* 28, 34. An anonymous work became attributed to Galen, because the preceding text in the manuscript had the name of Galen.

In fact, a close examination of the textual tradition of the text shows no links with well-established Galen manuscripts; instead, the work seems to have emerged from an astrological collection. But Weinstock made a case for an alternative authorship, and put forward the name of Imbrasius of Ephesus, otherwise unknown, as found in a fifteenth-century manuscript, the *Bodleian Cromwell* 12. This seductive and slightly sensationalist thesis made it into some prestigious library catalogues (such as the Wellcome library) and in the reference work that is the *Galen-Bibliographie* by G. Fichtner (see under n. 126). But, once

---

[8] René Chartier, vol. VIII, *concisae notae* p. 924. About René Chartier's attitude towards spurious and dubious texts by Galen, see C. Petit, 'René Chartier (1572–1654) et l'authenticité des traités galéniques', in G. Cobolet/ V. Boudon-Millot eds, *René Chartier éditeur des œuvres de Galien et d'Hippocrate*, Paris, 2012, 287–300 (esp. p. 296–300). About René Chartier's edition in terms of evolution of the Hippocratic and Galenic *corpora*, see P. J. van der Eijk, 'Le rôle de Chartier dans la constitution des canons des traités hippocratiques et galéniques', *CRAI expand* 154–3, 2010, pp. 1163–1178.

[9] S. Matton (art. cit. note 6) lists them and their works, highlighting the intellectual connections between them and L'Aigneau.

[10] S. Weinstock, 'The author of Ps.-Galen's *Prognostica de decubitu*', *Classical Quarterly*, 42, 1948, pp. 41–43.

again, the evidence is elusive: a late manuscript containing only part of the text among many important astronomical, Hermetic or astrological works, is MS *Cromwell* 12 a truly reliable witness? The manuscript has been studied by major specialists of ancient and Byzantine science, with mixed results: for Jean Lempire, this manuscript represents a minority group of manuscripts attributing Stephanus' astronomical commentary to Heraclius;[11] for Anne Tihon studying Ptolemy and Theon,[12] the manuscript is only a remote relative of earlier, more important manuscripts (notably MS *Vatican. Gr.* 175). Such studies shed indirect light on *Cromwell* 12 as a minor witness to the textual history of several important texts. What should we then make of the name of Imbrasius of Ephesus in a fifteenth-century manuscript, containing only part of the *Prognostica*, in the absence of a detailed study of the textual tradition of that text? Ms. *Cromwell 12* is currently the only source for the name of Imbrasius of Ephesus: it is otherwise not attested. Direct examination of the manuscript in Oxford did not lead to any additional clues: it is unclear when this name could have crept in and to what extent it could have been altered by scribes. In fact, this would not be the first example of a name created by the imagination of a scribe or a slip of the pen, and I would suggest treating Weinstock's hypothesis with appropriate caution for the time being. Meanwhile, most of the other manuscripts seem to clearly derive from the Laurentianus, so that the Galen attribution remains linked to that manuscript only. As we have seen, a typical mistake launched this misattribution. So, where to turn?

The *Prognostica* can tentatively be compared with other astromedical texts from antiquity, preserved in the Hermetic corpus. It also ties in well with a strand in ancient, post-Hellenistic medicine, offering to see links between the various levels of the cosmos, between the celestial bodies and the rest of the natural world: plants, animals, stones – an area of ancient knowledge that has been studied extensively by the likes of Festugière, Franz Cumont, and Jean-Pierre Mahé.[13] Further research is necessary to probe Cumont's investigations into the

---

[11] J. Lempire, 'D'Alexandrie à Constantinople. Le commentaire astronomique de Stéphanos', *Byzantion*, 81, 2011, pp. 241–266.

[12] A. Tihon (éd), *Le "petit commentaire" de Théon d'Alexandrie aux Tables faciles de Ptolémée*, Studi e Testi 282, Città del Vaticano, Biblioteca Apostolica Vaticana, 1978, 17–18.

[13] Franz Cumont also wrote on the pseudo-Galenic *Prognostica*: F. Cumont, 'Les *Prognostica de decubitu* attribués à Galien', *Bull. Inst. Hist. Belge Rome*, 1935, 119–132. Festugière's four-volume study *La révélation d'Hermès Trismégiste* (1942–1953) is still authoritative, as are the four volumes of the Nock-Festugière edition of the Hermetic corpus in the Budé series (1945–1954). Volume V of *Hermès Trismégiste* was recently completed by Jean-Pierre Mahé (2019) and includes crucial new evidence from various traditions.

language of the text, comparing it to extant material – indeed, dates ranging from the Hellenistic through to late antiquity have been suggested. This deserves re-examination. While I would not venture to risk a more precise dating at this stage in my research, I should invite cautiousness around early hypotheses on the authorship of the text. Clearly, a more convincing answer will come from studying the area of ancient astrological texts, rather than from medicine and the Galenic corpus.

What remains of this fascinating text, however, is its sheer plasticity: versions and quotations from it can be found throughout the medieval period, in the Oriental as well as the Western traditions – areas where, once more, crucial information could yet be found to understand the origins of the *Prognostica de decubitu infirmorum ex mathematica scientia*.

De urinis and *De urinis compendium*

Texts on uroscopy are notoriously difficult to handle: they are spread over countless (and poorly catalogued) manuscripts and early, unreliable editions. Among the works on uroscopy attributed to Galen in manuscripts, two at least never made it to the printing press and were studied only in the twentieth century.[14] A pivotal work is Theophilus Protospatharius's *De urinis*, yet the very dating of Theophilus' work is controversial (hypotheses range from the early 7th to the 9th century).[15] Later Byzantine works by the likes of Actuarius are in turn poorly edited: this has damaging consequences for the study of more obscure, perhaps earlier works such as the pseudo-Galenic works on uroscopy, because they often appear in the same medieval manuscripts, of which there are many.[16] Early editors of medical texts have further complicated matters by not citing their exact sources and often omitting crucial manuscripts. Kühn is not the only editor who is blameworthy: Ideler's *Physici et medici graeci minores* is another collection fraught with inaccuracies, partially overlapping with Kühn's

[14] See the excellent work by V. Lorusso, 'Il trattato pseudo-galenico *De urinis* del *Paris. Suppl. Gr.* 634', *Bollettino dei classici*, s. III, fasc. 26, 2005, 5–44; P. Moraux, 'Pseudo-Galen, *De signis ex urinis*', *ZPE* 60, 1985, 63–74 (Moraux focuses on ms. *Neap. Gerol.* XXI, 1 of the 15th c.).

[15] See M. Lamagna, 'Il trattato 'de urinis' di Stefano d'Atene e l'uroscopia alessandrina', in I. Garofalo & A. Roselli (eds), *Galenismo e medicina tardoantica. Fonte greche, latine e arabe*, Naples, 2003, 53–73 (p. 53–54); also the forthcoming volume on Theophilus Protospatharius edited by Alessia Guardasole and Caroline Magdelaine.

[16] Yet see Petros Bouras-Vallianatos, *Innovation in Byzantine Medicine. The Writings of John Zacharias Aktouarios (1275–1330)*, Oxford, 2020. On the use of pseudo-Galenic material on urine in Byzantium, see also his contribution in the present volume.

offerings.[17] In Kühn volume XIX, two texts stand out: a rather long *De urinis*, and a shorter *Compendium de urinis*. To those two works another should be added, a short compilation of minor texts on uroscopy: *De urinis ex Hippocrate, Galeno aliisque* (K. XIX, 607–628), the textual tradition of which is less complex.

The pseudo-Galenic *De urinis* has long raised the suspicion that the bulk of the text provided in Kühn was composed from the remains of the treatise *De urinis* by Magnus of Emesa.[18] One of the greatest authorities on uroscopy before Theophilus, Magnus' reputation was great in Alexandria. Yet there are doubts surrounding his exact dates and it is unclear whether we are dealing with the same iatrosophist as the one mentioned in Eunapius' *Lives*, 20.[19] If this is one and the same figure, Magnus was a medical authority and a celebrity in Alexandria, where he shone through his rhetorical mastery more than his technical abilities – according to both Eunapius and Actuarius.[20] Magnus is known for having systematised Galen's teachings on uroscopy, and it is probably fair to say he also relied on Hippocrates' *Prognostic*, the fundamental textbook on diagnostic and prognostic throughout antiquity and beyond. Magnus' focus was neatly theoretical and pedagogical, aiming at providing clear instructions about how to examine patients' urine. Special attention is given to the many hues of human urine, foreshadowing the famous medieval 'wheels' that practitioners carried with them in the Middle Ages. Later criticism by authors claiming to deliver the latest and most accurate knowledge on this topic may or may not be entirely sincere: both Theophilus and Actuarius aimed to dismiss previous writings on uroscopy. Magnus' work may thus be partially available in the text attributed to Galen in Kühn; it may also have passed into Latin at an early date: evidence of a late antique Latin translation was uncovered and analysed by Arsenio Ferraces Rodríguez. Several Latin manuscripts preserve a literal translation of the pseudo-Galenic text, under the name of a certain Athenagoras.[21] Once again, the authorship of the

---

[17] J. L. Ideler, *Physici et medici graeci minores*, 2 vols., Berlin, 1841. Reprint Hakkert, Amsterdam, 1963.

[18] See the classic study by U. Cats Bussemaker, 'Magnus von Emesa und dessen Buch vom Harne', *Janus* 2, 1847, 273–297.

[19] Richard Goulet, in his recent edition of Eunapius, seems to believe it is one and the same iatrosophist: *Eunape de Sardes. Vies de philosophes et de sophistes*, Les Belles Lettres, tome I, 2014, p. 545–548. *Contra*, Cats Bussemaker, *art. cit.* p. 297.

[20] R. Goulet, *op. cit.*, p. 546.

[21] A. Ferraces Rodríguez, '*Liber Athenagore de urinis*, una traducción latina de un compendio griego sobre semiótica de la orina', in *Il bilinguismo medico fra Tardoantico e Medioevo*, a cura di Anna Maria Urso, Messina, 2012, p. 87–103; *id.* 'Un anecdotum latino tardoantiguo: tentativa de edición crítica del pseudogalénico *Liber Athenagorae de urinis*', *Medicina nei secoli*, 25/3, 2013, pp. 715–764.

text is fluid and its origin obscure, untraceable. The existence of this translation, however, seems to demonstrate that, at an early stage, the text was neither attributed to Magnus nor to Galen. Is Athenagoras, otherwise unknown, the name of a translator, or is he a sophist and professor that we could compare to Agnellus of Ravenna? Or is the name Athenagoras yet another misunderstanding on the part of some scribe? The Latin manuscripts being quite late, it is difficult to settle on this name and draw conclusions about the author. The story is nevertheless typical of the formation of the Galenic corpus beyond the authentic works as an aggregate of medical works of dubious or difficult attribution. Galen as a default author name was given not only to medical works in the strict sense but also, as we have seen, to astro-medical works such as the *Prognostica*. The wandering fate of the *De urinis* shows however that late antiquity and the early medieval period were moments of unstable textual transition where practical compendia circulated under various guises and names. Strategies of attribution may have been motivated by circumstances that cannot be uncovered any more: the case of the mysterious Athenagoras shows that the name of Galen may not have always been the best selling point. The history of other early Latin translations of pseudo-Galenic works, such as the (partial) Latin translation of the pseudo-Galenic *Introductio sive medicus*, confirms that practical utility overcame any obstacles due to authorship.[22] In the case of the extant late antique translation of the *Introductio*, no author's name is definitely mentioned – the name of Galen is mentioned in a later annotation in one of the manuscripts. Since the translation is incomplete, it is adventurous to speculate any further. Whether authorship mattered at that point is unclear. But the translation is an interesting effort of adaptation for a new readership, complete with Latin glosses of difficult Greek words (*inter alia*).

In the case of the translation of the *Introductio* as in that of the *De urinis*, pragmatic use of the source text combines with literal rendering of the original to deliver a new text, usable by a fresh audience. While authorship may have mattered (a question that cannot be solved), those translations are, to an extent, repurposed adaptations of their models, and 'authentic' works of their own kind.[23]

---

[22] C. Petit, 'L'*introductio sive medicus* du Pseudo-Galien dans le Haut Moyen Age latin : problèmes d'édition posés par la tradition indirecte', in A. Ferraces Rodríguez (ed.), *Tradición griega y textos médicos latinos en el período presalernitano. Actas del VIII coloquio internacional: Textos médicos latinos antiguos*, A Coruña, 2007, 250–270; see also *ead.* 'The fate of a Greek medical handbook in the medieval West : the *Introduction, or the Physician* ascribed to Galen', in B. Zipser (ed), *Medical Books in the Byzantine World*, Eikasmos online, Bologna, 2013, 57–78 (pp. 61–63).

[23] See the penetrating remarks on various texts of the same period by K.-D. Fischer, 'Hoch-mittelalterliche redaktionelle Eingriffe in medizinischen Texten' in M. T. Santamaría Hernández (ed), *Textos médicos grecolatinos antiguos y medievales: estudios sobre composición y fuentes*, Cuenca,

Surprisingly enough, the Greek manuscripts transmitting the pseudo-Galenic *De urinis* are no earlier than the fourteenth century: there is a considerable gap in our sources between an early Latin translation (albeit transmitted in later manuscripts) and late medieval Greek manuscripts. Among those, promising witnesses include MSS *Parisin. Gr.* 1630 and *Vatican. Reg. gr.* 181 – but the overall tradition is slimmer than one could have expected, especially in comparison with the other pseudo-Galenic work on uroscopy, the *Compendium de urinis* (to which I intend to come back). In those manuscripts, however, the text is attributed either to Galen or to Magnus of Emesa – no trace of Athenagoras. The treatise *De urinis* appeared in print in the 1525 Aldine edition (vol. IV, f. 21r–23r) and was already relatively well-known in the Renaissance: by then, it was firmly established among Galen's works as the only (almost only) work dedicated to uroscopy in the corpus. The first Renaissance Latin translation appeared as early as 1535, by the same Josephus Struthius who translated the *Prognostica* (see above), and in the same diminutive volume. The young Polish physician who was soon to enjoy bookselling success with this treatise on the pulse (*Ars sphygmica*, 1550) started his medical career reading dubious Galenic works on prognostic matters whilst studying at Padua. His translation of *De urinis* remained a basis for all subsequent printings of the work, demonstrating widespread interest among Renaissance physicians. Thus René Chartier, once again, defended the opuscule as 'Galenic' in thought a few decades later. He published *De urinis* in volume VIII (p. 337–348), with brief comments in the *concisae notae* (p. 924):

> Galenus primo in librum de humoribus commentario dicit se librum unum de urinis conscripsisse : sed an hic ille sit, aliorum esto iudicium. Verumtamen codices vetusti & Graece scripti Germanum hunc esse Galeni foetum produnt, ut & quae in eo doctrina continetur.

> Galen in the first book of his commentary *On humours* says that he wrote one book *On urines*: but whether this is the same, let others decide. In any case, old Greek manuscripts give this as a genuine child of Galen, as does the doctrine expressed in it.

The reference in the commentary to *De humoribus* is dubious (as is the commentary itself), for, in contrast, no such reference is to be found in Galen's *De libris propriis.* But in this case, Chartier is also thrilled to say he has used 'old' Greek manuscripts that seem to confirm the venerable age of the treatise. But ultimately, he published the work as useful and 'Galenic' in a broad sense. Chartier's inclusive approach is, once again, what gave way to the confusion

2012, pp. 29–53.

that we find in Kühn between authentic and no-authentic works. As Chartier's indications were not carried forward in Kühn, the arrangement of texts by themes subsisted, but all sense of perspective was lost. Kühn thus erased all traces of (however perfunctory) textual criticism Chartier had included. In other words, Kühn made the situation seriously worse.

Let us now consider the shorter *Compendium de urinis*, whose relationship with *De urinis* is not easy to pin down. Like *De urinis*, and in fact more explicitly,[24] the *Compendium* is linked with the teaching of Magnus of Emesa. Unlike *De urinis* however, the *Compendium* is transmitted in at least one old manuscript, MS *BN Suppl. Gr.* 446 of the tenth century. Moreover, my investigations show that the archetype of the text predates that century.[25] It is thus extremely likely that we are in presence of a late antique text. This gives more weight to the hypothesis of a text based on Magnus's teaching – though I am not suggesting that this text may have been purely and simply written by the famous iatrosophist. It also makes it unlikely that the *Compendium* is a merely abbreviated *De urinis* – but it supports the antiquity of the latter. Its textual history makes it stand out, but we cannot rule out a connection with the longer text.

While MS *Suppl. Gr.* 446 is usually not considered important in the history of the texts it contains, it is striking that it was instrumental in preserving several important Pseudo-Galenic texts, such as the popular *Definitiones medicae* (about which see Marie Cronier's chapter in this volume) and the *Ad Antonium* (see below). As it happens, the *Compendium* is also preserved in a few very interesting medical collections, mixing up ancient and medieval material in Greek, some of which very rare (for example, MSS *Vatican. gr.* 279, 292, and 293). As the theme of prognostic is often prominent in those collections, the manuscripts generally offer not only texts on urine but also some works on other *excreta* and on the pulse, notably the *Ad Antonium de pulsibus*, a text whose history is tightly connected with that of the *Compendium de urinis*. There is also a strong late antique feel to collections that notably include commentaries to Hippocrates by the likes of Stephanus of Alexandria. But this was of little or no interest to later physicians, who much preferred to attribute those texts to a well-known figure, such as Galen. The *Compendium* did not appear until the Chartier edition, in the same volume VIII as *De urinis* and *Prognostica*. In his accompanying notes, the French editor adds the following information (p. 921):

---

[24] There is some variation in the title given by manuscripts, but MS *Corsinianus* 1410 for instance has Μάγνου Ἐμεσηνου σοφίστου ἀρχιητροῦ περὶ τῆς τῶν οὔρων θεωρίας καὶ διακρίσεως, which refers explicitly to Magnus the iatrosophist.

[25] The details will be available in my edition of the text (in preparation).

Hoc de urinis Galeni compendium quale hic subiicitur oculis, ex manuscriptis regiis codicibus deprompsimus, ac primum Graece Latineque dedimus, quod meus Pratellus primus vertit. Hocce libello paucissimis explicantur ea quae ad urinarum doctrinam spectant. An vero sit Galeni foetus, aut potius doctrinam Galenicam contineat, id iudicium lectori concedimus.

This *Compendium de urinis* by Galen that we hereby bring to public attention, was taken from manuscripts of the Royal library, and we are giving the first edition in Greek and in Latin, after my friend Pratel first translated it. The things that concern the doctrine of urines are explained in very brief words in this opuscule. Whether however this is Galen's child, or rather contains Galenic doctrine, we leave the reader to decide.

Here Chartier does not insist so much on the Galenic tone of the work – in fact, he prefers to leave that to the reader's judgment. Although (as ever!) he is not specific about which manuscript(s) he used, it is likely that he found the text in MS *Parisin. Gr.* 2316. A manuscript which was very close to this one on the shelves of the Royal library, the *Parisin. Gr.* 2315, is in all likeliness his source for the next work under scrutiny: the *Ad Antonium.*

Ad Antonium de pulsibus

The final work examined here is related to prognostic, but delves into the mysteries of the human pulse instead of looking at excrements. It was nevertheless often transmitted alongside the previously studied works. It is thus no surprise to find it in the same volume of the Kühn edition. A work of obscure origin, the short treatise on the pulse dedicated to an unidentified Antonius first appeared in the Chartier edition in Greek (vol. VIII, p. 333–336). Taking an unusual step, Kühn altered the text provided by Chartier by shortening it (removing the questions of this questions-and-answers-type text, thus ironing out one of the text's key features). It is clear which manuscript of Paris René Chartier used here (MS *Parisin. Gr.* 2315), because that is the only manuscript offering the same errors and problems in terms of contents and word order as the printed edition.[26] The fate of this text in Greek was thus marred by misunderstandings, and not just by its unclear authorship, which explains the lack of interest in its contents in our time. In his *concisae notae* (p. 920), Chartier describes the text as follows:

Hic libellus e regiis codicibus manuscriptis a me depromptus est, quem nondum prius editum Graece ac Latine edidimus, & Galeno adscripsimus, quum Galenicam redoleat doctrinam. In eo namque compendiosa de pulsibus doctrina recondita est.

---

[26] Details will be provided in my edition; in any case, neither Chartier nor Kühn can be used as a base text for an edition.

> This opuscule was taken by me from manuscripts of the Royal library; we gave the first Greek and Latin edition of this previously unpublished work, and attributed it to Galen, as it smells of Galenic doctrine. For it contains summary doctrine on the pulse.

To Chartier, the text was thus authentic, because it represents the Galenic doctrine on the pulse accurately. Indeed, the merit of this opuscule is to present in a synthetic manner teachings on the pulse that reflect Galen's doctrine, without the bulk of demonstrations, harangues, digressions and narratives that his genuine works on the pulse contain in abundance. The appeal of the text is understandable, especially as Chartier targeted an audience of students for his edition. Unfortunately for Chartier, who certainly used only one (very poor) manuscript, the text has a more complex history than he thought. *Ad Antonium* took various forms in extant manuscripts, from the tenth-century MS *BN Suppl. Gr.* 446 (already mentioned), in which it is split in two (but incomplete) due to mistakes in assembling the quires, to more recent versions displaying an extended text. Moreover, in some of these 'versions' (let us use this notion for the time being), Galen is mentioned in the third person, which seems to indicate a post-Galenic work. The manuscripts, as in the case of the *Compendium de urinis*, point to a late antique archetype, in any case an archetype much earlier than the oldest, tenth-century manuscript. Once again then, we are possibly faced with a late antique text in connection with diagnostic and prognostic skills; like the *Compendium de urinis*, the *Ad Antonium* could be linked to a professorial *milieu* in late antiquity – and where else than Alexandria could it emanate from? Although editing the text is a complex challenge due to the variations in the existing sources, it is, for the time being, the only legitimate approach to analysing a text whose authorial voice and intellectual milieu deserve fresh scholarly scrutiny. Among the few works on the pulse supposed to have emanated from late antique Alexandria, some may be attributed to John of Alexandria.[27] The text (in the

---

[27] The work of John of Alexandria is notoriously difficult to comprehend, due to frequent confusion with John Philoponos in the sources. Beyond his (scattered) extant works, Ibn Abī Usaybiʿa (*The Best Accounts of the Classes of Physicians*, 6.2 eds E. Savage-Smith, S. Swain and G. J. van Gelder, Leiden, 2020) lists commentaries on Galen's works on the pulse, as well as an opuscule on the pulse. Other accounts exist. On John of Alexandria and Galen, see S. Swain, 'Beyond the Limits of Greek Biography: Galen from Alexandria to the Arabs', in B. McGing and J. Mossman (eds), *The Limits of Ancient Biography*, Swansea, 2006, pp. 395–433, esp. pp. 400–403. See also the helpful introduction by John Duffy in his edition of John's commentary to Hippocrates' *Epid.* VI (CMG, XI, 1, 4, 1997). On the usefulness of John's testimony to assess the medical culture of late antique Alexandria, see C. Petit, 'Alexandrie, carrefour des traditions médicales au 7e s.: Les témoignages de Sophrone de Jérusalem, Alexandre de Tralles, Paul d'Egine, Stéphane d'Alexandrie et Jean d'Alexandrie' in J.-P. Caillet /S. Destephen/ B. Dumézil/H. Inglebert (eds.), *Des dieux civiques*

currently unpublished manuscript versions of it) is clearly reminiscent of the language of John of Alexandria in his few extant works – but is this sufficient evidence to pronounce the *Ad Antonium* as his own work, or could it simply reflect, in an indirect way, his teaching? This is an exciting hypothesis to explore further. Bringing together the faint evidence remaining of medical teaching in late antique Alexandria with those 'new' texts will no doubt refresh our knowledge and understanding of that chapter in medical history.

Ad Antonium is in itself a fascinating work. This is compounded by the now forgotten success this text enjoyed in the medieval period: despite recent suggestions that the Greek text has no genuine existence,[28] the *Ad Antonium* inspired a Latin version that was highly popular in the West from the twelfth century onwards, under the name of Philaretus. The Latin version was studied and edited in much detail by Piero Morpurgo, through his edition of Mauro de Salerno's commentary to the text.[29] The text made it into the *Articella*, which ensured a wide readership of the opuscule for centuries.

*

In retrospect, the pseudo-Galenic works contained in Kühn's volume XIX are well worth the time spent in early editions and manuscripts to reconstruct and illuminate their contents, composition and intellectual contexts. In the case of the above-studied works, as in the case of the *Definitiones Medicae* studied by Marie Cronier, a potential teaching milieu is appearing in the background. This is at least one of the possible lines of explanation for understanding the copying and gathering of student-friendly, short medical works, more detailed than summaries, but concise and systematic enough to facilitate memorisation. Talking of an actual *milieu* is not without its perils, because little or nothing allows us to join the dots between the surviving texts – if Magnus can be the ultimate source of both works on urine, and John of Alexandria that of the *Ad Antonium*, the only genuine links between the works remain the partially common textual transmission that they share. They do not further much our knowledge of the authoritative figures they

---

aux saints patrons, Paris, 2016, pp. 287–307.

[28] See I. Garofalo, 'Il De pulsibus di Philaretus e il [Peri sphygmōn] di Philaretos (con in Appendice l'edizione del *De pulsibus*)', in M. T. Santamaría Hernández (ed), *Textos médicos greco-latinos antiguos y medievales: estudios sobre composición y fuentes*, Cuenca, 2012, 55–94. Garofalo's analysis is based on a fraction of the Greek manuscripts. On the use of the text in a Byzantine manuscript, see Bouras-Vallianatos in this volume.

[29] P. Morpurgo, 'Il commento al *De pulsibus philareti* di Mauro Salernitano. Introduzione e edizione critica dal ms. Parisinus Latinus 18499', *Dynamis*, 7–8, 1987–88, pp. 307–346.

represent – as most late antique medical works, they let little come through of their authors or inspirations. If, however, further philological enquiries prove fruitful, it will be possible to unearth a set of medical texts from late antiquity that had been entirely neglected for the wrong reasons. Galen's *Prognostica*, on the other hand, are still difficult to date and contextualise, as they belong to a neighbouring, yet different intellectual sphere: astrology (or, astromedicine, as it were). The history of the text shows, however, that there is much to learn from the long history of pseudo-Galenic works to illuminate early modern medical thought. Therefore, like the case studies proposed by Vivian Nutton and Laurence Totelin in this volume, those texts prove intrinsically useful and valuable to the historian of medicine and of medical literature (ancient and modern). They are in fact relevant to intellectual history more broadly through their many contact points with bordering disciplines, such as alchemy and astrology.

A secondary conclusion to be drawn, is the value of an 'archaeology' of the Kühn edition. Through those case-studies, it becomes clear that the role played by Kühn added yet more confusion to the already unsatisfactory work left by René Chartier. It is prudent to emphasise once again how easily the Kühn edition, currently the standard reference edition for most Galenic works, can mislead and deceive modern readers. It should therefore be stressed, that a detailed history of the Galenic corpus (*inclusive* of inauthentic texts) is crucial to our understanding of Galen and ancient medical texts more generally.

Pseudonymity and Pseudo-Galen in the Syriac Traditions[1]

Siam Bhayro

Introduction

As is often the case when addressing a topic in Syriac medicine, it is necessary to divide an analysis of pseudonymity in Syriac medicine into three distinct periods: the age of Sergius in the early sixth century; the age of Ḥunayn in the ninth century; and, finally, the age of the encyclopedias in the early centuries of the second millennium – hence the use of the phrase 'Syriac traditions' in my title. Before doing this, I will attempt to provide some background information, on the issue of pseudonymity in late-antique eastern Christianity and in Syriac literature in general, that will help to explain the phenomena that we encounter in the medical literature.

Before Sergius

Our efforts to analyse the issue of pseudonymity in Syriac literature prior to the sixth century CE are hampered by the sources, or, rather, the relative lack of sources. The first three centuries of the Common Era is, in the words of Sebastian Brock, 'the most obscure period of Syriac literature'.[2] Aside from the Old Testament and the Old Syriac Gospels, which were translated into Syriac from Hebrew and Greek respectively, there is very little else.[3] When we come to the two great writers of the fourth century, Ephrem and Aphrahat, issues of authorship appear to be of marginal interest, although Ephrem does name theologians with whom he disagrees, such as Bardaisan, Marcion, and Mani. Thus Robert Murray writes, albeit in the context of a different discussion, 'If we look for

---

[1] I would like to thank Sebastian Brock for providing advice regarding the phenomenon of pseudonymity in Syriac sources, and Vivian Nutton and Caroline Petit for their advice about the Galenic sources and the *status quaestionis.*

[2] S. Brock, *A Brief Outline of Syriac Literature*, Kottayam, 1997, p. 13.

[3] The most prominent of the other Syriac texts from this period are the *Diatessaron* (a harmony of the four Gospels), Bardaisan's *Book of the Laws of the Countries*, the *Odes of Solomon*, and the *Acts of Thomas* – see Brock, *Brief Outline* (n. 2 above), pp. 13–19.

explicit references to earlier authors by name, we shall find very few. Aphrahat has none, while Ephrem refers thus only to opponents.'[4]

Judging from what we find in the Greek East, the problem of pseudepigraphy was certainly known in this period, particularly with reference to the New Testament Pseudepigrapha and pseudepigraphic patristic texts, which often played an important role in theological controversies in the East long after the dust had settled in the West.[5] The problem, of course, is that we have to wait until after the Council of Chalcedon (451 CE), and in particular until the reigns of Justin I (518–27 CE) and Justinian I (527–65 CE), for the resulting explosion in Syriac scholarship. This is because the accession of Justin I ushered in a new imperial policy that attempted to enforce Chalcedon on the eastern churches, which, in turn, hastened the schism between Chalcedonians and non-Chalcedonians.[6] It is not a coincidence, therefore, that the late fifth and sixth centuries witnessed a dramatic increase in Syriac scholarship and literature, particularly in terms of translations from Greek, in which Sergius of Resh ʿAina (d. 536 CE) played an important role.[7]

The Sixth and Seventh Centuries

When we come to the period in which Sergius flourished, we suddenly have much more information. A number of earlier texts circulated under false names—e.g., the Cave of Treasures, a sixth-century collection of tales relating to the Bible, was often attributed to Ephrem.[8] The problem of pseudepigraphy was often discussed, especially in the context of propagandist florilegia and in relation to the intense theological debates of the day.

For example, in the mid-seventh century, Athanasius of Nisibis translated the letters of Severus, the non-Chalcedonian Patriarch of Antioch who was a contemporary of Sergius, from Greek into Syriac. In one such letter, written to

---

[4] R. Murray, *Symbols of Church and Kingdom: A Study in Early Syriac Tradition*, Cambridge, 1975, p. 279.

[5] An excellent study is that of W. Speyer, *Die Literarische Fälschung im Heidnischen und Christlichen Altertum: Ein versuch ihrer Deutung*, Munich, 1971; see, e.g., p. 309.

[6] For an excellent assessment of the significance of the events of 451 CE and 518 CE, and their long-term consequences, see V. L. Menze, *Justinian and the Making of the Syrian Orthodox Church*, Oxford, 2008; see, e.g., pp. 275–6.

[7] See, e.g., the list in Brock, *Brief Outline* (n. 2 above), pp. 120–22; see also the useful (albeit dated and problematic in some respects) discussion in W. Wright, *A Short History of Syriac Literature*, London, 1894, pp. 65–133.

[8] Brock, *Brief Outline* (n. 2 above), p. 47.

a lady called Caesaria, Severus discussed the issue of forgeries, in respect of both himself and the fourth century Cappadocian bishop Basil of Caesarea:[9]

ܡܐܡܘܪܐ ܕܝܢ ܗܘ ܕܡܬܒܕܪ ܘܡܬܬܛܥܢܐ ܡܢ ܐܢܫܝܢ: ܗܘ ܕܐܡܪܬܝ ܕܪܫܝܡ
ܒܫܡܐ ܕܝܠܝ: ܘܡܫܩܠܐ ܦܘܫܩܐ ܕܐܝܟ ܗܢܐ: ܐܝܢܐ ܕܡܣܠܐ ܐܢܐ ܕܐܦ
ܒܣܦܘܬܐ ܕܝܠܝ ܐܝܬܘܗܝ: ܐܝܟ ܗܝ ܕܠܐ ܝܕܥܘܬܐ ܘܫܛܝܘܬܐ ܡܠܝܐ. ܕܥܝ
ܕܠܐ ܗܝ ܐܝܬܝܗ̇ ܕܒܨܝܪܘܬܐ ܕܝܠܢ. ܐܠܐ ܐܘ ܕܐܢܫܝܢ ܣܟܠܐ ܕܡܫܬܡܗܝܢ
ܐܪܬܕܘܟܣܘܣ ܐܝܬܝܗ̇ ܒܕܓܠܘܬܐ. ܐܘ ܕܗܪܛܝܩܘ ܕܒܥܝܢ ܕܢܟܣܘܢ ܠܒܗܬܬܗܘܢ
ܕܝܠܗܘܢ ... ܡܘܕܥ ܓܝܪ ܪܒܐ ܒܣܝܠܝܘܣ: ܒܐܓܪܬܐ ܗ̇ܝ ܕܪܫܝܡܐ ܠܘܬ
ܚܒܝܫܐ ܘܝܚܝܕܝܐ ܕܬܚܝܬܘܗܝ: ܗܢܘܢ ܕܒܐܘܪܘܒܝܢ ܘܒܚܠܐܠܢ. ܕܐܓܪ̈ܬܐ
ܒܥܠܬܐ ܘܢܘܟܪܝܬܐ ܡܒܕܪܝܢ ܗܘܘ ܐܢܫܝܢ ܥܠܘܗܝ ...

And the brief treatise that is being disseminated and carried around by certain people, which you said is inscribed with my name and carries a superscription like this, which I scorn even with my lips, as one that is full of ignorance and foolishness – know that it is not at all of our humble selves, but it is a forgery either of foolish people who are designated orthodox or of heretics who want to conceal their shame ... For the great Basil made known, in the letter that is inscribed to the ascetics and solitaries who were under him, those who were at Orobiane and at Chalane, that people were disseminating against him forged and strange letters ...

It is clear that, in such cases, forgeries were perceived as a problem, and those responsible for them were considered worthy of great condemnation. Before we move on to Sergius, however, it is worthwhile to consider an alternative type of forgery, or, at least, an alternative approach to analysing the phenomenon of pseudepigraphy.

Recently, Charles Stang has argued compellingly for the application to late-antique eastern Christianity of the 'religious' or 'psychological' approach to pseudepigraphy. In short, this approach:[10]

... argues that a pseudonymous author had a special kinship with the ancient sage or seer under whose name he wrote, and that pseudonymous writing served to collapse or 'telescope' the past and the present, such that the present author and the past luminary could achieve a kind of contemporaneity.

While this approach has come under some criticism, Stang's application of it specifically to the late-antique Christian East appears to have merit. This is because eastern Christianity, from the fourth to the sixth centuries, exhibits a 'peculiar understanding of time' in which 'the apostolic and sub-apostolic ages

[9] For the text, see E. W. Brooks, *The Sixth Book of the Select Letters of Severus Patriarch of Antioch in the Syriac Version of Athanasius of Nisibis*, 2 vols in 4 parts, London, 1902–4, vol. 1, part 2, pp. 504–5; the English translation is my own, but compare vol. 2, part 2, pp. 448–9.

[10] C. M. Stang, *Apophasis and Pseudonymity in Dionysius the Areopagite*, Oxford, 2012, p. 41.

are widely believed to exist in a "timeless communion" with the present age.'[11] This means that there is another category of pseudepigraphy that goes beyond a simple (and, perhaps, malicious) forgery. It is not simply that an anonymous author is sympathetic to the tradition of the ancient sage whose name he uses – he 'comes to understand himself as an extension of the personality of the ancient authority.'[12]

It is in this context that we should consider Sergius, who, famously, translated the Pseudo-Dionysian corpus into Syriac, within a few decades of its composition,[13] and then appended his own *Treatise on the Spiritual Life* as an introduction on account of how well it accorded with the Pseudo-Dionysian corpus.[14] Previous scholarship has wrestled with the problem of whether Sergius truly believed the text to have been written by Dionysius, the disciple of the apostle Paul (Acts 17:34). Thus Polycarpe Sherwood, who, among modern scholars, was probably best acquainted with the material, writes that Sergius 'accepted it as the genuine work of Denis the Areopagite,'[15] while, more recently, Stang leaves the question more open.[16] It seems likely that Sergius, one of the greatest scholars of his age,

---

[11] Stang, *Apophasis and Pseudonymity* (n. 10 above), p. 42. Stang's second chapter, 'Pseudonymous Writing in the Late Antique Christian East', pp. 41–80, gives an excellent summary of previous scholarship on pseudepigraphy and demonstrates well the value of the 'religious' or 'psychological' approach specifically to Sergius's context.

[12] Stang, *Apophasis and Pseudonymity* (n. 10 above), p. 201. See also pp. 71–8, which presents a detailed discussion of Margaret Mitchell's analysis of John Chrysostom's homilies, in which this contemporaneity is clearly in evidence, in this case between Chrysostom and the apostle Paul. Mitchell thus writes: 'In the verbal medium of his liturgical homilies Chrysostom himself in many ways became the very medium by which Paul was displayed, in his words and the content of his discourse on Paul, and in his own demeanor, diction and disposition, which were decidedly and emphatically in the Pauline mold, as the scribe quoted in the last chapter noted: "the mouth of Paul begot the mouth of Chrysostom." In Chrysostom's interpretations of Paul the identities, personalities and voices of the two men, like their faces in the miniature portrait, become conformed to one another. Thus in Chrysostom's discourse on Paul we have a complex interweaving of the two persons, the two selves, of Paul and Chrysostom.' – see M. M. Mitchell, *The Heavenly Trumpet: John Chrysostom and the Art of Pauline Interpretation*, Tübingen, 2000, p. 42. See also p. 33, where Mitchell quotes in full the eleventh-century copyist, who wrote: 'The mouth of Christ brought forth the mouth of Paul and the mouth of Paul the mouth of Chrysostom.'

[13] It has been suggested that Sergius was actually the author of the Pseudo-Dionysian corpus, but this is extremely unlikely – see, *inter alios*, R. A. Arthur, *Pseudo-Dionysius as Polemicist: The Development and Purpose of the Angelic Hierarchy in Sixth Century Syria*, Aldershot, 2008, p. 197.

[14] See P. Sherwood, 'Sergius of Reshaina and the Syriac Versions of the Pseudo-Denis', *Sacris Erudiri*, 4, 1952, pp. 174–84. Sergius's treatise on the spiritual life was published in a series of articles: P. Sherwood, 'Mimro de Serge de Rešayna sur la vie spirituelle', *L'Orient Syrien*, 5, 1960, pp. 433–57; 6, 1961, pp. 95–115, 121–56.

[15] Sherwood, 'Sergius of Reshaina' (n. 14 above), p. 180.

[16] From Stang, *Apophasis and Pseudonymity* (n. 10 above), p. 25: 'It is unclear whether Sergius

appreciated that the identity of the author was simply irrelevant – the text was Dionysius speaking to the present age.[17]

If this was indeed the prevailing attitude towards pseudepigraphy in Sergius's day, in respect of religious and philosophical texts, we are left with the possibility that the same attitude was held in respect of scientific texts. For Sergius, especially, this is likely to have been the case because, although he did distinguish between the medical, philosophical and theological genres, he viewed Aristotle as the foundation for a true understanding of all three and thus considered them together as a coherent system.[18] If a writer was able to achieve contemporaneity with an ancient philosopher or biblical character, then why not an ancient doctor as well?

Sergius and Galen

This brings us to Sergius's translations of Galen, for which our most important source remains Ḥunayn's رسالة حنين بن اسحق الى علي بن يحيى فى ذكر ما ترجم من كتب جالينوس بعلمه وبعض ما لم يترجم 'The Epistle of Ḥunayn Ibn Isḥaq to ʿAli Ibn Yaḥya concerning those of Galen's books that have been translated, to his knowledge, and some of those that are not translated.'[19] This source must be treated with caution—a sensible approach would be to accept Ḥunayn's statements on what Sergius *did* translate, as these are probably based on manuscripts that he

---

believed that the author of the CD was in fact Dionysius the Areopagite.' Stang notes that Sergius 'never explicitly calls the pseudonym into question,' but that other factors could suggest that 'he knew all too well and the CD was a pseudonymous work – perhaps even who the author was – but that he chose not to expose this fact.'

[17] Compare the remarks of John Watt: 'As an intelligent student of Neoplatonic philosophers in Alexandria, Sergius must surely have been aware of the similarities between Dionysius and the Neoplatonism of Plotinus and Proclus, whatever he thought about the identity of 'Dionysius the Areopagite'. While we have no evidence that he followed his Alexandrian teachers in considering Aristotle inferior or propaedeutic to Plato, in his enthusiasm for Dionysius evident in his translation of the corpus we have reason to suppose that he remained nevertheless to some extent true to those Alexandrian teachers in seeing Aristotle as inferior to a 'more divine' pedagogue. That pedagogue, however, was not Plato as interpreted by Plotinus or Proclus, but the Holy Scriptures as interpreted by Dionysius' – see J. Watt, 'From Sergius to Mattā: Aristotle and Pseudo-Dionysius in the Syriac Tradition', in *Interpreting the Bible and Aristotle in Late Antiquity: The Alexandrian Commentary Tradition between Rome and Baghdad*, eds J. Lössl and J. W. Watt, Farnham, 2011, pp. 239–57 (241).

[18] See, e.g., Brock, *Brief Outline* (n. 2 above), p. 204. This is a point I discuss in S. Bhayro, 'Galen in Syriac: Rethinking Old Assumptions', *Aramaic Studies*, 15, 2017, pp. 132–54 (150–52); see also S. Bhayro, 'Sergius of Reš ʿAyna's Syriac Translations of Galen: Their Scope, Motivation, and Influence', *Bulletin of the Asia Institute*, new ser., 26, 2016, dated 2012, pp. 121–8 (124–5).

[19] Published with German translation by G. Bergsträsser, *Ḥunain ibn Isḥāq über die syrischen und arabischen Galen-Übersetzungen*, Leipzig, 1925; a new edition with English translation was recently published by J. C. Lamoreaux, *Ḥunayn ibn Isḥāq on His Galen Translations*, Provo, 2016.

had consulted, while, at the same time, remaining open minded when Ḥunayn mentions nothing of Sergius in respect of a specific text. After all, Ḥunayn's knowledge was not exhaustive.[20]

We can now adduce another example, namely *In Hippocratis de Alimento*, which may also be spurious:[21]

تفسيره لكتاب الغذاء. هذا الكتاب جعله في اربع مقالات. وقد ترجمته انا الى السريانية لسلمويه وترجمت ايضا فص كلام بقراط لهذا الكتاب واضفت اليه شرحا وجيزا.

His commentary on the Book of Nutriment: He produced this book in four treatises. And I translated it into Syriac for Salmawayh, and I also translated Hippocrates' lemmas for this book, and I added to it a short commentary.

Ḥunayn was clearly unaware of any preceding Syriac translation of this work. We now know, however, that Sergius did indeed translate this work, because a Judaeo-Arabic translation of Sergius's Syriac translation has recently been discovered, complete with a translation of Sergius's introduction.[22]

An important feature of Sergius's introduction, for our present purposes, is how it follows the canonical formula of *accessores ad auctores*. In the case of *In Hippocratis de Alimento*, this consists of the following eight sections:[23]

1. the purpose/uses of the book
2. the reason for the book's title
3. the division of the Hippocratic corpus
4. the place of the book within the Hippocratic corpus
5. authenticity, in this case of the Hippocratic work upon which Galen's commentary is based
6. the book's contents
7. the book's lineage, in this case in terms of theory and practice
8. the book's mode of composition

[20] I discuss this point and the overall aims and scope of Sergius's translation project in Bhayro, 'Sergius of Reš 'Ayna's Syriac Translations of Galen' (n. 18 above).

[21] See Bergsträsser, *Ḥunain ibn Isḥāq* (n. 19 above), p. 35 (German translation) and ٤٣ (Arabic text).

[22] The Judaeo-Arabic כתאב אלגדא is equivalent to the Arabic كتاب الغذاء, both meaning 'Book of Nutriment'. The Judaeo-Arabic introduction has been analysed and published by G. Bos and Y. T. Langermann, 'The Introduction of Sergius of Rēshʻainā to Galen's Commentary on Hippocrates' *On Nutriment*', *Journal of Semitic Studies*, 54, 2009, pp. 179–204.

[23] See the discussion of the 'Alexandrian' introduction in Bos and Langermann, 'The Introduction of Sergius of Rēshʻainā' (n. 22 above), pp. 181–8.

As Gerrit Bos and Tzvi Langermann observe, this structure for an introduction is a 'tradition that developed in late antiquity among commentators to books of science and philosophy,' and 'continued by Syriac, Arabic, Hebrew and Latin authors.'[24]

The section on authenticity appears to have been a consistent feature of such introductions. We may suppose, therefore, that, whenever Sergius translated a Galenic text and added his own introduction, he would have addressed the issue of authorship – a tantalising prospect indeed. Unfortunately, due to the paucity of preserved Syriac medical texts, we are unable to test this supposition.[25]

The authenticity section of Sergius's introduction to Galen's *In Hippocratis de Alimento* deals with the authenticity of the original Hippocratic work rather than Galen's commentary, but it still contributes well to our present discussion as it gives us an insight into the criteria by which such things were assessed. The Judaeo-Arabic translation reads:[26]

פלדלך הדא אלכתאב הו אלראבע מן כתב אבקראט ובעדה יקרא. ואעלם אנה יסמי
באסם אבקראט סלתה נפר (?) וקד וצ'ע כתבא בעצ'הא יכאד ישבה בעצ'א" פלדלך
מא שך מן פסר כתבהם וכאדוא לא ימיזון בעצ'הא מן בעץ'. פאמא נחן פנקול והו
אלחק אן הדא אלכתאב הו לאבקראט אלדי וצ'ע כתאב תקדים אלעלם וכתאב אלפצול
וכתאב אלגבר וכתאב אלמפאצל וכתאב אפידימיא וכתאב אלעלל אלחאדה ואנמא
עלמנא דלך מן איגאזה וחד'פה אלתטויל מע גמוץ' תפהמה וקלה פצ'ולה ופי הדא מא
הו אצדק ואכד פי אלחג'ה. והו שהאדה גאלינוס ותפסירה איאה מן בינהא כלהא.

Therefore, this book is the fourth of Hippocrates' books, after which he reads. Know that it was called by the name Hippocrates... He composed books, some of which are almost like others. This is the reason why the commentators had some doubts and could hardly distinguish the one from the other. As for us, we say – and it is the truth – that this book is by the Hippocrates who wrote *On Prognosis*, the *Aphorisms*, *On Bone-Setting*, *On Joints*, *Epidemics*, and *Acute Diseases*. We know this, because of its conciseness and wariness of prolixity, along with the depth of understanding and the rarity of anything superfluous, yet concerning this, there is an argument that is

---

[24] Bos and Langermann, 'The Introduction of Sergius of Rēshʿainā' (n. 22 above), p. 181.

[25] The only other introductions to Galenic texts by Sergius that we do have, namely to books six, seven and eight of Galen's *De Simplicium Medicamentorum Temperamentis Ac Facultatibus*, do not possess such a structure. But these introductions only relate to the individual books – it is possible that Sergius wrote a general introduction to the entire work that did possess this structure. For the introduction to book six, see S. Bhayro and S. Brock, 'The Syriac Galen Palimpsest and the Role of Syriac in the Transmission of Greek Medicine in the Orient', in *Ancient Medical and Healing Systems: Their Legacy to Western Medicine*, ed. R. David, Manchester, 2013, pp. 25–43 (38–40).

[26] The text is not perfectly preserved and some issues remain. The text and translation given here is taken from Bos and Langermann, 'The Introduction of Sergius of Rēshʿainā' (n. 22 above), pp. 195–6, 202.

more correct and more firm. This is the testimony of Galen and his commentary to it, among all of them.

The criteria by which Sergius favoured the authenticity of the Hippocratic text, therefore, are two-fold and very straightforward: first, it is just like other Hippocratic works; and, second, the existence of Galen's commentary on it confirms its Hippocratic authorship. I would suggest that this very much reflects the same attitude towards authorship and pseudonymity that Sergius, reflecting the spirit of his age, displayed towards theological and philosophical works: the text accords properly with the canon of the ancient authority, in terms of both content and tone, and is also affirmed by a subsequent authority who very much represents both the mouthpiece of, and the true means of accessing, the more ancient authority.[27] In view of this, it is not surprising that Sergius would have translated a Pseudo-Galenic work. It is not that Sergius was not concerned with authenticity – rather, he understood authenticity in a completely different way to how we would do so today.[28]

Ḥunayn and Galen

It appears that Ḥunayn, on the other hand, possessed a different attitude towards authenticity. For example, consider Ḥunayn's description of the Pseudo-Galenic *In Hippocratis De Foetus Natura Librum Commentarius*:[29]

تفسيره لكتاب طبيعة الجنين. هذا الكتاب لم نجد له تفسيرا من قول جالينوس
ولا وجدنا جالينوس ذكر فى فهرست كتبه انه عمل له تفسيرا الا انه وجدناه
قد قسم هذا الكتاب بثلثة اجزاء فى كتابه الذى عمله فى علم ابقراط بالتشريح
وذكر ان الجزء الاول والثالث من هذا الكتاب منحول ليس هو لابقراط وانما
الصحيح منه الجزء الثانى وقد فسر هذا الجزء جاسيوس الاسكندرانى وقد وجدنا

[27] Returning to the way John Watt describes Sergius's theological and philosophical endeavours (see n. 17): 'Beginning with Sergius, the original Alexandrian 'program' was 'copied' with various additions and modifications over the years: the substitution of the Bible and Dionysius for Plato and pagan Neoplatonism ... ' – see Watt, 'From Sergius to Mattā' (n. 17 above), p. 257. In the case of medicine, there would be little need for a parallel substitution, so Sergius would be able to maintain the pattern of Hippocrates and Galen.

[28] See also the discussions of *In Hippocratis De Foetus Natura Librum Commentarius* and *De Remediis Parabilibus* below. It is also worth noting that, while Ḥunayn appears to have not known about earlier doubts as to the authenticity of Hippocrates' *On Nutriment*, Sergius is clearly aware of such doubts, even though he rejected them for the reasons just discussed.

[29] See Bergsträsser, *Ḥunain ibn Isḥāq* (n. 19 above), pp. 35–6 (German translation) and ٤٤-٤٣ (Arabic text).

لجميع الثلثة الاجزاء تفسيرين احدهما سريانى موسوم بانه لجالينوس وقد كان
ترجمه سرجس فلما فحصنا عنه علمنا انه لبالبس والاخر يونانى فلما فحصنا عنه
وجدناه لسورانوس الذى من شيعة الموثوذيقوا. [ترجم حنين فص هذا الكتاب
الا قليلا منه الى العربية فى خلافة المعتز.]

His commentary on the Book of the Nature of the Embryo: We have not found
concerning this book a commentary by Galen, neither did we find that Galen
mentioned in the list of his books that he produced a commentary on it. But we
found that he did divide this book into three parts, in his book that he produced
concerning Hippocrates' knowledge about anatomy, and he mentioned that the first
and third parts of this book are spurious – they are not by Hippocrates – and only
the second part of it is genuine. And Gesius the Alexandrian commented on this part.
And we have found for all three parts two commentaries. One of them is (in) Syriac
– it is ascribed to Galen. And Sergius translated it. But, when we inquired about it,
we learned that it is by Pelops. And the other is (in) Greek. And, when we inquired
about it, we found it is by Soranus, who was of the sect of the Methodists. [Ḥunayn
translated a section of this book except for a little bit of it into Arabic during the
Caliphate of Muʿtazz.]

In short, in the sixth century, as part of his comprehensive translation project,
Sergius translated a Pseudo-Galenic commentary into Syriac and declared it to
be of Galen. Given what we observed above, it could be that it was sufficiently
Galenic in tone and content to merit such an ascription. Such an approach to
pseudonymity, however, did not satisfy Ḥunayn, whose investigations established
its true author to be Pelops. As the above quotation suggests, Ḥunayn's suspicions
were probably aroused by Galen himself, who observed the spurious nature of the
Hippocratic text and stated that he never wrote a commentary on it.[30]

It is also clear that, for Ḥunayn, the pseudonymous nature of a text had very
little bearing on his decision on whether or not to translate it. This, in itself,
is not surprising – Ḥunayn was, after all, a professional translator and it stands
to reason that he would exploit any potential market. Thus, to adduce another
example, following a brief discussion of three books concerning the Empiricists,
Ḥunayn mentioned that he knew of one more book concerning them, adding:[31]

علمت انها مفتعلة الا انى قد ترجمتها على ما علمت منها الى السريانية
لبختيشوع

---

[30] Of course, this raises the question of whether Sergius could also have known this – if he did,
then his decision to ascribe the text to Galen would be a striking confirmation of the difference in
attitude towards authenticity.

[31] Bergsträsser, *Ḥunain ibn Isḥāq* (n. 19 above), p. 38 (German translation) and ٤٦ Arabic text).

I knew that it was spurious but I translated it, according to what I knew of it, into Syriac for Bukhtīshūʿ.

So it is not surprising that Ḥunayn would translate part of Soranus's commentary. It is significant, however, that he appears to have made serious investigations into the authorship of the original text and its commentaries in order to understand better the history of scholarship. In comparison to Sergius, Ḥunayn's approach would appear to be much more akin to what modern scholars do. Furthermore, in terms of sources, it would seem that Ḥunayn used much more than Galen's own statements.

It is clear, however, that Galen remained Ḥunayn's most important source for distinguishing the genuine from the spurious. Thus, in the case of *In Hippocratis de Humoribus*, Ḥunayn appears to have considered it genuine on account of Galen's description of the text:[32]

تفسيره لكتاب الاخلاط. ذكر انه جعله فى ثلث مقالات. ولم اكن رايتها فيما مضى باليونانية ثم وجدتها من بعد فترجمتها الى السريانية مع فص كلام بقراط.

His commentary on the *Book of the Humours*: He states that he produced it in three treatises. And I had not seen them in the past in Greek. Then afterwards I found them, and I translated them into Syriac with Hippocrates' lemmas.

Similarly, the genuine status of *De Optima Secta ad Thrasybulum* was established by means of Galen's allusion to it in another text:[33]

كتابه المسمى ثراسوبولس. هذا الكتاب مقالة واحدة وغرضه فيه ان يفحص هل حفظ الاصحاء على صحتهم من صناعة الطب ام هو من صناعة اصحاب الرياضة وهى المقالة التى اشار اليها فى ابتداء كتاب تدبير الاصحاء حين قال ان الصناعة التى تتولى القيام على الابدان واحدة كما بينت فى غير هذا الكتاب. وقد ترجمت انا هذه المقالة الى السريانية وترجمها حبيش الى العربية لابى الحسن احمد بن موسى.

His book which is named Thrasybulus: This book is one treatise, and his aim in it is that he will investigate whether the preservation of the healthy in their health is by the art of medicine or by the art of the adherents of physical exercise. And it is the treatise to which he alludes at the start of the Book of the Management of the Healthy, when he said that 'the art that displays concern for bodies is one, as I explained in

---

[32] Bergsträsser, *Ḥunain ibn Isḥāq* (n. 19 above), p. 35 (German translation) and ٤٢ (Arabic text).

[33] Bergsträsser, *Ḥunain ibn Isḥāq* (n. 19 above), p. 32 (German translation) and ٣٩ Arabic text).

this other book.' And I translated this treatise into Syriac, and Ḥubaysh translated it into Arabic for Abū'l-Ḥasan Aḥmad ibn Mūsā.

In other cases, it is clear that Ḥunayn was not aware of a text's spurious nature. For example, regarding the spurious *De Victus Ratione in Morbis Acutis ex Hippocratis Sententia*, he stated:[34]

كتابه فى تدبير الامراض الحادة على راى بقراط. هذا الكتاب مقالة واحدة وغرضه فيه يعرف من عنوانه. وقد ترجمته انا الى السريانية منذ قريب لبختيشوع وترجمته بعد ذلك الى العربية لمحمد بن موسى.

His book concerning the management of acute diseases according to the opinion of Hippocrates: This book is one treatise, and his aim in it is known from its title. And I translated it into Syriac recently for Bukhtīshūʿ, and I translated it afterwards into Arabic for Muḥammad ibn Mūsā.

A curious example is *De Theriaca ad Pamphilianum*, regarding which Ḥunayn stated:[35]

كتابه قى الترياق الى بمفوليانس. هذا الكتاب مقالة صغيرة. وقد رايته بالسريانية والاغلب على ظنى انى ترجمته فى حداثتى الا انى اعلم انى رايته فاسدا فلا ادرى افسده الوراقون او قصد لاصلاحه قاصد فافسده الا ان نسخته باليونانية فى كتبى.

His book concerning Theriac to Pamphilianus: This book is a small treatise. And I have seen it in Syriac and it is likely that I translated it in my youth. But I know that what I saw is corrupt but I do not know who corrupted it – the copyists or one who intended to improve it but corrupted it. Yet there is a copy of it in Greek among my books.

In this case, not only was Ḥunayn unaware that this work is spurious, but he was also very keen to disown his earlier translation of it.

Finally, Ḥunayn's comments on *De Remediis Parabilibus* prove to be very interesting for a number of reasons:[36]

كتابه فى الادوية التى يسهل وجودها. هذا الكتاب مقالتان وغرضه فيه بين من عنوانه. ولم اجد لهذا الكتاب نسخة باليونانية اصلا ولا بلغنى انه عند احد على انى قد كنت فى طلبه بعناية شديدة وقد ترجمه سرجس الا ان الحاصل فى

---

[34] Bergsträsser, *Ḥunain ibn Isḥāq* (n. 19 above), p. 30 (German translation) and ٣٦ (Arabic text).

[35] Bergsträsser, *Ḥunain ibn Isḥāq* (n. 19 above), p. 31 (German translation) and ٣٨ (Arabic text).

[36] Bergsträsser, *Ḥunain ibn Isḥāq* (n. 19 above), pp. 30-31 (German translation) and ٣٧-٣٨ (Arabic text); see also Laurence Totelin's paper in this volume.

ايدى السريانيين فى هذا الوقت فاسد ردىء. وقد اضيف اليه مقالة اخرى فى هذا
الفن نسبت الى جالينوس وما هى لجالينوس لكنها لفلغريوس. وقد رايت تلك
المقالة بل ترجمتها مع مقالات لفلغريوس لبختيشوع الى السريانية. ولم يقتصر
المفسرون للكتب على هذا حتى ادخلوا فى هذا الكتاب هذيانا كثيرا وصفات
بديعة عجيبة وادوية لم يرها جالينوس ولم يسمع بها قط ... كانت مضرته من
منفعته ... وسالنى بعض اصدقائى ان اقرا الكتاب السريانى واصححه على
حسب ما ارى انه موافق راى جالينوس ففعلت.

His book concerning Drugs that are Easy to Find: This book is two treatises and his
aim in it is clear from its title. And I have not personally encountered a copy of this
book in Greek, neither have I heard that it is with anyone even though I looked for it
with great care. And Sergius translated it, but the result in the hands of the Syrians
(i.e. Syriac speakers) at this time is corrupt (and) bad. And another treatise has been
added to it on this specific field – it is attributed to Galen, but what is (attributed)
to Galen is but to Philagrius. And I had seen this treatise and even translated it,
together with (other) treatises by Philagrius, for Bukhtīshūʿ into Syriac. And the
commentators of the books are not content with this until they have incorporated
into this book much folly and marvellous wonderful recipes and drugs concerning
which Galen had never seen nor heard ... it is more harmful than useful ... And one
of my friends asked me to read the Syriac book and to correct it in accordance with
what I consider is appropriate for the opinion of Galen – and so I did.

Ḥunayn was thus aware that only the first and second parts of *De Remediis
Parabilibus* are genuine. He identified the third part as spurious, despite it being
attributed by others to Galen, and instead attributed it to Philagrius on account of
his past experience translating Philagrius's works. It would seem, therefore, that
we have here a nice illustration of the two distinct approaches to pseudonymity
that we have already observed. Initially, the Galenic text was translated into
Syriac in the sixth century, and, in keeping with the prevailing attitude towards
authorship, it was probably not long afterwards supplemented with the similar
work by Philagrius. By the time of Ḥunayn, however, this attitude had changed.
Having said that, the appending of Philagrius to Galen appears to have not
detracted from Galen in the estimation of Ḥunayn—he just wanted to be clear
about who wrote what.

Ḥunayn's problem lay elsewhere. In his opinion, the interpolation of another
body of tradition, namely traditional 'folk' remedies, rendered the resulting Syriac
text dangerous. It was necessary for a 'clean' text to be produced, i.e. for these
'unscientific' aspects to be removed – a task Ḥunayn claimed to have accomplished.
Interestingly, the aim of producing a useful text was not accomplished by

removing everything that was not *by* Galen – instead, it was accomplished by removing everything that was not *in accordance with* Galen. Thus it appears that the consequences of the earlier attitude towards medical pseudepigraphy were acceptable, as long as the true authorship was determined.

Ḥunayn's description of the Syriac version of *De Remediis Parabilibus* very much accords with what we find in the Syriac *Book of Medicines*, to which we now turn and which contains what we could call the 'wrong' kind of medical pseudepigraphy that Ḥunayn disdained.

The Syriac *Book of Medicines*

In the Syriac *Book of Medicines* (c. twelfth century CE),[37] which seems to be simultaneously a product of the Syriac Renaissance (eleventh to thirteenth centuries CE)[38] and the age of the great encyclopedic compilations (tenth to thirteenth centuries CE),[39] all the Galenic quotations and paraphrases are drawn from genuine works:

List of Galenic works quoted or paraphrased in the Syriac *Book of Medicines*[40]

- *Ars Medica*
- *De Temperamentis*
- *De Symptomatum Causis*
- *De Locis Affectis*
- *De Methodo Medendi*
- *De Compositione Medicamentorum Secundum Locos*
- *De Compositione Medicamentorum per Genera*
- *De Remediis Parabilibus*

As Sergius alone translated all of the above works, it seems possible that these excerpts were based on the translations of Sergius rather than Ḥunayn.[41] Moreover, it may be that the *Book of Medicines* only quotes from the first two parts

---

[37] E. A. W. Budge, *The Syriac Book of Medicines. Syrian Anatomy, Pathology and Therapeutics in the Early Middle Ages*, 2 vols, London, 1913.

[38] For an introduction to the Syriac Renaissance, see H. Teule, 'The Syriac Renaissance', in *The Syriac Renaissance*, eds H. Teule et al, Leuven, 2010, pp. 1–30.

[39] For which, see H. D. Isaacs, 'Arabic Medical Literature', in *Religion, Learning and Science in the 'Abbasid Period*, eds M. J. L. Young et al, Cambridge, 1990, pp. 342–63 (347–8).

[40] For more details, see R. Degen, 'Galen im Syrischen: Eine Übersicht über die syrische Überlieferung der Werke Galens', in *Galen: Problems and Prospects*, ed. V. Nutton, London, 1981, pp. 131–66.

[41] This conclusion remains tentative at present, as the majority of quotations from *De Remediis*

of *De Remediis Parabilibus*, i.e. from the authentic parts, that Sergius translated, and not from the spurious third part that Ḥunayn discussed (see above).

Unfortunately, not knowing much about the production of the *Book of Medicines*, which remains in need of a thorough reediting and a fresh analysis in the light of new manuscript discoveries,[42] we are not in a position to say at this point whether its use of exclusively genuine works is entirely coincidental or whether scholars in the Syriac Renaissance consciously rejected the Pseudo-Galenic works that were translated in the early medieval period.

We can, on the other hand, note two rather interesting features of the use of Galen in the *Book of Medicines*. First, we can observe the rather free treatment of Galen's works, which were excerpted and adjusted according to contemporary needs and tastes, and the lack of an explicit ascription to Galen when quoting from his works.[43] Indeed, I have elsewhere discussed not only this phenomenon, but one instance in which Galen's voice is entirely removed from one such excerpt, thus showing little regard for the original author.[44]

Second, and conversely, we can also note that, when there is an ascription to Galen, it is often spurious and intended to lend authority to a practitioner or to an indigenous near eastern remedy. For example, the following is found in a list of prescriptions for the spleen:[45]

ܐܝܢܪ ܝ ܠܠܘܣܩ ܘܢܥܣ ܘܕ ܐܗܘܝ ܪܒܓܝܘܟ ܐܗܐ ܒܡܘܣ ܒܗܕ ܕܘܐ.
ܝܘܒ ܝܡܒ ܢܘܝ ܘܡܒܪ ܘܡܣܡܪ ܝܡ ܕܣܩ.

Parabilibus may derive from *De Compositione Medicamentorum Secundum Locos*, which Ḥunayn did translate. This point requires further investigation.

[42] See, most recently, the survey of manuscripts in the doctoral dissertation by Stefanie Rudolf: S. M. Rudolf, 'Die astraldivinatorischen Passagen des Syrischen Medizinbuches: Neu übersetzt und kommentiert', PhD diss., Free University Berlin, 2014; see also S. M. Rudolf, *Syrische Astrologie und das Syrische Medizinbuch*, Berlin, 2018. Stefanie Rudolf and I plan to publish a full edition of the Syriac *Book of Medicines* in due course; see S. Bhayro and S. M. Rudolf, 'Budge's Syriac Book of Medicines after One Hundred Years: Problems and Prospects', in *Mesopotamian Medicine and Magic: Studies in Honor of Markham J. Geller*, eds S. V. Panayotov and L. Vacín, Leiden, 2018, pp. 116–30.

[43] With one exception: a discussion of the use of white dog faeces in treating diseases of the colon; see Budge, *The Syriac Book of Medicines* (n. 37 above), vol. 1, p. 428 (text), vol. 2, pp. 504–5 (translation), which appears to be drawing on a passage from Galen's *Simples* (XII, 291 K.) – see R. J. Durling, 'Excreta as a Remedy in Galen, his Predecessors and his Successors', in *Tradition et traduction: Les textes philosophiques et scientifiques grecs au moyen age latin*, eds R. Beyers et al., Leuven, 1999, pp. 25–35 (29–30).

[44] See S. Bhayro, 'The Reception of Galen's *Art of Medicine* in the Syriac *Book of Medicines*', in *Medical Books in the Byzantine World*, ed. B. Zipser, Bologna, 2013, pp. 123–44.

[45] With the measurements removed; see Budge, *The Syriac Book of Medicines* (n. 37 above), vol. 1, p. 403 (text), vol. 2, p. 473 (translation).

Another of Galen, and it is very useful. Moist pitch, wax, sulphur, natron, small pieces of alum,[46] wine and oil as much as is sufficient. Mix and use as a plaster.

Of the seven ingredients in this prescription, four are listed using authentic Syriac terms: ܙܦܬܐ ܪܛܝܒܬܐ 'moist pitch', ܩܘܦܐ ܘܣܟܠܐ 'small pieces of alum', ܚܡܪܐ 'wine', and ܡܫܚܐ 'oil'. Furthermore, two of the remaining terms are probably Akkadian loanwords: ܟܒܪܝܬܐ 'sulphur' < Akk. *kibrītu*, and ܢܝܬܪܐ 'natron' < Akk. *nitiru*. In these latter cases, this is significant because the available Greek loanwords are not used: ܬܐܦܢ < θεῖον for sulphur, and ܢܝܛܪܘܢ < νίτρον for natron. The remaining term is a Greek loanword: ܩܝܪܐ 'wax' < κηρός. The balance of evidence, therefore, very much suggests that this is a near eastern prescription and nothing to do with Galen.

Further examples, relating to other authoritative figures from Greco-Roman antiquity (e.g. Archigenes, Hippocrates etc.), could be adduced. Elsewhere, I have already raised the issue of medical pseudepigraphy in the Syriac *Book of Medicines*, arguing that such instances are a consequence of the clash of two distinct medical systems: the encroaching Greco-Roman system, which possessed a highly theoretical framework, and the indigenous Mesopotamian system, which was much more empirical. I argued that pseudepigraphy was one of a number of strategies employed to ensure the persistence of the Mesopotamian system alongside the new science.[47]

Be that as it may, it is clear that medical pseudepigraphy was very much alive and kicking in the Syriac Renaissance. Later Syriac scholarship, like that of their forebears, was very much concerned with what worked in practice. The name of an ancient writer such as Galen may have been useful for lending authority to a medical practitioner or recipe, but Galen himself was usually not given credit when being quoted and he was easily tossed aside when convenient. As we saw above, it appears that Ḥunayn had already encountered such practices in the ninth century, and rejected them as resulting in useless and dangerous manuscripts – they exhibited the wrong type of pseudepigraphy.

---

[46] Budge translated ܩܘܦܐ ܘܣܟܠܐ as 'smelters' dross'; Philippe Gignoux would translate it as 'rock alum' – see P. Gignoux, *Lexique des termes de la pharmacopée syriaque*, Paris, 2011, p. 75. The translation given here is based upon M. Sokoloff, *A Syriac Lexicon. A Translation from the Latin, Correction, Expansion, and Update of C. Brockelmann's Lexicon Syriacum*, Winona Lake/Piscataway, 2009, p. 1284.

[47] See S. Bhayro, 'Theory and Practice in the Syriac *Book of Medicines*: The Empirical Basis for the Persistence of Near Eastern Medical Lore', in *In the Wake of the Compendia: Infrastructural Contexts and the Licensing of Empiricism in Ancient and Medieval Mesopotamia*, ed. J. C. Johnson, Berlin, 2015, pp. 147–58.

Pseudo-Galenic Texts on Urines and Pulse in Late Byzantium*

Petros Bouras-Vallianatos

Introduction

The circulation of Pseudo-Galenic texts in Byzantium has not so far been the subject of a comprehensive study. There are, for example, long Pseudo-Galenic treatises such as *Introduction, or the Physician,*[1] *Medical Definitions,*[2] and *Euporista* or *On Procurable Remedies,*[3] which have their origins in antiquity and apparently have undergone detectable stages of elaboration throughout the Byzantine period. Although today these texts are certainly Pseudo-Galenic, they were often considered genuine by their Byzantine readers, as is, for example, attested in the vast majority of the manuscripts preserving these works, which

* I am grateful to Orly Lewis and Caroline Petit for their useful comments on an earlier draft of this chapter. Special thanks also go to Georgi Parpulov and Sophia Xenophontos for their helpful remarks on the transcription of the texts.

[1] The most recent edition of the text is by C. Petit, *Galien. Le Médecin. Introduction*, Paris, 2009. The date of this treatise is not certain; C. Petit, 'What does pseudo-Galen tell us that Galen does not? Ancient medical schools in the Roman Empire', in *Philosophical Themes in Galen*, eds P. Adamson, R. Hansberger and J. Wilberding, London, 2014, pp. 269–90, has shown that it could have been written during the second half of the 2nd century AD – when Galen was still alive – or even later, providing us with a *terminus ante quem* not later than the 5th or 6th century, i.e. a probable date for its early Latin translation, although she is in favour of the earlier date. About traces of Byzantine reelaboration of the Greek text, see Petit, *Galien. Le médecin*, Notice p. LXV-LXXX.

[2] *Medical Definitions* is only available in K. G. Kühn's edition: *Claudii Galeni Opera omnia*, 20 vols, Leipzig, 1821–33, vol. 19, pp. 346–46. A comprehensive study of the text was published by J. Kollesch, *Untersuchungen zu den pseudogalenischen 'Definitiones medicae'*, Berlin, 1973, pp. 60–66, who considers that it was written in the late 1st century AD, thus before Galen's time. This was a popular text in Byzantium and circulated in various versions. For example, Kollesch, ibid. p. 143, informs us that the version in *Palatinus gr. 297* (14th century) includes extracts from the Byzantine treatise *On the Constitution of Man* by Meletios the monk (9th century [?]). On the transmission of this text, see Cronier in the present volume.

[3] On this text, see the chapter by L. Totelin, 'The Third Way: Galen, Pseudo-Galen, Metrodora, Cleopatra and the Gynaecological Pharmacology of Byzantium', in *Collecting Recipes: Byzantine and Jewish Pharmacology in Dialogue*, eds L. Lehmhaus and M. Martelli, Berlin, 2017, pp. 103–22. There is an edition of the text by Kühn, XIV, 311–581 K., in which we can see Byzantine interpolations; in particular, there are recipes of clearly oriental influence, attested only in late Byzantine pharmacological works. See, for example, the recipe for a julep (ζουλάπιον) for spitting (περὶ πτύσεως), XIV, 563.12–564.11 K., which among other ingredients includes sugar (σάκχαρ) and *zūfā* (ζουφά), the Arabic for hyssop (ὕσσωπος). About the transmission of the *Euporista*, see Totelin in this volume.

display Galen's name in the title.[4] Additionally, we can see some very short works, some as brief as a single paragraph, also ascribed to Galen. These texts usually focus on something very practical, such as uroscopy,[5] sphygmology,[6] venesection,[7] or even on weights and measures.[8] Some of them, although composed many centuries after Galen's death and having no relationship with any Galenic material, may regularly be attributed to the author. In other cases, although not assembled in their present form by Galen, these texts could be the product of several successive processes of compilation based on content and ideas originating in a Galenic text.[9]

In this chapter, I shall examine a group of Pseudo-Galenic texts on urines and pulse, as presented in *Wellcomensis* MS.MSL.60. I would like to explore the sources of these brief treatises, confirm their spurious status, and also whether any part of them derives from Galen's works or ideas. Close textual analysis will be accompanied by a concluding discussion on the intended audience of these treatises in the attempt to demonstrate how conscious late Byzantine and post-Byzantine medical authors and practitioners were of the circulation of Pseudo-Galenic material.

[4] For example, according to C. Petit, 'The Fate of a Greek Medical Handbook in the Medieval West: the *Introduction, or the Physician* ascribed to Galen', in *Medical Books in the Byzantine World*, ed. B. Zipser, Bologna, 2013, pp. 57–77 (59), all forty Byzantine and post-Byzantine manuscripts of the *Introduction, or the Physician* give Galen's name in the title of the work.

[5] Examples of Greek treatises on urines ascribed to Galen are included in Kühn's edition, XIX, 574–601, 602–6, and 607–28 K. Another brief treatise on urines ascribed to Galen and surviving in three 15th-century codices was published by E. T. Moraux, 'Anecdota Graeca Minora VI. Pseudo-Galen, De signis ex urinis', *Zeitschrift für Papyrologie und Epigraphik*, 60, 1985, pp. 63–74. See also the treatise edited by V. Lorusso, 'Il trattato pseudogalenico *De Urinis* del Parisin. Suppl. gr. 634', *Bollettino dei classici*, 25, 2004, pp. 5–43.

[6] The most well-known example is the treatise *On the Pulse to Antonius, a Man of Learning and Philosopher*, XIX, 629–42 K. On this text, see H. A. Lutz, 'Leitfaden der Pulse, dem Galen zugeschrieben. Galens Schrift über die Pulse an Antonius, den Freund der Wissenschaften und der Philosophen', PhD diss., Ludwig-Maximilians-Universität Munich, 1940. On this treatise, see also Petit's contribution in this volume.

[7] See, for example, the short treatise edited by Kühn, XIX, 519–28 K.

[8] Among the various texts of this kind ascribed to Galen, see the long treatise edited by Kühn, XIX, 748–81 K.; the text was re-edited by F. Hultsch, *Metrologicorum scriptorium reliquiae*, vol. 1, Leipzig, 1864, pp. 218–44.

[9] On compilation methods in Byzantine medical literature, see the study by P. van der Eijk, 'Principles and practices of compilation and abbreviation in the medical "encyclopaedias" of Late Antiquity', in *Condensing Text – Condensed Texts*, eds M. Horster and C. Reitz, Stuttgart, 2010, pp. 519–54; in particular, on late Byzantine medical texts, see P. Bouras-Vallianatos, *Innovation in Byzantine Medicine: The Writings of John Zacharias Aktouarios (c.1275–c.1330)*, Oxford, 2020, pp. 105–76.

I have chosen to focus on a single manuscript, i.e. *Wellcomensis* MS.MSL.60, as I consider it an exceptional case, since it is obviously connected with contemporary medical practice.[10] The manuscript dates to the second half of the fifteenth century and it may be situated in a late Byzantine or slightly post-Byzantine environment in the Eastern Mediterranean. The main scribe was identified by Georgi Parpulov with a certain Ioannes, and apart from the fact that he was also one of the scribes of another medical manuscript (*Harleianus* 6295 [fols 117^r–308^v]),[11] we know nothing about him. There are a few marks of ownership, none belonging to the earliest history of the manuscript. The codex was acquired by Euthymios, the abbot of the monastery of Dionysios on Mount Athos, from Gallipoli in 1628,[12] and it was then brought to England, most probably, by either Richard Mead (1673–1754) or Anthony Askew (1722–1774), both famous English physicians and bibliophiles, after one of their trips to the Levant.[13]

Wellcomensis MS.MSL.60 contains several brief treatises or collections of opuscules with a clear diagnostic, prognostic, and therapeutic focus. The vast majority of the content had a practical orientation, as is substantiated by the fact that the manuscript preserves a large number of non-scribal, marginal annotations in vernacular Greek, including comments on the use of particular simple and composite drugs mentioned in the manuscript,[14] or even synonyms for plant substances in Greek and Turkish.[15] There are also occasionally recipes added by later hands on blank pages or in the space between the end of one treatise and the beginning of another.[16] Although it is impossible to identify or date these non-

---

[10] A detailed physical description and list of contents of the codex is available by P. Bouras-Vallianatos, 'Greek Manuscripts at the Wellcome Library in London: A Descriptive Catalogue', *Medical History*, 59, pp. 275–326 (293–302).

[11] *Repertorium der griechischen Kopisten, 800–1600*, ed. H. Hunger, 3 vols in 9 parts, Vienna, 1981–97, vol. 1A, no. 204.

[12] *Wellcomensis* MS.MSL.60, fol. 205^v: 'Τὸ παρὸν ἰατροσόφιον ὑπάρχη κτῆμα τῆς ἱερᾶς μονῆς τοῦ ἁγίου Διονυσίου καὶ ἀγωράστη παρ' ἐμοῦ Εὐθυμίου ἱερομονάχου καὶ προηγουμένου τῆς αὐτῆς μονῆς τὸ ,αχκη´ ἤ ἐν τῇ Καλιούπολη τῆς Θράκης.' On Euthymios, see S. K. Kadas, Τὰ σημειώματα τῶν χειρογράφων τῆς Μονῆς Διονυσίου Ἁγίου Ὄρους, Mount Athos, 1996, 144, no. 435.

[13] On the provenance of the manuscript and the history of the Wellcome collection, see P. Bouras-Vallianatos, 'Greek Manuscripts' (n. 10 above), pp. 276–7, 302.

[14] See, for example, the long annotation in vernacular Greek on fol. 129^v, which refers to the effectiveness of a certain recipe in the main text: inc. Τὸ ἐμπλάστρι ὅπου γένεται εἰς τὸν πόνων τῶν ποδαρίων, des. καὶ θετις το εἰς τὸν πόνον; and the comment on how beneficial it is to eat onions, which corresponds to the relevant chapter in Symeon Seth's dietetic treatise: τα κρομίδια να τα βραξης να τα τρογεις ἤνε καλα.

[15] E.g. *Wellcomensis* MS.MSL.60, fol. 79^r: 'τὸ ὀξιφίνικον τὸ λεγη καὶ τουρκικά μηρχέντι'.

[16] Among the various recipes added by later hands, the most notable example is an excerpt from a long recipe for theriac in fol. 72^r: inc. Ὁ περὶ τῶν ἀντιδότων ... ἀντίδοτος ἡ θηριακή, des. μετὰ

scribal additions, there can be no doubt that the codex was used by one or more medical practitioners.

In brief, we can see two Hippocratic texts (an excerpt from the *Aphorisms* and the *Prognostic*, fols 1ʳ–19ʳ), excerpts from or short works by well-known Byzantine authors (such as Nicholas Myrepsos's recipes for composite drugs, fols 20ʳ–45ᵛ; Paul of Aegina on the substitution of drugs, fols 50ᵛ–53ʳ; Symeon Seth on dietetics, fols 142ᵛ–162ᵛ; Theophilos on fevers, urines, and pulse, fols 138ᵛ–142ᵛ, 171ʳ–177ʳ, 199ʳ–205ᵛ), two collections of recipes with very varied content and a definite and easily observable influence from the Arabic pharmacological tradition (one is anonymous, fols 73ʳ–124ᵛ; while the other is attributed to the late Byzantine practising physician and medical author Demetrios Pepagomenos, fols 125ʳ–138ʳ), excerpts from the aforementioned Pseudo-Galenic works *Medical Definitions* (on the pulse, fols 198ᵛ–199ʳ), *Euporista* or *On Procurable Remedies* (fols 206ʳ–220ᵛ), and *On Weights and Measures* (fols 56ʳ–57ʳ), brief prognostic and diagnostic treatises attributed to Arab and Persian physicians (fols 58ʳ, 191ʳ⁻ᵛ), various anonymous recipes for drugs (fols 62ᵛ, 63ʳ, 220ʳ-222ᵛ) and opuscules on anatomy, physiology, urines, pulse, and excrements (fols 53ʳ–56ʳ, 138ʳ⁻ᵛ, 163ʳ–169ᵛ, 177ʳ–185ᵛ, 191ᵛ–192ᵛ), a lexicon of medical synonyms (fols 48ʳ–50ᵛ) and even a bilingual glossary of plant names (fol. 71ᵛ) in Greek and Arabic (in Greek transliteration). The contents are indicative of the high degree of pluralism in terms of available material in late Byzantium, where Greek and Byzantine medical knowledge was interwoven with introduced Arabic medical lore,[17] in particular, in the fields of diagnostics and pharmacology.

Uroscopy

The examination of urine did not occupy a central role in the interpretation of a patient's clinical condition in the ancient world. On the other hand, manuals on the examination of the pulse were constantly being produced and this was a subject that was studied in great detail. The first references to the value of uroscopy as a diagnostic and prognostic tool may be found in the Hippocratic

συμφύτου ῥίζης.'

[17] For an overview of Arabo/Persian-Byzantine medical translations, see A. Touwaide, 'Arabic Medicine in Greek Translation: A Preliminary Report', *Journal of the International Society for the History of Islamic Medicine*, 1, 2002, pp. 45–53; and more recently A. Touwaide, 'Agents and Agencies? The Many Facets of Translation in Byzantine Medicine,' in *Medieval Textual Cultures*, eds F. Wallis and R. Wisnovsky, Berlin, 2016, pp. 13–38. See also D. Gutas, 'Arabic into Byzantine Greek: Introducing a Survey of the Translations', in *Knotenpunkt Byzanz: Wissensformen und kulturelle Wechselbeziehungen*, eds A. Speer and D. Wirmer, Berlin, 2012, pp. 246–64, (252–4).

corpus, in texts such as *Aphorisms, Prognostic* and *Epidemics*.[18] Colour gradually became the index of digestive power and thus an important element in the diagnosis of humoral excess. Galen identified various urinary characteristics as an outcome of partial digestion and he also describes the colour of healthy urine as yellowish (ὑπόξανθον) or reddish-yellow (ὑπόπυρρον).[19]

Uroscopy was further developed in the next few centuries and started to play a more important role in the examination of the patient. Magnos (ca. fourth/fifth century AD) was most probably the first author to write a treatise focusing solely on uroscopy.[20] The most influential work was written by Theophilos (ca. seventh or ninth century AD).[21] The spectrum of colours extends to a total of nineteen, providing considerable detail in terms of variation as, for example, in the case of white.[22] In Byzantium, interest in uroscopy never ceased, with several anonymous short treatises or synopses of earlier works being compiled.[23] Among them, we

---

[18] [Hippocrates], *Aphorisms*, 4.69–83 and 7.31–9, ed. É. Littré, *Oeuvres complètes d'Hippocrate*, 10 vols, Paris, 1839–61, vol. 4, 526.7–532.8 and 584.8–588.7 = ed. W. H. S. Jones, *Hippocrates, with an English Translation*, Cambridge, MA, 1931, vol. 4, 152.18–156 and 198.10–200; *Prognostic*, 12, ed. Littré, *Oeuvres*, vol. 2, 138.15–142.15 = ed. J. Jouanna, *Hippocrate: Pronostic*, Paris, 2013, 32.5–37.2; *Epidemics*, 1.1.3, ed. Littré, *Oeuvres*, vol. 2, 610.5–9 = ed. J. Jouanna, *Hippocrate: Épidémies I et III*, Paris, 2016, 6.5–7; *Epidemics*, 3.1.2, 3.1.3, ed. Littré, *Oeuvres*, vol. 3, 34.2–38.6, 40.2–44.6, = ed. Jouanna, *Épidémies I et III*, 63.10–65.3, 65.9–68.12; *Epidemics*, 4.1.14, ed. Littré, *Oeuvres*, vol. 5, 152.7–15; and *Epidemics*, 7.1.92, ed. Littré, *Oeuvres*, vol. 5, and 448.10–11 = ed. J Jouanna, *Hippocrate: Épidémies V et VII*. Paris, 2000, 104.15–105.1. For a survey of Hippocratic uroscopy, see G. Marketos, 'Hippocratic Medicine and Nephrology', *American Journal of Nephrology*, 14, 1994, pp. 264–9.

[19] On Galen's theories about digestion and nutrition, see F. Cirenei, *La fisiologia di Galeno*, Genoa, 1961, pp. 29–37; and A. Debru, 'Physiology', in *The Cambridge Companion to Galen*, ed. R. J. Hankinson, Cambridge, 2008, pp. 263–82 (273–5). On Galen's remarks about the colour of healthy urine, see *On Crises*, 1.12, IX, 595.4–6 K. = ed. B. Alexanderson, Περὶ κρίσεων: *Überlieferung und Text*, Gothenburg, 1967, 97.18–22.

[20] U. C. Bussemaker, 'Über Magnus von Emesa und dessen Buch vom Harne', *Janus*, 2, 1847, pp. 273–97 argues that chapters 1–28 and 30–6 of the treatise ascribed to Galen and edited by Kühn, XIX, 574–601 K. contain Magnos's work. There is also a synoptic version of this work edited by J. L. Ideler, *Physici et medici Graeci minores*, 2 vols, Berlin, 1841–2, vol. 2, 307–16. On the identification of Magnos, see Nutton in *DNP*, s.v. Magnus, (1) and (5). There is one more uroscopic treatise that should probably be dated to the early Byzantine period and that is attributed to Stephanos, see M. Lamagna, 'Il trattato *De urinis* di Stefano d'Atene e l'uroscopia Alessandrina', in *Galenismo e medicina tardoantica fonti Greche, Latine e Arabe*, eds I. Garofalo and A. Roselli, Naples, 2003, pp. 52–73; the text was published by U. C. Bussemaker, 'ΣΤΕΦΑΝΟΥ ΠΕΡΙ ΟΥΡΩΝ. Traité d'Etienne sur les urines, publié pour le première fois d'après un manuscrit de la Bibliothèque royale', *Revue de Philologie* 1, 1845, pp. 415–38 (423–8), pp. 545–60.

[21] The work is available in Ideler, *Physici* (n. 20 above), vol. 1, 261–83.

[22] Theophilos, *On Urines*, 7.1, ed. Ideler, *Physici* (n. 20 above), vol. 1, 268.7–8.

[23] See for example, ed. Ideler, *Physici* (n. 20 above), vol. 2, 323–7. For a study of Byzantine uroscopy, see K. Dimitriadis, 'Byzantinische Uroskopie', PhD diss., Rheinische Friedrich-Wilhelms-

can see a number of texts attributed to Syrian, Persian, and Arab physicians.[24] The most notable example is the treatise ascribed to Ibn Sīnā, of which one version was revised by John Zacharias Aktouarios.[25] This provides the first reference to a 'ring' (στεφάνη), which might be present in the urine and, depending on its colour and location in the urine vial, could indicate various states of health. The most substantial Byzantine work on uroscopy is the extensive treatise by John Zacharias Aktouarios (ca. 1275–ca. 1330) in seven books, entitled *On Urines*.[26] John discusses for the first time in great detail a large number and variety of urinary characteristics, including a considerable number of case histories, in which he describes his experience in treating his patients. He also introduced his own graduated urine vial divided into eleven areas, which enjoyed a considerable afterlife in Byzantium and the West. Above all, he managed to give a proper scientific profile to the art of examining urine, since the vial's great popularity had led to its often being exploited by charlatans or practitioners with inadequate education and background.[27]

Having provided a background to Greek and Byzantine contributions to the examination of urine, I now turn to the two brief uroscopic texts attributed to Galen on fols 170ʳ–171ʳ and 191ʳ of *Wellcomensis* MS.MSL.60. The first is entitled *On Galen's Division of Urines* (Appendix A) and deals with the various possible colours of urine with occasional references to the size, morphology and place of various kinds of particles, both basic features of uroscopic treatises. It can be divided into three parts according to its structure and contents.[28] The first part

Universität Bonn, 1971.

[24] See, for example, ed. Ideler, *Physici* (n. 20 above), vol. 2, 303–4, 305–6. See also A. Touwaide, 'Arabic urology in Byzantium', *Journal of Nephrology*, 17, 2004, pp. 583–9.

[25] On the various versions of the treatise, see M. Lamagna, 'Per l'edizione del *De Urinis* attribuito ad Avicenna: studio complessivo della tradizione manoscritta', *Revue d'Histoire des Textes*, 6, 2011, pp. 27–59. John Zacharias Aktouarios's version has been critically edited by M. Lamagna, *Giovanni Attuario. L'eccellent trattato sulle urine di Avicenna*, Cuenca, 2017, pp. 25–82.

[26] John Zacharias Aktouarios, *On Urines*, ed. Ideler, *Physici*, (n. 20 above), vol. 2, pp. 3–192. The first book has been critically edited and translated into French by S. Georgiou, 'Edition critique, traduction et commentaire critique du livre 1 'De Urinis' de Jean Zacharias Actouarios', Thèse de doctorat, École Pratique des Hautes Études (Paris), 2013.

[27] On John's uroscopic theories and his detailed case histories, see P. Bouras-Vallianatos, *Innovation in Byzantine Medicine* (n. 9 above), pp. 39–104.

[28] The first part is almost identical to Chapter 5 of a brief uroscopic treatise, which was edited by Ideler and is entitled *On Urines from a Syriac Book*, ed. Ideler, *Physici* (n. 20 above), vol. 2, 303–4. The structure shows also occasional similarities with some Latin Pseudo-Galenic uroscopic texts edited by H. Leisinger, *Die lateinischen Harnschriften Pseudo-Galens*, Zurich, 1925, pp. 17–51. Chapters 1–3 of the treatise *On Urines from a Syriac Book* are also very similar to the first three paragraphs (A.14–32) of the second part of our text.

(A.1–13) has an aphoristic structure and various colours are directly connected with diseases; for example, 'white (λευκόν) urine without sediment indicates indigestion and dysuria' (A.2) or 'yellow (ὠχρόν) and thicker urine indicates gout' (A.6). The second part (A.14–35) consists of four paragraphs with various details on reddish and white urine, which may show the quality of the blood, and is also related to seasons. We can also find advice on venesection (A.18, 22, 34) and the use of various purgatives in the event that the disease becomes more serious, including references to traditional purgatives (A.31), such as θεοδώρητος, but also juleps (A.20, 27–8).[29] The last part (A.36–83) contains several paragraphs on various colours and particles; the focus is clearly diagnostic and prognostic, and it has no therapeutic recommendations.

It is impossible to provide an approximate date of composition for the first part, since it uses no unique terms and no content related to any edited, dated uroscopic work. However, the reference to juleps clearly points to a late Byzantine environment for the second part of the text. The julep was imported into Byzantium from Arabic medicine and attained great popularity. The word *julāb*, originally comes from the Persian *gul* (rose) and *āb* (water).[30] The original julep was made of sugar, water, and rosewater, obtained by the distillation of roses. The first mention of julep in the surviving Byzantine medical literature can be found in the *Syntagma Peri Trophōn Dynameōn* (*Treatise on the Capacities of Foodstuffs*) written by Symeon Seth for the Emperor Michael VII Doukas (r. 1071–1078).[31] Julep is also found in the Greek translation of Ibn al-Jazzār's (fl. tenth century) *Zād al-musāfir wa-qūt al-ḥāḍir* (*Provisions for the Traveller and Nourishment for the Sedentary*/Gr. Ἐφόδια τοῦ Ἀποδημοῦντος) that was completed by 1130/40,[32]

---

[29] In the treatise edited by Ideler, *Physici* (n. 20 above), vol. 2, 304.14, 22–3, we see χεράβιν instead of ζουλάπιν. Χεράβιν refers to syrup (Ar. *sharāb*), which is also found in Byzantine works as σεράβιν or σεράπιν and refers to a more viscous form of a julep, containing a larger quantity of sugar (see also n. 30, below); in this case the initial sibilant consonant sigma (σ) has been changed into the labial chi (χ).

[30] On juleps in the Arabic medical tradition, see M. Levey, *Early Arabic pharmacology*. Leiden, 1973, p. 77; and I. Fellmann, *Das Aqrābāḏīn al-Qalānisī*, Beirut, 1986, p. 201.

[31] Symeon Seth, *Syntagma Peri Trofōn Dynameōn*, ed. B. A. Langkavel, *Simeonis Sethi Syntagma de alimentorum facultatibus*, Leipzig, 1868, 30.7, 41.4–13, and 66.17–19.

[32] See, for example, *Ephodia tou Apodēmountos*, Vaticanus gr. 300 (AD1130/40), fol. 220ᵛ, l.25- fol. 221ʳ, l.1: '… καὶ πιέτω τὸ σεράβιν τῶν ῥοῶν ἢ ζουλάβιν καφοράτον…'. In this case the tenue, non-fricative labial pi (π) σεράπιν or ζουλάπιν, has been changed into its medial fricative version, beta (β). Vaticanus gr. 300 was copied, most probably in the area of Messina, around 1130/40, which constitutes the *terminus ante quem* for the Greek translation of the work itself. On the dating of this manuscript, S. Lucà, 'I Normanni e la "Rinascita" del sec. XII', *Archivio Storico per la Calabria e la Lucanica*, 60, 1993, pp. 1–91 (36–63).

and that of Abū Bakr al-Rāzī's (d. ca. 925) *Kitāb fī al-judarī wa-al-ḥaṣbah* (*On Smallpox and Measles*/ Περὶ Λοιμικῆς).[33] Julep became particularly popular from the thirteenth century onwards and references to it were included in almost all late Byzantine medical works with a therapeutic focus.[34]

To return to our treatise, the last part is the product of an even more complicated textual tradition. Here, in contrast to the first two parts, the vast majority of the contents coincide with some chapters from the first and longest Pseudo-Galenic treatise *On Urines* edited by Kühn,[35] the third treatise *On Urines* edited by Kühn and ascribed to Galen, Hippocrates *et alii* physicians,[36] some chapters from the anonymous *Synopsis on Urines* edited by Ideler,[37] and the uroscopic material in the edition of Aetios of Amida's (fl. first half of the sixth century AD) *Tetrabiblos* edited by Olivieri.[38] A detailed *apparatus* of *loci paralleli* between our text and the abovementioned treatises is provided in Appendix A. Although an examination of the relationship between the aforementioned works is beyond the scope of this chapter, it is noteworthy that Ideler's anonymous text and some chapters of Kühn's first Pseudo-Galenic treatise have been identified as parts of Magnos's uroscopic work and thus should be dated to the early Byzantine period.[39] Furthermore, some ideas presented in the text (A.83), such as, for example, the connection between pale green (χλωρός) urine and a malignant condition (κακοήθεια) may also be found in Galen, but are clearly not directly derived from Galen in this case.[40] The version of these in our manuscript is the product of a combination of a long, ongoing process of compilation and synthesis

---

[33] *Peri Loimikēs*, 5, ed. A. Kousis, Ῥαζῆ Λόγος Περὶ Λοιμικῆς. Athens, 1909, 17.8. The translator of this work is not known. M.-H. Congourdeau, 'Le traducteur grec du traité de Rhazès sur la variole', in *Storia e ecdotica dei testi medici greci*, eds A. Garzya and J. Jouanna, Naples, 1996, pp. 99–111, suggested that the work might have been translated by Symeon Seth in the 11th century, but there is not sufficient evidence to confirm this identification.

[34] On the introduction and dissemination of sugar-based medical potions in Byzantium, see P. Bouras-Vallianatos, 'Cross-Cultural Transfer of Medical Knowledge in the Medieval Mediterranean: The Introduction and Dissemination of Sugar-Based Potions from the Islamic World to Byzantium', *Speculum*, 96, 2021 (forthcoming).

[35] Pseudo-Galen, *On Urines*, XIX, 574–601 K.

[36] Pseudo-Galen, *On Urines*, XIX, 607–28 K.

[37] Anonymus, *Synopsis on Urines*, ed. Ideler, *Physici* (n. 20 above), vol. 2, 307–16.

[38] Aetios of Amida, *Tetrabiblos*, 5.28–44, ed. A. Olivieri, *Aetii Amideni libri Medicinales*, 2 vols, Leipzig/Berlin, 1935–50, vol. 2, 19.4–25.23.

[39] On Magnos's work, see n. 20, above. It is worth noting that *Wellcomensis* MS.MSL.60 preserves the synoptic version of Magnos's work as edited by Ideler on fols 171ʳ–177ʳ, i.e. right after the first Pseudo-Galenic uroscopic work, and is entitled: Ἰατρὸς περὶ οὔρων Μάγνου ἀπὸ φωνῆς Θεοφίλου.

[40] Galen, *On Crises*, 1.12, IX, 604.10–11 K. = Alexanderson, Περὶ κρίσεων (n. 19 above) 103.16–17.

from a variety of available sources – some of which were regularly ascribed to Galen – and several anonymous contributions.

The next short uroscopy work in *Wellcomensis MS.MSL.60* is entitled *Galen's Interpretation of the Urine Vial* (Appendix B). This text is less than a folio long and focuses on diagnosis and prognostication of disease. For example, thick sediment indicates an excess of bile (B.93–4). Unfortunately, we cannot establish a direct relation to any other edited work on urines as in the case of the first Pseudo-Galenic uroscopic treatise, but we can at least see one element which indicates a late date. There are two references to τζίπα, that is a distinct film of oil that may appear in the upper part of the urine vial (B.90, 92).[41] According to the text, if the τζίπα remains on the upper part, it indicates an imminent death (B.89–91); later on, the text provides even more precise prognostic information referring to death within twelve days for those patients with a τζίπα that covers the entire upper surface of their urine (B.91–3). Descriptions of various kinds of oily urine may be found in the majority of Byzantine uroscopic treatises.[42] The earliest dated use of this term is found in a Greek lexicon of synonymous medical terms surviving in a manuscript (*Holkhamicus gr.* 112) dating to the early twelfth century and originating in the area of Reggio di Calabria.[43] The use of the same term in a uroscopic context is found once in the short uroscopic treatise in the form of an ecclesiastical canon attributed either to Nikephoros Blemmydes (1197–ca. 1269) or Maximos Planoudes (ca. 1255–ca. 1305).[44] Lastly, as we have already shown in the case of the first Pseudo-Galenic uroscopic treatise (third part) of our manuscript, we can again see some details given similar mentions in some of Galen's works,[45]

[41] Τζίπα or τσίπα is commonly used in medieval Greek to define a light coat or membrane. D. Dimitrakos, *Μέγα Λεξικὸν Ὅλης τῆς Ἑλληνικῆς γλώσσης*, 9 vols, Athens, 1936–51, s.v. τσίπα.

[42] For example, Theophilos, *On Urines*, 17, ed. Ideler, *Physici* (n. 20 above), vol. 1, 278.34–280.2, refers to the topic in one chapter, while John Zacharias Aktouarios, *On Urines*, 2.18, ed. Ideler, *Physici* (n. 20 above), vol. 2, 48.11–49.16; and 6.8, vol. 2, 156.15–157.3, devotes an entire chapter to oily urines in the books on diagnosis and prognosis respectively.

[43] P. Bouras-Vallianatos, 'Enrichment of the Medieval Vocabulary in the Greek-Speaking Medieval Communites of Southern Italy: The Lexica of Plant Names', in *Life Is Short, Art Long: The Art of Healing in Byzantium, New Perspectives*, eds B. Pitarakis and G. Tanman, Istanbul, 2018, pp. 155–84 (182 and nn. 103–4).

[44] Nikephoros Blemmydes/Maximos Planoudes, *Canon on Urine Vials*, ed. Ideler, *Physici* (n. 20 above), vol. 2, 319.9–12 = ed. A. P. Kousis, 'Les oeuvres médicales de Nicéphoros Blémmydès selon les manuscrits existants', Πρακτικὰ Ἀκαδημίας Ἀθηνῶν 19, 1944, 56–75 (61.4–6). This treatise is also found in *Wellcomensis MS.MSL.60* (fols 187ᵛ–189ʳ) where it is ascribed to Blemmydes. I am currently preparing a critical edition, English translation, and commentary of this text in collaboration with Dimitrios Skrekas.

[45] Galen, *On Black Bile*, 8, V, 142.6 K. = ed. W. De Boer, *Galeni De propriorum animi cuiuslibet affectuum dignotione et curatione, De animi cuiuslibet peccatorum dignotione et curatione, De atra bile,*

such as the existence of clouds (νεφέλαι) in the upper part of urine vials, which are connected with a healthy condition (B.87). However, a direct connection with genuine Galenic material or, as above, with a uroscopic treatise consistently ascribed to Galen cannot be established.

Sphygmology

In contrast to uroscopy, Galen gave considerable importance to the study of the pulse. He emphasized the importance of the examination of the pulse in diagnosing and prognosticating his patients and described several categories according to the various characteristics of the pulse in his specialized treatises (i.e. *On the Function of the Pulse, On Differences of the Pulse, On Diagnosis by the Pulse, On Causes of the Pulse, On Prognosis by the Pulse, On the Pulse for Beginners*).[46] The most popular Byzantine text on the subject is that by Theophilos[47] and specific parts on sphygmology were included in the medical works of Aetios of Amida,[48] Paul of Aegina (fl. first half of the seventh century AD),[49] and Michael Psellos (1018–ca. 1076).[50] In addition to the aforementioned works, a revised, condensed version of the Pseudo-Galenic *On the Pulse to Antonius, a Man of Learning and Philosopher*, attributed to the otherwise unknown Philaretos appeared at some point before the tenth century, and became very popular in its Latin translation.[51] Meanwhile, several anonymous shorts works, in part derived from one of the above mentioned Byzantine treatises, were produced to cover contemporary practical needs.[52]

Leipzig/Berlin, 1937, 90.23–4.

[46] Galen, V, 149–80 K.; VIII, 493–765 K.; VIII, 766–961 K.; IX, 1–204 K.; IX, 205–430 K.; and VIII, 453–92 K., respectively. On Galen's theory of the pulse, see C. R. S. Harris, *The Heart and the Vascular System in Ancient Greek Medicine*, Oxford, 1973, pp. 397–431; and L. M. Pino Campos, 'Observaciones al tratado de Galeno *Acerca de la diferencia de los pulsos*', *Fortunatae*, 17, 2006, pp. 99–115.

[47] Theophilos, *On the Pulse*, ed. F. Z. Ermerins, *Anecdota medica Graeca e codicibus MSS. Expromsit*, Leiden, S. and J. Luchtmans, 1840, pp. 3–77.

[48] Aetios of Amida, *Tetrabiblos*, 5.27, ed. Olivieri, *Aetii Amideni* (n. 38 above), vol. 2, 18.15–19.4.

[49] Paul of Aegina, *Epitome*, 2.11, ed. J. L. Heiberg, *Paulus Aegineta*, 2 vols, Leipzig/Berlin, 1921–24, vol. 1, 81.16–93.25.

[50] Michael Psellos, *On Medicine*, 9, ed. L. Westerink, *Michaelis Pselli Poemata*, 283–425. Leipzig, 1992, pp. 200–204. Michael Psellos also appears as the author of a brief unedited work on the pulse in *Parisinus gr.* 1630 (14th century, fols 198ʳ–199ʳ), which has many similarities with the section on the pulse in his above-mentioned poem *On Medicine*.

[51] Philaretos, *On the Pulse*, ed. J. A. Pithis, *Die Schriften 'Περὶ σφυγμῶν' des Philaretos*, Husum, 1983, pp. 84–144. See also the discussion by O. Temkin, 'Geschichte des Hippokratismus im ausgehenden Altertum', *Kyklos*, 4, 1932, pp. 1–80 (56–66).

[52] See, for example, the opuscule edited in Ideler, *Physici* (n. 20 above), vol. 1, 317; the anonymous treatise in *Palatinus gr.* 199 (13th century) edited by A. Mavroudis, 'Τὸ ἀνώνυμο ἔργο *Περὶ Σφυγμοῦ*

The text on the pulse (Appendix C) in our manuscript (fols 193^r–198^r) is significantly longer than the uroscopic ones and is entitled *Galen's on the Pulse*. It is followed by a brief anonymous text on the qualities of the pulse (fols 198^{r-v}) and two excerpts on the pulse from the Pseudo-Galenic *Medical Definitions* (fols– 198^v–199^r).[53] It is divided into seven parts as follows: a) general introduction on the pulse and its basic characteristics (C.96–115), b) on the function of the pulse and how to diagnose by the pulse (C.116–46), c) on how to examine the pulse (C.147–90), d) on the various classes of the pulse and their differences (C.191–239), e) on causes of the pulse (C.240–338), f) on opposite kinds of the pulse (C.339–60), and g) on the pulse of those who are exercising and suffering from fatigue (C.361–469). We cannot identify any substantial parts of the text that are common to any published Greek or Byzantine text on the pulse.[54] Furthermore, one particular section on the examination of the pulse (c) is rare in Greek and early Byzantine sphygmological treatises, with the exception of a chapter in the treatise by Marcellinus (second century AD[?]) and a brief section in the Latin treatise *On the Pulse* ascribed to Soranus.[55]

There are various ideas and terms in the text that relate to certain characteristics of the pulse, which may help us to place our text in the development of medical thought on the pulse in Byzantium. For example, the treatise (C.241ff) refers to Galen's three retaining (συνεκτικαί) causes of the production of the pulse, as described in *On Causes of the Pulse*,[56] although this particular chapter is not directly drafted from the Galenic original. On the other hand, the anonymous author uses the term ὠφέλεια (C.116) to introduce a chapter on the function of the pulse rather

στον κώδικα Vaticanus Palat. Gr. 199 και το *Περὶ τῆς τοῦ Ἀνθρώπου Κατασκευῆς* του Μελετίου', *Ἑλληνικά*, 41, 1990, pp. 235–65 (242–7). Another brief opuscule is either ascribed to Ibn Sīnā or to the so-called monk Merkourios, ed. R. Masullo, 'Sul Περὶ Σφυγμῶν attribuito a Mercurio monaco', in *Ecdotica e ricezione dei testi medici greci*, eds V. Boudon-Millot, A. Garzya, J. Jouanna and A. Roselli, Naples, 2006, pp. 335–46 (344–6).

[53] Pseudo-Galen, *Medical Definitions*, 74, 110–12, 205–6, XIX, 375.16–376.13, 402.18–403.8, 365.16–366.6, 376.15–378.2 K.

[54] Some brief phrases may have been derived from genuine Galenic works after several stages of composition. Cf., for example, C.376, which deals with the pulse related to distress (λύπη) and Galen, *On Causes of the Pulse*, 4.4, IX, 160.5–6 K.

[55] Marcellinus, *On the Pulse*, ed. H. Schöne, 'Markellinos' Pulslehre. Ein griechisches Anekdoton', in *Festschrift zur 49. Versammlung deutscher Philologen Schulmänner*, Basel, 1907, pp. 448–72 (459.114–460.171). On Marcellinus, see the study by O. Lewis, 'Marcellinus' De pulsibus: a Neglected Treatise on the Ancient "Art of Pulse"', *Scripta Classica Israelica*, 39, 2015, pp. 195–214. Pseudo-Soranus, *On the Pulse*, ed. V. Rose, *Anecdota Graeca et Graecolatina*, Berlin, 1864, 276.1–13.

[56] Galen, *On the Causes of the Pulse*, 1.2–4, IX, 4.6–9.2 K. Our treatise uses the term καθεκτικαί (C.141) to refer to the retaining causes rather than the Galenic συνεκτικαί.

than the common Galenic term χρεία;[57] later on, ὠφέλεια and χρεία may be used interchangeably (C.120–2). It is worth noting that the only Byzantine edited work in which we can see a similar use of ὠφέλεια is that by Philaretos.[58] Furthermore, the use of διάπυρον (C.128), i.e. extremely hot, in relation to innate heat (ἔμφυτον θερμόν) is only found in early Byzantine works, such as Palladios's synopsis on fevers or the redaction ascribed to Stephen and Theophilos.[59] However, a careful examination of section (d) on various classes of the pulse may provide us with an opportunity to discuss further noteworthy terms. For this reason, I have prepared Table 1, in which we can see the distinguishing features of various classes of the pulse according to Greek and Byzantine authors listed in chronological order; for purposes of comparison, our text is in the first column.

Ancient medical authors considered various classes of the pulse. In referring to the subject in his *On Differences of the Pulse* Galen provides us with a variety of terms used by past authorities to define the various kinds of the pulse, i.e. γένη, εἴδη, ποιότητες, and διαφοραί.[60] He then proceeds to describe the classes concerning a single beat, of which – according to an explicit statement at the end of his account – there are five (πέντε γένη).[61] In addition to these, Galen refers to at least four more classes, two concerning different characteristics of a sequence of beats and another two that compare one beat to another.[62] It is notable, however,

[57] See, for example, Galen's work *On Function of the Pulse* (Περὶ χρείας σφυγμῶν), V, 149–80 K. On χρεία in Galen, see L. M. Pinos Campos, 'La polisemia de χρεία y su aplicación en Galeno', *Fortunatae*, 24, 2013, pp. 117–40. It is worth pointing out that in Galen's *On the Function of the Parts of the Body* the terms χρεία and ὠφέλεια are often interchangeable, but this is related to the use of the parts not to physiological processes as in the case of the pulse.

[58] Philaretos, *On the Pulse*, ed. Pithis, *Die Schriften* (n. 51 above), 88.31.

[59] Palladios, *On Fevers*, 26.2, ed. Ideler, *Physici* (n. 20 above), vol. 1, 118.25; Stephen and Theophilos, *On Differences of Fevers*, 42, ed. D. Sicurus, *Theophili et Stephani Atheniensis de febrium differentia ex Hippocrate et Galeno*, Florence, 1862, 32.13–14. On the complicated textual transmission of the above-mentioned treatises on fevers, see I. Garofalo, 'Note sulla tradizione alessandrina del *De Differentiis Febrium* di Galeno', in *Trasmissione e ecdotica dei testi medici greci*, eds A. Garzya and J. Jouanna, Naples, 2003, pp. 149–64.

[60] Galen, *On Differences of the Pulse*, 1.2, VIII, 498.15–17 K.

[61] Galen, *On Differences of the Pulse*, 1.5, VIII, 509.13 K. According to Orly Lewis's interpretation, 'Galen against Archigenes on the Pulse and what it Teaches us about Galen's Method of Diairesis', in *Galen's Epistemology*, eds M. Havrda and R. J. Hankinson, Cambridge, forthcoming, the variations in the pulse related to a single beat relate to the time of the motion, the quantity of the distension, the strength which the fingers perceive at the peak of the *diastole*, the texture of the arterial walls, and the contents of the arteries.

[62] The first two concern the rest/interval in the artery and the rhythm and the next two are with regard to evenness/unevenness and regularity/irregularity. On these, see Lewis, 'Galen against Archigenes' (n. 61 above).

that he does not enumerate all the classes and is not always very clear in his text.[63] Although our text refers explicitly to ten classes (C.192),[64] a division which first appears in a definite structure in the Pseudo-Galenic work *On the Pulse to Antonius*,[65] it ultimately lists just seven. Interestingly, the terms used in our text for the first four classes are almost identical to those used by Galen in four out of his five classes concerning a single beat, while the fifth is in part the same as Galen's fourth class.

The first Byzantine example of the above-mentioned model of ten classes appears in the relevant chapter in Paul of Aegina, which – although it is not derived directly from an authentic Galenic work – is ascribed to Galen; Paul may have been partly influenced by the Pseudo-Galenic *On the Pulse to Antonius*.[66] Our treatise shows many similarities with the Pseudo-Galenic *On the Pulse to Antonius* and follows closely Paul of Aegina's and Theophilos's terminology. On the other hand, our treatise refers explicitly to the cold (ψυχρός) and hot (θέρμος) pulse (C.201, 218), a distinction which is not found in Galen and is alluded to briefly in Pseudo-Galen *On Pulse to Antonius* and by Paul of Aegina; it is clearly mentioned in the Pseudo-Galenic work *Medical Definitions* and the lists of classes by Byzantine authors such as Philaretos and Michael Psellos.[67] The most unusual terms used to describe the pulse regarding the extent to which the arteries expand

[63] Galen, *On Differences of the Pulse*, 1.3–9, VIII, 500.6–522.18 K.

[64] The text refers to the movement of the vein (φλεβός) rather than the artery (ἀρτηρίας), but there is an overall confusion between veins and arteries throughout the treatise.

[65] Pseudo-Galen, *On the Pulse to Antonius, a Man of Learning and Philosopher*, XIX, 634.2–637.8 K. It is notable that according to a brief treatise preserved in *Laurentianus Plut.* 75.7 (12th century) and ascribed to Ruphus, *On the Pulse*, 8, eds C. Daremberg and C. É. Ruelle, *Oeuvres de Rufus d'Ephèse*, Paris, 1879, 231.14–232.5, the theory of ten classes goes back to Archigenes, although this is not confirmed by Galen or any other author. On this, see also the comment by Daremberg/Ruelle, *Oeuvres de Rufus*, 641. See also the Pseudo-Galenic *Medical Definitions*, XIX, 404.1–412.15 K., in which we can see the all terms referring to the ten categories, although there are no numbers allotted to them at this stage.

[66] The ten categories also appear in the so-called *Tabulae Vindobonenses*, in the section dealing with Galen's *On the Pulse for Beginners*, and seem to be related to the teaching of medicine in early Byzantine Alexandria. See B. Gundert, 'Die *Tabulae Vindobonenses* als Zeugnis alexandrinischer Lehrtätigkeit um 600 n. Chr.', in *Text and Tradition: Studies in Ancient Medicine and Its Transmission; presented to Jutta Kollesch*, eds K. D. Fischer, D. Nickel and P. Potter, Leiden, 1998, pp. 91–144 (128–9); and P. Bouras-Vallianatos, 'Diagrams in Greek Medical Manuscripts', in *The Diagram as Paradigm: Cross-Cultural Approaches*, eds J. Hamburger, D. Roxburgh and L. Safran, Cambridge MA, forthcoming. On the function of the *Tabulae*, see O. Overwien, *Medizinische Lehrwerke aus dem spätantiken Alexandria: Die 'Tabulae Vindobonenses' und 'Summaria Alexandrinorum' zu Galens 'De sectis'*, Berlin, 2019, pp. 98–107.

[67] A clear reference to θερμός pulse is also made in the above-mentioned treatise on fevers attributed to Stephen and Theophilos, 26, ed. Sicurus, *Theophili et Stephani* (n. 59 above), 27.1–4.

and contract and the time taken for the expansion (διαστολή) are κοντός[68] (short) (C.189, 193, 206, 215, 217) and κοντότητος[69] (shortness) (C.196) respectively, as opposed to μακρός (long) and μακρότητος (lengthiness). The terms usually employed for such a pulse and the time taken for the expansion in the Greek and Byzantine medical literature are βραχύς[70] and βραχύτης[71] respectively.

Thus, we can see that this text seems to follow, at least, some Galenic ideas (e.g. retaining causes) and terminology (e.g. classes of the pulse), and that it shows a stronger connection with genuine Galenic works than that attested in the uroscopic texts. Furthermore, the text follows the model of the ten classes (although in an incomplete fashion), which is found in the Pseudo-Galenic work *On the Pulse to Antonius* and uses terms that are common to another Pseudo-Galenic text, i.e. *Medical Definitions*, which also suggest a connection with pseudepigraphic works consistently ascribed to Galen throughout the Byzantine era. On the other hand, there are terms (e.g. κοντός) that are peculiar to the author/compiler of our treatise and clearly alien to Galen or Pseudo-Galen.

Table 1. Classes of the pulse.[72]

[Table notes are found after the table.]

---

[68] See G. Babiniotis, Ὁ διὰ συνθέσεως ὑποκορισμὸς εἰς τὴν ἑλληνικήν. Athens, 1969, pp. 202–8, who shows that the introduction of κοντός in place of βραχύς is only attested from the 4th century AD onwards.

[69] This is a *hapax legomenon*. Georgios Babiniotis, in a personal communication, confirmed that he has never attested the derivative κοντότης before. However, he considers the use of the word unsurprising in an informal linguistic environment.

[70] See, for example, Galen, *On Differences of the Pulse*, 1.4, VIII, 504–6 K.; Pseudo-Galen, *Medical Definitions*, 215, XIX, 407.2–3 K.; and Theophilos, *On Pulse*, ed. Ermerins (n. 47 above), *Anecdota*, 17.4–5.

[71] See, for example, Galen, *On Differences of the Pulse*, 4.10, VIII, 745.18 K.; and *On Prognosis by the Pulse*, 2.10, IX, 276.15 K.

[72] Numbers are given when the text provides a numerical reference to a particular class, e.g. πρῶτον γένος.

Pseudo-Galen, On the Pulse, Well.MS.MSL.60 (C.191-239)	Pseudo-Galen,[73] Medical Definitions (XIX, 404.1-412.15 K.)	Galen,[74] On Differences of the Pulse (VIII, 500.6-526.8 K.)	Marcellinus,[75] On the Pulse (Schöne, 458.90-113, 460. 173-461.221)	Pseudo-Galen, On the Pulse to Antonius (XIX, 634.2-637.8 K.)	Paul of Aegina, Epitome (Heiberg, I, 82.4-88.18)	Theophilos,[76] On the Pulse (Ermerins, 11.14-33.12)	Philaretos,[77] On the Pulse (Pithis, 110.138-118.175, 132.245-136.282)	Michael Psellos, On Medicine (Westerink, 200.283-204.425)
(1) μακρός, κοντός, σύμμετρος, πλατύς, στενός, σύμμετρος, ὑψηλός, σύμμετρος, ταπεινός, σύμμετρος, μέγας, μικρός, σύμμετρος	(1) μέγας, μικρός, μέσος	μακρός, βραχύς, σύμμετρος, πλατύς, στενός, σύμμετρος, ὑψηλός, σύμμετρος, ταπεινός, σύμμετρος, μέγας, μικρός, σύμμετρος	μέγας, μικρός, μέσος	(1) μέγας	(2) μακρός, βραχύς, πλατύς, στενός, ὑψηλός, ταπεινός, μέγας, μικρός, σύμμετρος	μακρός, βραχύς, σύμμετρος, πλατύς, στενός, σύμμετρος, ὑψηλός, ταπεινός, σύμμετρος, μέγας, μικρός, σύμμετρος	(1) μέγας, μικρός, σύμμετρος	(2) μακρός, μικρός, πλατύς, στενός, ὑψηλός, ταπεινός
(2) σφοδρός, σφοδρός, σύμμετρος, ἀμυδρός, σύμμετρος	(2) σφοδρός, σφοδρός, ἀμυδρός, σύμμετρος	(3) σφοδρός, σφοδρός, σύμμετρος, ἀμυδρός, σύμμετρος	σφοδρός, σύμμετρος, ἀμυδρός	(3) σφοδρός, σύμμετρος, ἀμυδρός	(3) σφοδρός, σύμμετρος, ἀμυδρός	σφοδρός, σύμμετρος	(3) ἰσχυρός, σύμμετρος, ἀμυδρός	(3) σφοδρός, σύμμετρος, ἀμυδρός
(3) ταχύς, σύμμετρος, βραδύς, σύμμετρος	(3) ταχύς, βραδύς, σύμμετρος	ταχύς, σύμμετρος, βραδύς, σύμμετρος	ταχύς, βραδύς	(2) ταχύς, βραδύς, σύμμετρος	(1) ταχύς, βραδύς, σύμμετρος	ταχύς, βραδύς, σύμμετρος	(2) ταχύς, βραδύς, σύμμετρος	(1) ταχύς, βραδύς, σύμμετρος
(4) πυκνός, σύμμετρος, ἀραιός, σύμμετρος	(4) πυκνός, ἀραιός, σύμμετρος	πυκνός, ἀραιός, σύμμετρος	πυκνός, ἀραιός	(5) πυκνός, ἀραιός	(7) πυκνός, ἀραιός, σύμμετρος	πυκνός, ἀραιός, σύμμετρος	(5/7) πυκνός, ἀραιός, σύμμετρος	(7) πυκνός, ἀραιός, σύμμετρος
(5) ψυχρός, θερμός, σύμμετρος	(5) ψυχρός, θερμός, σύμμετρος			(10) τὸ παρὰ τὴν θερμασίαν τὴν ἀναδιδομένην διὰ τοῦ σώματος διὰ σφυγμίας	(6) κατὰ τὴν καρδίαν θερμασίας ἔοικέ πως μᾶλλον κατὰ τὴν ἀρτηρίαν		(10/6) ψυχρός, θερμός, σύμμετρος	(6) ψυχρός, θερμός, σύμμετρος

Consistency	Fullness	Evenness	Intermittence	Rhythm	Order
(4) σκληρός μαλακός σύμμετρος	(5) πλήρης κενός σύμμετρος	(9) ὁμαλός ἀνώμαλος		(8) εὔρυθμος ἄρρυθμος	(10) ἄτακτος τεταραγμένος
(4) σκληρός μαλακός σύμμετρος	(8/5) πλήρης κενός σύμμετρος	(6/9) ὁμαλός ἀνώμαλος	(9/8) ἐμπίπτων παρεμπίπτων	(-/10) εὔρυθμος ἄρρυθμος	(7/-) ἄτακτος τεταραγμένος
σκληρός μαλακός σύμμετρος	πλήρης κενός σύμμετρος	ὁμαλός ἀνώμαλος κατὰ μίαν πληγήν / ὁμαλός ἀνώμαλος κατὰ περιόδους		εὔρυθμος	ἄτακτος τεταγμένος
(4) σκληρός μαλακός σύμμετρος	(5) πλήρης κενός σύμμετρος	(9) ὁμαλός ἀνώμαλος	διαλείπων παρεμπίπτων	(8) εὔρυθμος ἄρρυθμος / παράρρυθμος ἑτερόρρυθμος ἔκρυθμος	(10) ἄτακτος τεταγμένος
(4) σκληρός μαλακός σύμμετρος	(8) πλήρης κενός	(6) τὸ παρὰ τὴν ὁμαλότητα καὶ τὴν ἀνωμαλίαν	(9) διαλείπων παρεμπίπτων		(7) ἄτακτος
	πλήρης κενός μέσος	ὁμαλός ἀνώμαλος			ἄτακτος τεταγμένος
(4) σκληρός μαλακός (ἀνώνυμος)	πλήρης κενός (ἀνώνυμος)	ὁμαλός ἀνώμαλος **	διαλείπων παρεμπίπτων	εὔρυθμος ἄρρυθμος (παράρρυθμος ἑτερόρρυθμος ἔκρυθμος)	ἄτακτος τεταγμένος
σκληρός μαλακός μέσος / ὑγρός αὐχμηρός μέσος	πλήρης κενός μέσος	ὁμαλός ἀνώμαλος	διαλείπων παρεμπίπτων	εὔρυθμος ἄρρυθμος κακόρρυθμος παράρρυθμος ἑτερόρρυθμος ἔκρυθμος	ἄτακτος τεταγμένος
(6) σκληρός μαλακός σύμμετρος	(6) πλήρης κενός σύμμετρος	(7) ἴσος ἄνισος / ὁμαλός ἀνώμαλος			

113

Concluding Remarks

It has been shown that both texts on urines and pulse are products of a long process of composition. In the case of urines, material common to what are usually held to be Pseudo-Galenic treatises was elaborated further in the late Byzantine period and especially after the introduction of Arabic medical knowledge. The latter provides evidence of the great variety of knowledge available to late Byzantine medical audiences. Another issue which this chapter has raised is that, among the Pseudo-Galenic texts in Byzantium, we must make a distinction between those that show at least some partial similarity with Galenic works and those which have little or no relationship with any genuine Galenic work. Thus, for example, in the case of our text on the pulse, readers who considered they were reading a Galenic text were not totally wrong, since they were actually coming into indirect contact with various Galenic notions filtered and developed through several stages of compilation.

Many Byzantine practitioners would probably not have been able to identify what was likely to be Galenic and what not. For example, in the case of late Byzantine *iatrosophia*, a group of texts intended for everyday practice, we can see that Galen could be arbitrarily invoked – invariably to give authority to the text.[78] The large number of linguistic infelicities in the treatises and annotations

---

[73] The author does not refer explicitly to classes, but provides a list of definitions of various kinds of pulse, which roughly corresponds to the usual classes.

[74] Galen refers explicitly to numbers in only two cases concerning the five classes with regard to a single beat. In one case I have marked two terms by using **, thus indicating that, although the terms are found in Galen, they do not form a separate class. Ἀνώνυμος in brackets denotes another pulse between these two, which is described by Galen, but for which he does not give a name. See, for example, *On Differences of the Pulse*, 1.5, VIII, 508.15–16 K.: 'τὸ γὰρ μέσον ἀμφοῖν ἀνώνυμον κἀνταῦθα'.

[75] Marcellinus neither mentions the total number of classes nor numbers them, but he makes some distinctions between various classes ('τῷ δὲ σφυγμῷ αἵ λέγονται παρέπεσθαι ποιότητες αἱ κοινόταται ἐπὶ πάντων θεωρούμεναι αἵδε· μέγεθος, σφοδρότης, ἀμυδρότης, τάχος, πυκνότης, πληρότης, τάξις, ὁμαλότης, ῥυθμός· ἅπασαι γὰρ αἱ τοιαῦται διαφοραὶ εἰς ταύτας ὑπαχθήσονται', ed. Schöne, 'Markellinos' Pulslehre' (n. 54 above), 458.90–3).

[76] Theophilos refers explicitly to ten classes ('γένη μὲν οὖν σφυγμῶν εἰσι δέκα', ed. Ermerins (n. 47 above), *Anecdota*, 23.15), but he does not give an arithmetical reference in the description of each class.

[77] Philaretos provides first a description of the various classes and then a list; there are some slight differences in numbering between these two parts of his work and, where applicable, these are indicated by two numbers corresponding to lines 138–75 and 245–82 of Pithis's, *Die Schriften* (n. 51 above), edition respectively (e.g. 9/8).

[78] See, for example, the *iatrosophion* attributed to John Archiatros, *John the Physician's Therapeutics: A medical handbook in vernacular Greek*, ed. B. Zipser, Leiden, 70.3–5 and 255.6. Cf. P.

contained in *Wellcomensis* MS.MSL.60 suggest an audience of poorly educated practitioners, who would probably have been unaware of Galen's actual medical contribution to the topic. This theory is substantiated by the fact that we do not really have evidence of a large number of educated physicians or even an established centre of medical education in late Byzantium, apart from the *Katholikon Mouseion* of the Kral *xenon*, annexed to the monastery of St John the Baptist in Constantinople, under John Argyropoulos (ca. 1393/4 or 1415–1487) and his circle of students, which existed for a few years before the city fell to the Ottoman Turks in 1453.[79] Yet even intellectuals such as these were not always as well informed as we might think, as for example in the case of the long Pseudo-Galenic *Introduction, or the Physician*,[80] which seems to have been considered authentic by John Argyropoulos's circle. However, in this case, unlike with our treatises, the text had a long textual tradition and was in most cases included in manuscripts that transmitted a large number of other genuine Galenic works. When all is said and done, short, diagnostic and prognostic, Pseudo-Galenic texts served a practical purpose and therefore it did not much matter to Byzantine practitioners when it came to actual medical practice why some anonymous compiler or scribe had consciously or unconsciously connected them with the name of Galen.

Pseudo-Galenic Texts in *Wellcomensis* MS.MSL.60[81]

Appendix A

[170ʳ] Περὶ οὔρων Γαληνοῦ διαίρεσις

Οὖρον λευκὸν μὴ ἔχον ὑπόστασιν, ἀπεψίαν σημαίνει καὶ δυσουρίαν.

Bouras-Vallianatos, 'Galen in Byzantine Medical Literature', in *Brill's Companion to the Reception of Galen*, eds P. Bouras-Vallianatos and B. Zipser, Leiden, 2019, pp. 86–110 (97–8); and B. Zipser, 'Galen in Byzantine *iatrosophia*', in *Brill's Companion* (n. 78), pp. 111–23.

[79] On Argyropoulos and his students, see B. Mondrain, 'Jean Argyropoulos professeur à Constantinople et ses auditeurs médecins, d'Andronic Eparque à Démétrios Angelos', in Πολύπλευρος νοῦς: *Miscellanea für Peter Schreiner zu seinem 60. Geburtstag*, eds G. Makris and C. Scholz, Munich, 2000, pp. 223–50.

[80] See Petit, 'The fate' (n. 4 above), pp. 66–8, who informs us that a large number of the 15th-century witnesses of the Pseudo-Galenic *Introduction, or the Physician*, in which the work is consistently ascribed to Galen, are connected with late Byzantine intellectuals associated with the circle of John Argyropoulos.

[81] Transcriptions from Greek retain the punctuation used in the codex. The text is orthographically normalized, the iota subscription has been supplied, and accents and breathings have been tacitly corrected.

Οὖρον ἐν πυρετοῖς, μέλανι ἐοικὸς οἴνῳ αὐστηρὸν ἡπατικὸν σημαίνει.

Οὖρον τεθολωμένον ἐοικὸς κοκκίνῳ ἐλαίῳ θάνατον σημαίνει.

5　Οὖρον ξανθὸν μὴ ἔχον ὑπόστασιν, θάνατον ἐξαπιναῖον σημαίνει.

Οὖρον ὠχρὸν παχύτατον, ποδαλγίαν σημαίνει.

Οὖρον ἐρυθρὸν μὴ ἔχον ἐναλλαγήν, ἐλεφαντίασιν σημαίνει.

Οὖρον κροκῶδες μὴ ἔχον ἀλλοίωσιν περιπνευμονικὸν καὶ βηχικὸν σημαίνει.

Οὖρον μελαντήριον στίλβον, κωλικὸν σημαίνει.

10　Οὖρον μαῦρον πελιδνόν, ἄνευ πυρετοῦ καὶ ἱδρώτου κεφαλαλγίαν σημαίνει.

Οὖρον κρυσταλλοειδὲς μὴ ἔχον ἐναλλαγὴν ὕδρωπα σημαίνει.

Οὖρον ἐν τριταίῳ πυρετῷ μὴ ἔχον ὑπόστασιν μαρασμὸν σημαίνει.

Οὖρον ὑποκείμενον ὑδαρὸν παροξυσμὸν σημαίνει.

Τὸ οὖρον τὸ ῥούσιον καὶ παχύ, δηλοῖ ἀπὸ αἵματος εἶναι τὸ δὲ αἷμά ἐστι θερμόν,
15　καὶ ὑγρὸν αὔξει δὲ τὸ ἔαρ ἀπὸ κα′ Μαρτίου ἕως κδ′ Ἰουνίου· καὶ εἰ μὲν ἔχει
τὸ τοιοῦτον οὖρον ἀφρόν, δηλοῖ ἄνεμον καὶ κεντισμόν· καὶ βηχὸς γένεσιν καὶ
λαγόνες κεντοῦνται καὶ ὠμοπλάται βαρύνονται· καὶ ἡ καρδία σφίγγεται· καὶ εἰ
μέν ἐστι νέος ἐνδέχεται ἵνα ἀφαιμάξῃ, κάτωθεν, τῶν ζ′ ἡμερῶν ἐὰν ἔχῃ δύναμιν·
ἐπεὶ σὰν διαβῇ τὰς ζ′, οὐκ ἐνδέχεται διὰ τὸ ἀδύνατον τοῦ σώματος αὐτοῦ· χρεία
20　γοῦν ἵνα ἐπιδώσῃς αὐτῷ τὰς βιόλας· καὶ τὸ ζουλάπιν αὐτὸ ἢ τὸ διὰ κρόκον καὶ
τὸ μάννα μεθ᾽ ὕδατος ἢ φοίνικα ἰνδικά· καὶ εἰ μέν ἐστιν ἔαρ, καὶ εἰ γέρων ἐστί, ἃς
ἀφαιμάξῃ αἷμα· εἴπερ ἔχει αὐτό, ἐκ συνηθείας.

Τὸ δὲ ῥούσιον καὶ λεπτὸν οὖρον, δηλοῖ ξανθὴν χολήν· καὶ θερμὴν καὶ ξηράν, τὸ
δὲ λεπτὸν οὖρον, δηλοῖ φρίκην· καὶ κατακλασμὸν καὶ πικρότητα τοῦ στόματος·
25　καὶ σκοτισμὸν εἰς τὴν κεφαλήν· καὶ πόνον εἰς τὴν ῥάχην καὶ δίψαν· καὶ πόνον
εἰς τὰς λαγόνας· ἐνδέχεται οὖν ἵνα κινήσῃ τὴν γαστέρα καὶ καθαίρειν· ὥσπερ τὰ
μυροβάλανα τὰ κίτρινα· καὶ τὸ ζουλάπιν τῶν δαμασκήνων· καὶ τῶν ῥόδων· καὶ
τὸ ζουλάπιν τὸ ῥοδόστακτον, καὶ τὰ τοιαῦτα.

Τὸ δὲ ἄσπρον καὶ λεπτὸν οὖρον, δηλοῖ μέλαιναν χολήν· δηλοῖ δὲ τὸ τοιοῦτον
30　οὖρον, ληθαργίαν· καὶ πόνων λαγόνων· ὄκνον ἀγρυπνίαν· ἐρυγμοὺς κακοὺς
κτύπον καρδίας· πρέπει δὲ ἵνα πίῃ τὴν θεοδώρητον· καὶ τὴν λογάδιον καὶ τὰ
τοιαῦτα.

Καὶ ὁποῖον ἔχει τὸ οὖρον ἀφρόν, δηλοῖ, ἀνέμους εἰς τὰ σπλάγχνα· καὶ χρὴ
καθαίρειν τὸ σῶμα, ἢ ὅταν πλεονάζῃ τὸ αἷμα, [170ᵛ] ἵνα ἀφαιμάξῃ· ὅταν δὲ
35　πλεονάζουσι τὰ ἄλλα καθαίρειν αὐτόν.

Τὸ ἐρυθρὸν οὖρον, ἀπεψίαν σημαίνει, καὶ οὐ θάνατον· ἀλλὰ χρόνου δεῖται εἰς
πέψιν· ἔστι γὰρ ἐξ αἵματος ἰχωροειδοῦς· μήπω τελείαν πέψιν λαβόντος· μὴ δὲ τὴν
ἰδίαν χώραν καὶ διὰ τοῦτο χρονιώτερον σημαίνει τὸ νόσημα· ἐπὶ δὲ τῶν συνεχῶν
πυρετῶν, ἐπὶ πλῆθος αἵματος συνιστάμενον ἐκκρίνεται οὖρον ἐρυθρὸν καὶ παχύ·

καὶ δῆλον ὅτι τοιοῦτόν ἐστι τῷ χρώματι καὶ τῇ συστάσει τοῦ χύματος· καὶ τὸ   40
παρυφιστάμενον ἄπεπτον.

Τί δηλοῖ τὸ ὠχρὸν καὶ λεπτὸν οὖρον· τὸ λεπτὸν καὶ εὔωχρόν ἐστι τῇ συστάσει·
πεττόμενον μετρίως τῆς χρόας ασθένειαν, τοῦτο δηλοῖ τῆς φύσεως· τὸ μὲν γὰρ
χρώματι· ἔπεψεν ὡς ἀνδρεῖον ὑπάρχον· οὐκ ἔστι δὲ καὶ τῇ συστάσει· διὰ τοῦτο
δυσκολώτερον.   45

Οὖρον λεπτὸν τῇ συστάσει· καὶ πυρὸν τῷ χρώματι, βέλτιον τοῦ ὠχροῦ· ὅμως
ἄπεπτον διὰ τὴν σύστασιν.

Τὸ λεπτὸν οὐρούμενον καὶ μετὰ ταῦτα ἀναθολώμενον, ἄπεπτόν ἐστι διὰ
παρουσίαν πνεύματος παχέος· δηλοῖ δὲ τὴν φύσιν, ἄρχεσθαι πέττειν.

Οὖρον ἐλαιῶδες. Πόσαι διαφοραὶ τοῦ ἐλαιώδους οὔρου· καὶ τί σημαίνουσιν·   50
εἴωθεν ὁ πυρετός· πρότερον τὴν πιμελὴν ἐκτήκειν· εἶτα τὴν σάρκα ὕστερον δέ,
καὶ αὐτῶν τῶν στερεῶν σωμάτων καθάπτεσθαι· τῆς μὲν οὖν πιμελῆς τηκομένης,
τὰ ἐλαιώδη οὖρα ἐκκρίνεται, κατὰ βραχὺ ἡ πιμελὴ τήκεται· ὅθεν καὶ ἀρχὴν ἔχει·
καὶ ἀνάβασιν καὶ ἀκμήν· {ἐν ἀρχῇ} ἐν ἀρχῇ μὲν οὖν τῆς συντήξεως, ὅλα διόλου
τὰ οὖρα, καὶ ἐν χρώματι καὶ ἐν συστάσει, οἷον ἔλαιόν ἐστιν ἐπεὶ αὐτὴ ἡ τηκομένη   55
πιμελὴ ἢ τῶν νεφρῶν μόνον ἐστὶν ἀθρόως ἐκκρίνεται πλῆθος τοιοῦτον· ἐπεὶ καὶ
θερμασίας πλείονος αἴσθησις περὶ τοὺς νεφροὺς γίνεται· εἰ δὲ ἐκ τοῦ παντὸς
σώματός ἐστι, κατὰ βραχύ, τὴν προσθήκην ποιεῖται.

Οὖρον κριμνῶδες. Τί δηλοῖ τὸ κριμνῶδες, ἐν τοῖς οὔροις· ἐπειδὰν ὁ πυρετὸς
μετὰ τὸ κατειληφέναι τὸ βάθος, καὶ μεῖζον πλάτος ἐπιλάβῃ καὶ μῆκος, ἁδρότερα   60
γίνεται τὰ τοιαῦτα τῶν πιτύρων· καὶ καλεῖται κριμνώδη· ἀλλὰ τὰ κριμνώδη δύο
σημαίνουσιν ἢ γὰρ ὑπερόπτησιν αἵματος δηλοῦσιν, ἢ σύνταξιν ἰσχυρὰν τῶν
στερεῶν· εἰ μὲν οὖν ἦν τὰ τοιαῦτα κριμνώδη τῶν στερεῶν σωμάτων ἐστὶ τὸ πάθος·
εἰ δὲ ἐρυθρὰ τοῦ αἵματος.

Τὸ δυσῶδες οὖρον, σῆψιν δηλοῖ, καὶ τῆς φύσεως νέκρωσιν μέλουσαν.   65

Πάντα τὰ μελανὰ τῶν οὔρων, εὐθὺς καὶ παχέα πάντως ἐστί· σπάνιον γὰρ ἢ
οὐδόλως εὑρεθῆναι λεπτὸν καὶ μέλαν· τὸ γὰρ μέλαν χρῶμα πρὸς γίνεται τοῖς
οὔροις ἐκκαθαιρομένου τοῦ μελαγχολικοῦ χυμοῦ· ἢ αὐτῆς τῆς μελαίνης [171ʳ]
χολῆς· τῆς τε διὰ ψῦξιν γινομένης· καὶ παχύτητας κέκτηται τὰς συστάσεις· ἐξ
ἀναγκαίου καὶ παχέα εὑρεθήσεται τὰ μέλανα τῶν οὔρων ἐπὶ μὲν τῶν ὀξέων   70
νοσημάτων, ὀλεθριώτατόν ἐστι σύμπαν τὸ οὖρον μελανθὲν καὶ μάλιστα ὅταν τε
δυσῶδες ὑπάρχῃ· καὶ παχύ· καὶ ὑπόστασιν ἔχον μέλαινα· ἀδύνατον γὰρ ὀξέως
νοσοῦντα τοιοῦτον οὐρήσαντα σωθῆναι καὶ εἰ μὲν ἡ ὑπόστασις εἴη μέλαινα,
ὀλεθριώτατον· εἰ δὲ ἐναιώρημα μέλαν, ἧττον κακόν· ὁμοίως δὲ εἶναι κακὸν
ἐπιπλέον εἰ νεφέλη μέλαινα.   75

Τὸ δὲ μέλαν, ποτὲ μὲν ἐνδείκνυται ψῦξιν· ποτὲ δὲ θερμότητα· εἰ μὲν οὖν
πρότερον οὐρηθείη πελιδνόν, εἶθ' οὕτως γένηται, μέλαν, ψῦξιν ἔχει τὴν αἰτίαν·

εἰ δὲ τὸ ξανθὸν, προηγήσοιτο, ἔπειτα μέλαν εὑρεθείη, δῆλον ὅτι ἀπὸ θερμότητος
πλείονος μέλαν γέγονεν· γνωστέον μέντοι ὅτι καὶ ἐπὶ τῇ παρακμῇ τοῦ τεταρταίου
80 πυρετοῦ· καὶ ἐπὶ τῆς μελαγχολικῆς παρανοίας λυομένης, οὖρά φαμεν εἶναι ταῦτα
φαίνεται μέλανα καὶ παχέα· ἡμεῖς δὲ ὀλέθρια ἔφαμεν εἶναι ταῦτα ἐπὶ τῶν ὀξέων,
νοσημάτων.

Τὸ χλωρὸν οὖρον, δηλοῖ θερμασίαν πλείστην· καὶ κακοήθειαν τοῦ σώματος.

2-4 Ideler, *Physici*, 2, 304.18–22 || 6–12 Ideler, 2, 304.23–34 || 14–32 cf. Ideler, 2, 303.4–
304.3 || 36 cf. XIX, 586.14–15 K. || 36–41 Ideler, 2, 312.23–30; Olivieri, *Aetii Amideni*, 2,
21.26–22.5; XIX, 620.3–10 K. || 42–45 Ideler, 2, 312.14–18; Olivieri, 2, 21.16–20; cf. XIX,
598.16–599.3 K.; cf. XIX, 619.9–13 K. || 46–47 Ideler, 2, 312.20–21; Olivieri, 2, 21.24–25;
XIX, 599.4–5 K.; cf. XIX, 619.18–620.2 K. || 48–49 Ideler, 2, 313.2–4; Olivieri, 2, 22.6–9;
XIX, 599.15–18 K.; XIX, 620.13–15 K. || 50–55 cf. XIX, 588.5–13 K. || 50–58 cf. Ideler, 2,
314.1–17; cf. Olivieri, 2, 23.9–22 || 59–64 Ideler, 2, 315.10–17; Olivieri, 2, 24.17–23; XIX,
590.16–591.5 K.; XIX, 624.12–625.2 K. || 65 Ideler, 2, 315.19–20; Olivieri, 2, 24.24–25; XIX,
591.10–11 K.; XIX, 625.3 K. || 66–82 cf. Ideler, 2, 315.22–316.13; cf. Olivieri, 2, 24.26–25.23;
cf. XIX, 625.5–626.7 K., 10–11 || 76–82 cf. XIX, 587.11–14 K. || 79–80 cf. XIX, 582.3–4 K.

Appendix B

[191ʳ] Ἑρμηνεία τοῦ Γαληνοῦ περὶ κλοκίου

85 Ἔπαρε τὸ κλοκίον, καὶ θὲς αὐτὸ εἰς ἀσφάλειαν διὰ μιᾶς ὥρας τῆς νυκτός, καὶ τὸ
πρωὶ ἰδὲ αὐτό· καὶ διάκρινε ὡς φησὶν ὁ Γαληνός· καὶ εἴπερ ἐστὶ τεταραγμένον,
οἷον ὑποζυγίου, ὑγείαν σημαίνει· εἰ δὲ νεφέλη κρεμᾶται, ὑγείαν σημαίνει· εἰ δὲ
ἐναιώρημα ἢ ὑπόστασις, πλεονασμὸς φλέγματός ἐστι, ἐὰν ὡς πυροειδὴς ᾖ καὶ
αἱματοειδής, φλεβοτομίαν δηλοῖ, καὶ γαστρὸς κένωσιν· ἐὰν δὲ ποιήσῃ ἐπάνω
90 τζίπαν, τὸ διὰ μέσου, πρὸς τὴν φύσιν ἐστί· ὅτι ἰσχυροτέρα οὖσα ἡ φύσις, ὑγείαν
σημαίνει· εἰ δὲ καὶ ὑπερισχύσῃ ἡ νόσος, θάνατον δηλοῖ· ἐὰν δὲ ποιήσῃ ἐπάνω
τζίπαν, καὶ σκεπάσῃ τὴν ἐπιφάνειαν ὅλην τοῦ ὑελίου, καὶ κάτω ἔστι καθαρόν,
θάνατον σημαίνει μέχρι τῶν ιβ′ ἡμερῶν· ἐὰν δὲ ὑπόστασις παχεῖα οὖσα, κάτω εἰς
τὸν πυθμένα τοῦ ὑελίου, πλεονασμὸν χολῆς δηλοῖ· ἄριστος λόγος καὶ ἀληθής·
95 καὶ δόκιμος καὶ ἀδιάψευστος.

Appendix C

[193ʳ] Γαληνοῦ περὶ σφυγμῶν

Ὁ σφυγμὸς κίνησίς ἐστιν ἀρτηριῶν ἀπὸ καρδίας ἀρχομένη· ἕκαστον δὲ σφυγμῶν
διὰ β′ κινήσεων καὶ β′ ἠρεμιῶν τέλειος γίνεται· καὶ ἡ μὲν πρώτη κίνησις καλεῖται

διαστολὴ καὶ ἠρεμία ὄπισθεν αὐτῆς· ἡ δὲ β΄ κίνησις καλεῖται συστολὴ καὶ ἠρεμία
ὄπισθεν αὐτῆς ὅτι ἀδύνατόν ἐστι τῷ ποιοῦντι ἐπὶ τίνι κίνησιν καὶ ἐπιφθάσει εἰς τὸ 100
τέλος ἐκείνου τοῦ ἄκρου μέρους· καὶ πάλιν τραπῇ ἐξ αὐτοῦ ἐπὶ τὸ ἕτερον ἄκρον
μέρος καὶ ἀναμέσων τῶν β΄ κινήσεων γενήσεται ἠρεμία ὅτι δύο κινήσεις ἐναντίαι
συνεχεῖς μία μὲν μετὰ τῆς ἄλλης, ἀδύνατόν ἐστι γενέσθαι· ἀνάγκη ἢ δεῖ ἐστιν
ὅτι ἀναμεταξὺ τῆς φθανούσης τῶν ἄκρων τῆς κινήσεως τῆς διαστολῆς καὶ τῆς
ἐνάρξεως τῆς κινήσεως τῆς συστολῆς, ἠρεμία γένηται· τὸν αὐτὸν οὖν τρόπον 105
ἀναμέσον τῆς ἐπιφθάσεως τοῦ ἄκρου τῆς συστολῆς καὶ τῆς ἀρχομένης κινήσεως
τῆς διαστολῆς γενέσθαι ἠρεμίαν· τὶ γὰρ ἐὰν αἱ δύο ἠρεμίαι οὐκ εἰσὶ φανεραί· ἡ γὰρ
κίνησις τῆς διαστολῆς, φανερωτέρα ἐστὶν ὡς φυσικὴ καὶ ἀεὶ δυνάμεθα εὑρίσκειν
ἐπὶ τοῖς δακτύλοις· χωρὶς δὲ ὅταν ἐστὶν ἡ δύναμις εἰς ἄκρον ἀσθενής· ὑπ᾽ ἐνίων δέ
ἐστιν ὅτι τὴν κίνησιν τῆς συστολῆς ἀδύνατον εὑρίσκεσθαι· οὐκ ἔστι δὲ ἀληθές· 110
ὅτι ἐν τῷ μεγάλῳ σφυγμῷ καὶ ἐν τῷ σκληρῷ καὶ ἐν τῷ δυνατῷ καὶ πυκνῷ καὶ ἐν
τῷ ἀραιῷ δύναται· καὶ ταύτῃ εὑρεθῆναι· οὕτως δὲ εὑρίσκεται ἐν τῷ μεγάλῳ καὶ
σκληρῷ σφυγμῷ ὅτι ἡ νεῦσις τῶν β΄ κινήσεων τῶν διαστολικῶν διὰ τὴν αἰτίαν
τῆς μεγαλειότητος καὶ τῆς σκληρότητος· μαλακότητα καὶ ἰσότητα μὴ ποιούντων,
φανεροῦται. 115

Περὶ τοῦ τί ἐστιν ὠφέλεια τοῦ σφυγμοῦ καὶ διατί διαγινώσκεται ἀπὸ τοῦ σφυγμοῦ

Χρὴ γινώσκειν ὅτι ἡ καρδία ὁμοιά ἐστι τῶν ἀρτηριῶν ὅλου τοῦ σώματος· ἑκάστη
δὲ ἀρτηρία ἤτοι σφυγμὸς ὥσπερ ἡ καρδία ἕν μέρος ἐστὶ καὶ ὥσπερ τὸ πνεῦμα
τὸ ὂν ἐν τῇ καρδίᾳ χρείαν ἔχει ψυχροῦ καὶ καθαροῦ ἀέρος ἀπὸ τοὺς πόρους τοῦ 120
πνεύμονος, καὶ αἱ ἀρτηρίαι τὴν αὐτὴν χρῄζουσι χρείαν ἀπὸ τῶν διεξόδων τῶν
ἀδήλων πόρων· λοιπὸν ἡ ὠφέλεια τοῦ σφυγμοῦ ἀὴρ ἐστὶ καθαρὸς καὶ ψυχρὸς
εἰσερχόμενος ἐπὶ τὸν πνεύμονα καὶ ἀπὸ τοῦ πνεύμονος ἐπὶ τὴν καρδίαν· ἐξωθῶν
τὸν λιγνυώδη καὶ θερμὸν καπνὸν ἀπὸ τῆς καρδίας καθὼς διεγνώσθη ἐν τῷ ἰδίῳ
τόπῳ αὐτῶν· καὶ ὅτι ἡ κίνησις τῶν ἀρτηριῶν καὶ ἡ κίνησις τῆς καρδίας ἅμα 125
γίνονται· ἀρχὴ δὲ τῆς ζωτικῆς δυνάμεως καὶ τοῦ ἐμφύτου θερμοῦ ἡ καρδία ἐστί·
καὶ ἅπαν τὸ σῶμα διὰ τῆς ζωτικῆς δυνάμεως ζωογονεῖται· καὶ διὰ τοῦ ἐμφύτου
θερμοῦ ἐστι τὸ σῶμα διάπυρον· καὶ αὐτὴ ἡ ζωτικὴ δύναμις κατὰ πάντα τὰ μέρη
τοῦ σώματος διὰ τῆς δυνάμεως τοῦ ἐμφύτου θερμοῦ διαβαίνει καὶ διασώζεται·
καὶ κατὰ πάσας τὰς δυνάμεις· τάς τε σωματικὰς καὶ τὰς ψυχικὰς καὶ αὐτὴ ἡ 130
σύστασις ὅλου [193ᵛ] τοῦ σώματος διὰ τούτων τῶν δύο δυνάμεων συνίσταται τοῦ
ζωτικοῦ φημι καὶ τοῦ ἐμφύτου θερμοῦ· πηγὴ δὲ τούτων ἐστὶν ἡ καρδία· διὰ ταύτην
οὖν τὴν αἰτίαν τὴν κατάστασιν πάντων τῶν δυνάμεων· ἐκ τῆς καταστάσεως τῆς
καρδίας δυνάμεθα γνωρίσαι· καὶ τὴν κατάστασιν τῆς καρδίας ἀπὸ τὴν κίνησιν
τῶν ἀρτηριῶν δυνάμεθα γινώσκειν· ἀναγκαῖον οὖν ἐστι τῷ ἰατρῷ ἵνα γινώσκει 135

119

τὴν κατάστασιν τῆς ζωτικῆς δυνάμεως· καὶ ἡ ἐνέργεια αὐτῆς ἐστιν οἱ σφυγμοί·
ἡ δὲ καρδία καὶ αἱ ἀρτηρίαι ὄργανά εἰσι τῆς ζωτικῆς δυνάμεως· ἐν αὐταῖς δὲ
ταῖς κοιλότησι τῆς καρδίας καὶ τῶν ἀρτηριῶν αἷμά ἐστι καὶ πνεῦμα· λοιπὸν
ἁπτόμενος χεῖραν ὁ ἰατρὸς ἐν ταῖς ἀρτηρίαις ἐκ τῆς ἐνεργείας τῆς δυνάμεως δεῖ
140 ζητεῖν· καὶ ἐκ τῆς ἐνεργείας τῆς ταχύτητος, καὶ βραδύτητος· καὶ ἐκ τῆς ἰσότητος
καὶ ἀνισότητος· καὶ ἀπὸ τῆς χρονήσεως τοῦ καιροῦ τοῦ διαστήματος· καὶ ἀπὸ τῆς
ταχύτητος· καὶ ἀπὸ τοῦ ὀργάνου τὴν θερμότητα καὶ τὴν ψυχρότητα· καὶ ἀπὸ τῆς
σκληρότητος καὶ ἀπὸ τῆς μαλακότητος καὶ ἀπὸ τῶν φλεβῶν τῶν εὑρισκομένων
ἐν ταῖς κοιλότησι τῆς καρδίας καὶ τῶν ἀρτηριῶν· πλήρης ὄντων ἢ καὶ κενῶν· ὅτε
145 γὰρ ταύτας ὑποθέσεις εὕροι ὁ ἰατρός, τότε εὑρίσκει καὶ πάσας τὰς ὑποθέσεις τοῦ
ὅλου σώματος ἤτοι τὰς καταστάσεις.

Περὶ τοῦ πῶς δεῖ ζητῆσαι ὁ ἰατρὸς τὸν σφυγμὸν

Ζητῆσαι ἀπὸ τοῦ δεξιοῦ καρποῦ τῆς χειρὸς διὰ τὴν ταχεῖαν αὐτῆς εὕρεσιν καὶ
διὰ τὸ ἔστι κατὰ τὴν ἐπιφάνειαν τοῦ δέρματος τῆς χειρὸς καὶ διὰ τὸ ἔστιν
150 ἀνεπαίσχυντος· καὶ διὰ τὸ ἔστι κατέναντι τῆς καρδίας καὶ πλησίον· διὰ τὸ
οὐκ ἔστι κεκαλυμμένη ὑπὸ σαρκὸς καθῶς τῆς ῥάχης καὶ μηρῶν καὶ οὐκ ἔστι
πεπληρωμένη ἀπὸ τῶν ἀτμῶν αἱ ἀρτηρίαι διὰ τῶν μηνίγγων· ἅπτεσθαι δὲ δεῖ
τὸν σφυγμὸν διὰ τῶν δʹ δακτύλων τοῦ λιχανοῦ καὶ μέσου καὶ παραμέσου καὶ
μικροῦ· καὶ τὸν καρπὸν τοῦ βραχίονος πλαγιάζειν δεῖ καὶ μὴ ἀνασκελίζειν·
155 αἱ δὲ χεῖρες τοῦ ἰατροῦ ἁπαλαὶ καὶ μᾶλλον αἱ κορυφαὶ τῶν δακτύλων· καὶ
πρῶτον μὲν οὖν ζητεῖν χρὴ τὸν σφυγμὸν σφοδρός ἐστι καὶ δυνατός· ἢ ἀσθενὴς
καὶ ἀδύνατος· καὶ εἰ μὲν εὕροι τὸν σφυγμὸν ἰσχυρὸν σφοδρῶς, χρὴ ἅπτεσθαι
τοῦτον ἐν συμμετρίᾳ· ἐὰν δὲ ἀσθενῆ καὶ ἀδύνατον χρὴ ἅπτεσθαι ἐλαφροτέρως
καὶ ἐν ἠρεμίᾳ· καὶ ὅτε θήσει χεῖραν ὁ ἰατρὸς ἐπὶ τὸν σφυγμὸν τοῦ ἀρρώστου δεῖ
160 ἐπιτηρεῖν ἕως οὗ παρέλθωσι σφυγμοὶ τῶν ἀριθμῶν λʹ· ἐν τούτῳ γὰρ τῷ χρόνῳ
δύναται διαγνῶναι τὴν κατάστασιν τοῦ σφυγμοῦ· οὕτω δὲ ποιήσας μεγάλως
ὠφεληθήσεται ἀπὸ τὸν σφυγμὸν καὶ τελείως διαγνώσεται· ἀδύνατον γάρ ἐστιν
ὅτι ὁ σφυγμὸς ἐν τούτῳ τῷ χρόνῳ ἐκ τῆς καταφάσεως τῆς μαλακότητος γενέσθαι
ἐν σκληρότητι· ἢ ὄπισθεν τῆς πληρώσεως ἤγουν γεμώσεως γενέσθαι κενὸς ἢ
165 ὄπισθεν τῆς κενότητος γενέσθαι πλήρης· ἀλλὰ δυνατόν ἐστιν ὅτι ἐν τῇ ψυχρότητι
καὶ ἐν τῇ θερμότητι καὶ ἐν τῇ μεγαλειότητι καὶ ἐν τῇ μικρότητι· [194ʳ] καὶ ἐν τῇ
ἀραιότητι καὶ ἐν τῇ πυκνότητι, τρόπον ποιῆσαι· καὶ ἐν τῇ πρώτῃ καὶ ἐν τῇ ὑστάτῃ·
καὶ ἐν τῇ δυνάμει καὶ ἐν τῇ ἀδυναμίᾳ· καὶ ἡ διάγνωσις τούτων ὄφελος μέγα ἐστί·
καὶ ὅτε θήσει τὴν χεῖραν ὁ ἰατρὸς κατὰ τὴν ἀρτηρίαν· ἐν εἶδος ἀπὸ τῶν εἰδῶν τῶν
170 σφυγμῶν ὅπερ ἔχει ἕκαστος ἄνθρωπος κατὰ τὴν οἰκείαν αὐτοῦ κρᾶσιν καὶ ἔστιν
ἐπιτήδεια καὶ ἁρμόζουσα τῆς καταστάσεως αὐτοῦ τοῦ νοσοῦντος ταύτην χρὴ
ζητεῖν ὅπως εὕροι τοῦ αὐτοῦ ἀνθρώπου ὃν εἶχε τὸν κατὰ φύσιν σφυγμὸν αὐτοῦ

ὅταν ὑπῆρχεν ὑγιής· ὅτι ἀπὸ τῶν παραφύσιν εὑρίσκεται ὁ καταφύσιν· ζητεῖν δὲ
χρὴ τὸν σφυγμὸν ὅτε οὐκ ἔστιν ὁ ἄνθρωπος ἐν θυμῷ ἢ ἐν περιχαρίᾳ ἢ ἐν φόβῳ· ἢ
ἐν κόπῳ ἢ ἀπὸ λουτροῦ· ἢ ἀπὸ ἀμέτρου ὕπνου· ἢ ἀπὸ ἀγρυπνίας· ἢ ἀπὸ ἀσιτίας   175
ἢ ἐν κόρῳ· καὶ ὥσπερ ἐστὶν ἡ φύσις καὶ ἡ κρᾶσις ἑκάστου ἄλλη καὶ ἄλλη, οὕτως
ἐστὶ καὶ ὁ σφυγμὸς ἑκάστου ἄλλος καὶ ἄλλος· κατὰ γὰρ τὴν κρᾶσιν ἑκάστου καὶ
τὴν κατάστασιν τῆς ἡλικίας αὐτοῦ καὶ κατὰ τοὺς χρόνους αὐτοῦ καὶ κατὰ τὴν
κατάστασιν τῆς ἐναλλαγῆς τῶν δ΄ καιρῶν τοῦ ἐνιαυτοῦ καὶ κατὰ τὴν κατάστασιν
τῆς φύσεως καὶ κατὰ τὴν κατάστασιν τοῦ ἀέρος καὶ κατάστασιν τῶν χώρων·   180
χρὴ οὖν τὸν ἰατρὸν ὅταν ἅπτεται ἑκάστου τὸν σφυγμὸν μετὰ πολλῆς ἀκριβείας
δεῖ ἅπτεσθαι πολυμαθὴς ὑπάρχων καὶ ἔμπειρος καὶ οὕτως ἅπτεσθαι· ὕστερον δὲ
πάντων τῶν κινήσεων καὶ καταστάσεων ἅπερ ἀνεμνήσθημεν προγινώσκον καὶ
τὰ ἤθη τοῦ σφυγμοῦ αὐτοῦ ἐν ἑκά[στῃ] καταστάσει· ὅτι ὅτε ἐν καιρῷ τραπῇ ὁ
σφυγμὸς ἐκ τοῦ ἤθους αὐτοῦ αὐτὴν τὴν τροπὴν ἣν ἐτράπη εὕροι· καὶ ζητήσει   185
τὴν αἰτίαν τῆς παρατροπῆς τοῦ σφυγμοῦ πρὸς τὸ δυνηθῆναι πρᾶξαι ὁρισμὸς ἐπὶ
τοῦτο· ἰστέον δὲ ὅτι ἀπὸ τὰ εἴδη καὶ ἀπὸ τὰς διαφορὰς τοῦ συμμέτρου σφυγμοῦ
πρότερον χρὴ ζητεῖν· ἵνα εὑρεθῇ ὁ μικρὸς καὶ ὁ μέγας καὶ ὁ πυκνὸς καὶ ὁ ἀραιὸς
καὶ ὁ μακρὸς καὶ ὁ κοντὸς καὶ οἱ λοιποί· ὅτι ἀπὸ τοῦ ζητεῖν τὸν σύμμετρον
σφυγμόν, εὑρίσκονται οἱ ἄλλοι σφυγμοί.   190

Περὶ τὰ γένη καὶ τὰ εἴδη τῶν σφυγμῶν καὶ περὶ τὰς διαφορᾶς αὐτῶν

Γένη σφυγμῶν εἰσι ι΄· τὸ α΄ χρὴ ζητεῖν ἀπὸ τὸν ἀριθμὸν τοῦ διαστήματος καὶ ἀπὸ
τῆς κινήσεως τῆς φλεβός· διαφοραὶ αὐτῶν θ΄· μακρός· κοντός· πλατύς· στενός·
μέγας· μικρός· ὑψηλός· ταπεινός· καὶ σύμμετρος· β΄ ον γένος ἐκ τῆς δυνάμεως τῆς
κινήσεως τῆς φλεβός· διαφοραὶ αὐτοῦ τρεῖς· σφοδρός· ἀμυδρός· καὶ σύμμετρος·   195
γ΄ γένος ἐστὶν ὅπερ χρὴ ζητεῖν ἀπὸ τῆς κοντότητος καὶ ἀπὸ τῆς μακρότητος
τῆς κινήσεως τῆς διαστολῆς· διαφοραὶ αὐτοῦ γ΄· ταχύς· βραδύς· σύμμετρος·
τέταρτον γένος ὃ χρὴ ζητεῖν ἀπὸ τὸν χρόνον τῆς ἠρεμίας τῆς φλεβός· αὕτη δὲ
ἡ ἠρεμία ἐστὶν ὅτι ἀναμέσον τῶν β΄ κινήσεων τῶν διαστολικῶν καὶ συστολικῶν
καὶ διαφοραὶ αὐτῶν εἰσι γ΄· πυκνός· ἀραιός· σύμμετρος· [194ᵛ] ε΄ γένος ἐστί· ὃ   200
χρὴ ζητεῖν ἀπὸ τὴν κατάστασιν τῆς φλεβός διαφοραὶ αὐτοῦ ε΄· ψυχρός· θερμός·
σκληρός· μαλακός· σύμμετρος· ἕκτον γένος ὃ χρὴ ζητεῖν ἀπὸ τοῦ πνεύματος
ὅπερ ἐστὶν ἀναμέσον τῶν φλεβῶν καὶ ἀπὸ αἵματος ὅπερ ἐστὶν ὄχημα αὐτοῦ·
διαφοραὶ αὐτοῦ γ΄· πλήρης· κενός· σύμμετρος· ζ΄ γένη ἐστί· ἴσος· ἄνισος· ὁμαλός·
καὶ ἀνώμαλος· τάξις καὶ ἀταξία· μακρὸς σφυγμός ἐστι· ὁ πλήττων τοὺς δ΄   205
δακτύλους· κοντὸς ὁ πλήττων τὸν ἕνα δάκτυλον· πλατύς ἐστιν ὅτε ὁ δάκτυλος
ἀπὸ τῆς κινήσεως τῆς παχύτητος τῆς φλεβός· δίδει τελείαν ἀγγελίαν· στενός
ἐστιν ὁ ἐναντίος τοῦ πλατέος· μέγας ἐστὶν ὅτε ἡ κίνησις τῆς φλεβὸς ἐν τῇ
μακρότητι αὐτῆς τὸ πλάτος τῆς φλεβὸς ὅλον ἐγείρεται καὶ συστέλλεται· ὁ δὲ

210 μικρὸς σφυγμὸς ἐναντίος ἐστὶ τοῦ μεγάλου· ὑψηλὸς σφυγμός ἐστιν ὁ τέλειος
ὑψηλὸς ταπεινὸς ὁ πίπτων ἀεὶ καὶ οὐδέποτε ὑψοῦται καὶ ἔστιν ἐναντίος τοῦ
ὑψηλοῦ· σφοδρῶς ὁ πλήττων μετὰ δυνάμεως τοὺς δακτύλους καὶ κινήσεως τῆς
διαστολῆς αὐτοῦ δὲ διὰ δυνάμεως τῶν δακτύλων· ὁ δὲ ἀσθενὴς ἐναντίος τοῦ
σφοδροῦ· πυκνός ἐστι {ὅταν} ὅταν ὁ χρόνος τῆς κινήσεως τῆς διαστολῆς αὐτοῦ
215 πάνυ ἐστὶ κοντὸς ὁ δὲ ἀραιὸς ἐναντίος τοῦ πυκνοῦ· συνεχὴς σφυγμός ἐστιν
ὅτι ὁ χρόνος τῆς ἠρεμίας ὁ ἀναμέσον τῶν β΄ κινήσεων τῶν διαστολικῶν πάνυ
κοντὸς γινόμενος· ἐναντίος δὲ τοῦ συνεχῆ ἐστιν ὁ πλήττων μίαν καὶ ἵσταται καὶ
πάλιν πλήττει· σφυγμὸς ψυχρὸς καὶ θερμὸς χρείαν σαφηνείας οὐκ ἔχει· σφυγμὸς
μαλακός, ποτὲ μὲν γίνεται ὅταν τὴν δύναμιν εἰς τοὺς δακτύλους πλήττει· ὥσπερ
220 τὸν ἀσθενῆ σφυγμὸν καὶ ἡ δύναμις ἡ διαστολικὴ ταύτην ὠθεῖ καὶ κάθηται κάτω·
καὶ ἔστιν ἐναντίος τοῦ μαλακοῦ ὁ σκληρός· σφυγμὸς γέμων ἤγουν πλήρης ἐστί·
ὅταν ἡ θερμασία τῆς ὑγρότητος εἰς τὴν αἴσθησιν τῶν δακτύλων ἀποδίδοται· ὁ
δὲ κενὸς ἤγουν εὔκαιρος ἐναντίος ἐστὶ τοῦ πλήρους ἰστέον δὲ ὅτι ὁ σφοδρὸς
σφυγμὸς μετὰ τὴν δύναμιν τὴν διαστολικὴν ὠθεῖ τοὺς δακτύλους· καὶ τὴν ἐλπίδα
225 τῶν δακτύλων ἀποκρούεται· καὶ μετὰ τὴν ἠρεμίαν τὴν γινομένην ὄπισθεν τῆς
διαστολῆς καὶ μετὰ τὴν κίνησιν τῆς συστολῆς ἀνατρέπεται ἡ δὲ σκληρὰ ἀφανὴς
γίνεται· καὶ αὐτὴ ἡ δύναμις τοῦ σκληροῦ σφυγμοῦ ἐκ τῆς δυνάμεως τῆς κινήσεως
τῆς {ἀρ} ἀρτηρίας οὐκ ἔστι· καὶ ἡ κίνησις αὐτοῦ τοὺς δακτύλους οὐ διώκει καὶ
ἐν τῇ ἀποκαταστάσει τῆς ἠρεμίας οὐκ ἀνατρέπεται· ἰστέον δὲ ὅτι ἐν τῷ πυκνῷ
230 σφυγμῷ ὁ χρόνος τῆς κινήσεώς ἐστι κοντός· ἐν δὲ τῷ συνεχεῖ σφυγμῷ ὁ χρόνος
τῆς ἠρεμίας ἐστὶ κοντός· ὁ ἴσος {σφυγμὸς} σφυγμός ἐστι· ὅτι ἐν τῇ κινήσει αὐτοῦ,
πάλιν ὁ ἐρχόμενος ὄπισθεν· ὅμοιός ἐστι τῆς προτέρας κινήσεως κατὰ πάντα· ἡ
κίνησις τῆς φλεβὸς ἐν τῷ ἑνὶ δακτύλῳ· ἡ μία μετὰ τὴν ἄλλην ἐναντία οὐκ ἔστι
γίνεται δὲ ὅτι πλήττει τὸν ἕναν δάκτυλον. [195ʳ] πλήττει δὲ καὶ εἰς τὸ ἥμισυ τοῦ
235 δακτύλου· διὰ ταύτην οὖν τὴν αἰτίαν ὁ ἐναντίος σφυγμὸς τρία εἰσὶν εἴδη· ἕν μὲν
εἶδός ἐστιν ὅτι ἡ ὕστερος πληγὴ ἐναντία ἐστὶ τῆς πρώτης κατὰ πάντα δεύτερον
δὲ ὅτι ἡ πληγὴ τοῦ ἑνὸς δακτύλου ἐναντία ἐστὶ τοῦ ἑτέρου δακτύλου· ἰστέον δὲ
ὅτι ἀναμέσον τῶν σφυγμῶν ὀρθῶν ἤγουν ἴσων, εἰς σφυγμὸς ἐμπίπτειν ἐναντίος·
ἢ ἐπὶ πέντε σφυγμοὺς ἐμπίπτουσι δύο ἐναντίοι σφυγμοί.

240 ## Περὶ τῶν σφυγμῶν τὰς αἰτίας

Πᾶσαι αἰτίαι τῶν σφυγμῶν γ΄ εἰσίν· καλοῦνται δὲ αἰτίαι καθεκτικαί, καὶ πρώτη
μὲν αἰτία ἐστὶν ἡ καρδία καὶ αἱ ἀρτηρίαι καλοῦνται ὄργανα· δευτέρα ἐστὶν ἡ
ζωτικὴ δύναμις καλεῖται ἐνέργεια· τρίτη αἰτία ἐστὶν ἡ ἑλκτικὴ δύναμις ἡ ἕλκουσα
ἀπὸ τῆς καρδίας καὶ ἀπὸ τῶν ἀρτηριῶν ψυχρὸν ἀέρα ἐκ τῆς κινήσεως τῆς
245 διαστολῆς καὶ ἐκβάλλουσα τὸν θερμὸν καὶ λιγνυῶδες ἀέρα διὰ τῆς κινήσεως
τῆς συστολῆς καὶ καλεῖται χρεία· ταῦτα οὖν τὰ γ΄ αἴτιά εἰσιν ἅπερ τίκτουσι

285 ὅτι ὅταν τραπῇ ἡ δύναμις ἐκ τῆς μεγαλειότητος, ὁ σφυγμὸς πάλιν ἀπομένει
καὶ εἰς λεπτότητα ῥέπει· καὶ ὅταν τὸ ὄργανον οὐδὲν ἀκολουθεῖ εἰς λεπτότητα
ῥέπει εἰς πυκνότητα· καὶ ὅταν ἐστὶν ἡ δύναμις ἰσχυρὰ καὶ ἡ χρεία μεγάλη καὶ τὸ
ὄργανον μαλακόν, ἐπὶ τὴν μεγαλειότητα αὐξάνεται ἐὰν δὲ ἔστιν ἡ χρεία πολλὴ
καὶ ὁ σφυγμὸς εἰς μεγάλην λεπτότητα ἔρχεται· εἰ δὲ ἔστιν ἡ χρεία πολλὴ μέγας
290 καὶ πυκνὸς ὁ σφυγμὸς γίνεται· καὶ ἐκ τούτων οὐκ ἔστιν ἄλλη τις ἀφορμή· ἢ
ἄλλος σφυγμὸς ἵνα ἐμπέσῃ ἐν αὐτῇ σπουδῇ καὶ ἀγὼν δυνάμεως χρεία δεῖ· ἡ
ἀγανάκτησις γίνεται· ἢ χρεία ὀλιγοτέρα γίνεται· ἡ δὲ ἔστιν ἡ χρεία μεγάλη
καὶ ἡ δύναμις ἀσθενὴς καὶ τὸ ὄργανον σκληρὸν ὁ σφυγμὸς εἰς μεγαλειότητα
οὐ δύναται ἐγερθῆναι· ἀλλ᾽ ἡ πυκνότης εἰς τόπον τῆς μεγαλειότητος γίνεται
295 λοιπὸν ἡ αἰτία τοῦ πυκνοῦ σφυγμοῦ καὶ λεπτοῦ, ἡ αὔξησίς ἐστι τῆς χρείας καὶ
ἡ ασθένεια τῆς δυνάμεως· ἢ πλῆθος τῆς χρείας καὶ σκληρότης τοῦ ὀργάνου· ἡ
δὲ δύναμίς ἐστιν ἀσθενὴς καὶ ἡ χρεία πολλή· ὁ σφυγμὸς πυκνὸς γίνεται· ἰδοὺ ἡ
αἰτία τῆς πυκνότητος τοῦ σφυγμοῦ διὰ τὴν ἀσθένειάν ἐστι τῆς δυνάμεως καὶ διὰ
τὴν αὔξησιν τῆς χρείας καὶ διὰ τὴν σκληρότητα τοῦ ὀργάνου· ὅθεν δὲ οὐκ ἔστιν
300 ἡ δύναμις ἀσθενὴς καὶ τὸ ὄργανον σκληρὸν καὶ ἡ χρεία ὀλίγη, σφυγμὸς ἀραιὸς
γίνεται· λοιπὸν ἡ ἀραιότης τοῦ σφυγμοῦ, δι᾽ ἔνδειαν τῆς χρείας γίνεται· καὶ ἡ
δύναμις εἰ μὴ οὖσα εἰς ὑπερβολὴν ἀσθενής· ὅτι ὅπου ἐστὶν ἡ δύναμις ὀλιγοτέρα
ταχύτης καὶ πυκνότης οὐ γίνεται· καὶ ὅταν οὐκ ἔστιν ἡ δύναμις εἰς ὑπερβολὴν
ἀσθενής, ἐπὶ τὴν μεγαλειότητα ἀγωνίζεται· διὰ ταύτην οὖν τὴν αἰτίαν· εἰς τόπον
305 τῆς λεπτότητος καὶ πυκνότητος ἡ κίνησις ἡ διαστολικὴ γαληνοτέρα [196ʳ]
ἔρχεται καὶ ἡ γαληνότης μετὰ ἀραιότητος γίνεται· καὶ ὅπου αἱ τοιαῦται αἰτίαι
γίνονται πολλαί, σφυγμὸς ἀραιὸς γίνεται· ὅτι ὁ ἀραιὸς χρόνος ὁ γινόμενος
ὄπισθεν τῆς συστολῆς κοντότερός ἐστι καὶ ἐν τῷ ἀργῷ μακρότερος· καὶ ὅπου
διὰ τὴν ὀλιγότητα τῆς χρείας ἔστι καὶ ἀσθένεια τῆς δυνάμεως καὶ σκληρότης τοῦ
310 ὀργάνου· σφυγμὸς μικρὸς γίνεται· ἰδοὺ τὸ αἴτιον τοῦ μικροῦ σφυγμοῦ δια τρεῖς
καταστάσεις γίνεται· δι᾽ ἔλλειψιν τῆς χρείας· καὶ δι᾽ ἀσθένειαν τῆς δυνάμεως
καὶ διὰ τὴν σκληρότητα τοῦ ὀργάνου· αὕτη δὲ ἡ σκληρότης τοῦ ὀργάνου, εʹ
εἰσὶν εἴδη· ξηρότης ἀπὸ τῆς θερμασίας τοῦ καυσώδους πυρετοῦ· καὶ ἀπὸ τὴν
διαφόρησιν καὶ ἀνάλυσιν τῶν ὑγρῶν· δεύτερον διὰ τὴν ἀσθένειαν τοῦ ἐμφύτου
315 θερμοῦ καὶ διὰ τὴν κατάψυξιν καὶ ἀπογείλωσιν τῶν χυμῶν διὰ τὴν αἰτίαν τῶν
ἐργαζομένων τινὰ τῶν ψύξιν ποιούντων καὶ λουομένων ὑδάτων ψυχρῶν· γʹ διὰ
ξηρότητα καὶ τεινεσμὸν τῶν φλεβῶν δι᾽ αἰτιῶν τῶν ἁπλῶν κενώσεων· δʹ διὰ
φλεγμονὴν ἰσχυρὰν γενομένην κατὰ τὰ σπλάχνα· εʹ διάμετρον ἀγρυπνίαν καὶ
ἀλουσίαν καὶ διαλημμάτων ξηρῶν τρεφομένων· ἢ διολιγοτροφίαν καὶ νηστείαν·
320 πολλάκις δὲ γίνεται σκληρὸς σφυγμὸς ὅτε πλησιάζει ἐπικρίσιμος ἡμέρα διὰ τὴν
αἰτίαν τῆς πέψεως τῆς γενομένης· διαγανάκτησιν τῆς φύσεως· πλὴν ἡ μέλουσα
γενέσθαι κρίσις μετὰ ἰδρώτων· ἐκεῖ ὁ σφυγμὸς κυματώδης γίνεται· τὸ δὲ αἴτιον

τῆς μαλακότητος τοῦ ὀργάνου δύο εἰσὶν εἴδη· φυσικὸν καὶ παραφύσιν· τὸ μὲν
φυσικὸν γίνεται διὰ τροφῶν ὑγρῶν καὶ δια πόσεις ἅπερ ἀπογεννῶσιν ὑγρότητα·
καὶ λουτρὰ σύμμετρα· παρὰ φύσιν δὲ γίνεται ὁ ἀσκητὴς ὕδερος καὶ ληθαργία καὶ   325
σπασμὸς διὰ τὸ φλέγμα τὸ δὲ αἴτιον τῆς ἀσθενούσης δυνάμεως τρία εἰσὶν εἴδη·
α′ διὰ κένωσιν καὶ ἔλλειψιν τροφῶν καὶ πωμάτων· β′ ἑκτικὸς πυρετὸς καὶ κόπος
ἄμετρος καὶ ἀραιότης τῶν ἀδήλων πόρων· γ′ διὰ νόσων καὶ διὰ ὀδύνην πόνων
χαλεπῶν φερόντων λυποθυμίας· τὸ δὲ αἴτιον ἑκάστου τῶν τριῶν διαφόρησίς
ἐστιν ἄμετρος· τὰ δὲ αἴτια τὰ ἀνασώζοντα τὴν δύναμιν ἐν τοῖς νοσήμασιν,   330
ἡ πέψις ἐστὶ βοήθειαν ἀγαθὴ καὶ ἡ χρηστὴ κρίσις καὶ ἐν τῇ ἱλαρότητι τοῦ
στόματος περιχαρία σύμμετρος· θυμὸς σύμμετρος κόπος σύμμετρος· βρῶσις καὶ
πόσις σύμμετρος· τὰ δὲ αἴτια τοῦ μακροῦ σφυγμοῦ αὐτὰ εἰσὶν αἴτια τοῦ μεγάλου
σφυγμοῦ· αἴτια δὲ τοῦ πλατέως σφυγμοῦ εἰσι β′, μαλακότης καὶ εὐκαίρεσις
γινομένης τῆς φλεβὸς ἤγουν κουφότης καὶ κενότης· τὸ δὲ αἴτιον τοῦ μικροῦ   335
σφυγμοῦ ἀσθένειά ἐστι τῆς δυνάμεως καὶ ἔλλειψις τῆς χρείας καὶ σκληρότης
τοῦ ὀργάνου· ἰστέον ὅτι ὁ ὀμφαλὸς φλέβα ἐστί· οὗ ἡ ἀρχὴ αὐτοῦ ἐστιν ἐκ τῆς
ὑστέρας.

Περὶ τὰ εἴδη τῶν ἐναντίων σφυγμῶν καὶ αἰτίας αὐτῶν

Ἑκάστον εἶδος ἀπὸ τῶν εἰδῶν τῶν ἐναντίων σφυγμῶν δυσκρασίαν κατὰ τὴν   340
καρδίαν καὶ κατὰ τὰς ἀρτηρίας γινομένη τὴν κατὰ φύσιν κατάστασιν τῆς
δυνάμεως τρέπουσι καὶ διὰ ταύτην τὴν αἰτίαν [196ᵛ] ὁ σφυγμὸς ἐναντίος γίνεται·
καὶ ὅτε καθόλου τὸ σῶμα γένηται πλήρωσις, ἢ ἔμφραξις τῆς παρὰ φύσιν ἀπὸ τῶν
ψυχικῶν παθῶν, ὁ σφυγμὸς τρέπεται· καὶ ὅταν δὲ ἔστιν ἡ δύναμις ἰσχυρὰ ὁ δὲ
σφυγμὸς ἐναντίος, καὶ τοῦτο δι' αἰτίαν πληρώσεως ὅλου τοῦ σώματος γίνεται· ἢ   345
διὰ τὸ βάρος τοῦ στομάχου ἕνεκεν πολυφαγίας· ὁπότε δέ ἐστιν ἡ δύναμις ἀσθενὴς
ὁ δὲ σφυγμὸς ἐναντίος, αἴτιον τοῦτο ἐστὶν ὑπαγωγὴ τῆς κοιλίας ἄμετρος καὶ
ἀγανάκτησις τῆς φύσεως γίνεται δὲ ἐναντίος σφυγμὸς καὶ διὰ τὸ πλῆθος τοῦ
αἵματος καὶ τρέπει τοὺς σφυγμούς· λύεται δὲ τὸ τοιοῦτον διὰ φλεβοτομίας· εἰ
δὲ ἔστι τὸ αἷμα παχὺ καὶ γλίσχρον, τὸ πνεῦμα ἐπὶ τὰς ἀρτηρίας ἀποπνίγεται·   350
μᾶλλον δὲ ἐὰν ἡ πλήρωσίς ἐστι κατὰ τὰ χωρία τῆς κάρδίας· ἤγουν κατὰ τὰ
παραπλήσια αὐτῆς· ἐὰν δὲ οὐκ ἐγένετο τὸ φλεβοτομίας κατὰ τὸν ἐπιτήδιον
αὐτῆς καιρόν· καὶ ἡ κατάστασις τοῦ αἵματος ἐπὶ τὴν συμμετρίαν αὐτοῦ οὐκ
ἀπεκατεστάθη, πνιγμὸς καρδιακὸς τίκτεται καὶ κατάστασις γίνεται παραπλήσια
τῆς ἀποπληξίας καὶ γίνεται ἀπώλεια τοῦ πάσχοντος· αὕτη δὲ ἡ πλήρωσις γίνεται   355
τοῖς οἰνοπόταις καὶ τοῖς ἀδεῶς διαιτουμένοις· ἀπὸ δὲ τὰ εἴδη τῶν ἐναντίων εἰδῶν
τῶν σφυγμῶν, ἓν εἶδός ἐστι λεγόμενον μύουρον ὁ γὰρ τοιοῦτος σφυγμὸς ποτὲ μὲν
εἰς ἕνα σφυγμὸν ἐμπίπτει ποτὲ δὲ εἰς πολλὰς ἀλλ' ὅπερ ἐμπίπτει εἰς σφυγμοὺς
πολλοὺς γίνεται οὗτος· ὅτι πρότερον ἔρχεται σφυγμὸς σφοδρὸς ἢ μέγας ἢ πυκνὸς
καὶ ὕστερον κατὰ μικρὸν γίνεται ἀμυδρός· ἢ μικρός· ἢ ἀραιός.   360

Περὶ σφυγμῶν γυμναζόντων ἤγουν κοπιόντων

Ἀπὸ κόπου συμμέτρου ὁ σφυγμὸς κατὰ μικρὸν ἰσχυρότερος καὶ μεγαλύτερος γίνεται· διότι τὸ ἔμφυτον θερμὸν ἐξεγείρεται καὶ ἡ ζωτικὴ δύναμις ἰσχυροτέρα γίνεται καὶ ἐπὶ τὸ τέλος τοῦ κόπου γίνεται ὁ σφυγμὸς ταχὺς καὶ πυκνὸς διότι ἡ
365 θερμασία ταχέως ἀποπνίγεται καὶ ἡ χρεία εἰς τὸ βάθος εἰσδύνει· ὅτε δὲ ὁ κόπος ἄμετρος γένηται ὁ σφυγμὸς γίνεται μικρὸς καὶ ἀμυδρὸς καὶ ἀσθενής· ἐὰν δὲ ἔστιν ἡ δύναμις εἰς ἄκρον ἰσχυρὰ γίνεται ὁ σφυγμὸς πυκνὸς καὶ ἔστι τὸ αἴτιον τῆς μικρότητος· καὶ τῆς ἀμυδρότητος διότι ἀνοίγονται οἱ ἄδηλοι πόροι διὰ τὸ γίνεσθαι ἀραιοὺς γίνεται διαφόρησις πολλὴ καὶ κόπτεται ἡ δύναμις εἰ δὲ ὁ κόπος
370 γένηται εἰς ὑπερβολὴν ὁ σφυγμὸς γίνεται σκωληκίζων καὶ μυρμηκίζων· ἔστι δὲ καὶ τοῦτο τὸ αἴτιον πολλὴ διαφόρησις· καὶ ἔλλειψις τῆς δυνάμεως· σφυγμὸς τῶν ψυχικῶν παθῶν ἅ εἰσι περιχαρία· λύπη· φόβος σύντονος· φροντίς· ἡδονὴ· τῦφος· ἀδημονία· ἀγωνία· δειλία· χαρά· θυμός· ὁ σφυγμὸς τῆς περιχαρίας μέγας γίνεται καὶ ἄνισος· ἤγουν πλήττει μίαν καὶ ἵσταται καὶ πάλιν πλήττει· ἔστι δὴ αἴτιον
375 τῆς μεγαλειότητος αὐτοῦ διὰ τὴν ἔξωθεν κίνησιν τοῦ ψυχικοῦ πνεύματος καὶ τοῦ ἐμφύτου θερμοῦ· τῆς λύπης ἀμυδρὸς καὶ μικρὸς καὶ ἀραιὸς καὶ ἀσθενής· καὶ χρόνιος ἤτοι ἀργὸς διὰ τὴν ἀποφυγὴν καὶ κατάδυσιν τοῦ ψυχικοῦ πνεύματος ἐπὶ τὸ βάθος· τοῦ θερμοῦ φρενίτου ὁ σφυγμὸς μικρὸς καὶ ἀμυδρὸς καὶ ἀσθενὴς συσφίγγων καὶ σκληρός· ὅταν δὲ γένηται [197ʳ] πυρετὸς θερμὸς γίνεται μέγας καὶ
380 πυκνὸς καὶ συνεχὴς διὰ τὸ εἶναι τὴν φλεγμονὴν κατὰ τὴν κοιλίαν τοῦ ἐγκεφάλου· τοῦ λουτροῦ μέγας καὶ σφοδρὸς καὶ μαλακός· ὕστερον δὲ ψηλὸς γίνεται ἢ καὶ συνεχὴς διὰ τὴν αἰτίαν τῆς κινήσεως τῆς θερμασίας καὶ διὰ τὴν χρείαν· εἰ δὲ χρονήσει ἐν τῷ λουτρῷ καὶ διαφορηθῇ ἡ θερμασία, ὁ σφυγμὸς γίνεται ἀμυδρὸς καὶ ἀσθενὴς καὶ ἀραιὸς εἰ δὲ λουθῶσιν ἐν ὕδασι ψυχροῖς καὶ διαπεράσει ἡ
385 ψυχρότης τοῦ ὕδατος κατὰ τὸ βάθος τοῦ σώματος· ὁ σφυγμὸς γίνεται μικρὸς καὶ ἀμυδρὸς καὶ ἀραιὸς καὶ ἀσθενής· εἰ δὲ ψυχρανθῇ ἔξω τὸ σῶμα καὶ ἡ θερμασία ὅλη συναχθῇ εἰς τὸ βάθος τοῦ σώματος, ὁ σφυγμὸς γίνεται σφοδρὸς καὶ μέγας καὶ πυκνὸς τὰ δὲ αὐτοφυᾶ ὕδατα ξηραντικὰ ὄντα καὶ στυπτηριώδη, τὸν σφυγμὸν σκληρὸν ποιοῦσιν· ὅσα δὲ τῶν ὑδάτων εἰσὶ θερμαντικὰ οἷά εἰσι τὰ θειώδη καὶ
390 αὐτοφυᾶ τὸν σφυγμὸν μικρὸν ποιοῦσι· σφυγμὸς τῆς ὀδύνης λεπτός ἐστι καὶ συνεχὴς εἰ δέ ἐστι ἡ ὀδύνη μεγάλη ἀλλὰ ἀνίσχυρος ὁ σφυγμὸς γίνεται μικρὸς ἀμυδρὸς σκωληκίζων καὶ μυρμηκίζων· ὁ σφυγμὸς τῆς φλεγμονῆς τῶν νεφρῶν· θερμὸς καὶ ἐμπρίων καὶ τρομώδης· καὶ τρέπεται εἰς συνεχῆ καὶ πυκνόν· διότι ἡ φλεγμονὴ πιέζει τὴν φλέβα καὶ ὁ πιεσμὸς ἀνάγκην ποιεῖ σκληρύνεσθαι τὴν
395 φλέβα· καὶ ἡ φλεγμονὴ καὶ ἡ ὀδύνη διὰ τὴν βίαν ταράττουσι τὴν φύσιν τῶν νευρωδῶν μορίων διὰ ταύτην γοῦν τὴν αἰτίαν ἐμπρίων καὶ τρομώδης καὶ συνεχὴς καὶ πυκνός· ὁ σφυγμὸς τῆς σκληρᾶς φλεγμονῆς ἤγουν τῶν νεύρων, ἐμπρίων ἐστὶ καὶ ὅσον ἐστὶν ἡ φλεγμονὴ σκληροτέρα τοσοῦτον γίνεται ἐμπριότερος·

ὁ σφυγμὸς δὲ τῆς μαλακῆς φλεγμονῆς, κυματώδης ἐστὶ διὰ τὴν μαλακότητα
τοῦ ὀργάνου· τῆς δὲ ψυχρᾶς φλεγμονῆς· ἀραιός ἐστι· ὅτι ἡ ψυχρὰ δυσκρασία   400
τὴν σκληρότητα ἀναγκάζειν ποιεῖ τοὺς σφυγμούς· σφυγμὸς τῆς πεμφθείσης
φλεγμονῆς κυματώδεις γίνεται ὅτι ὅταν πεμφθῇ ἡ φλεγμονὴ ὁ τεινεσμὸς αὐτῆς
λύεται· καὶ τὸ ὄργανον μαλθακὸν γίνεται καὶ ὁμαλὸν καὶ ἡ μαλακότης ἀναγκάζει
γενέσθαι κῦμα· τοῦ δὲ ψυχροῦ φρενίτου διὰ τὴν αἰτίαν τῆς ψυχρᾶς δυσκρασίας·
γίνεται ἀργὸς καὶ διὰ τὴν φλεγματικὴν ὕλην γίνεται κυματώδης· ἡ δὲ ἀρτηρία   405
διὰ τὴν αἰτίαν τοῦ πολλοῦ φλέγματος γίνεται στενή· σφυγμὸς τῆς θερμῆς
κεφαλαλγίας συνεχὴς γίνεται καὶ πυκνός· τῆς δὲ ψυχρᾶς κεφαλαλγίας διὰ τὴν
αἰτίαν τῆς ψυχρᾶς δυσκρασίας, γίνεται ἀραιὸς καὶ ἀργός· τῶν ἐρώντων μέγας
γίνεται· μᾶλλον δὲ ὅταν ἀκούσωσι τὶ περὶ τῶν ἐρωμένων· ἢ ὅταν αὐτοὺς ἴδωσιν
τῆς διαστροφῆς τοῦ προσώπου καὶ τοῦ στόματος σκληρός· τῶν δ' ἑπομένων   410
κυματώδης καὶ ἄνισος ἀμυδρὸς καὶ ἀργός· εἰ δέ ἐστιν ἡ δύναμις ἀσθενὴς
καὶ ὁ σφυγμὸς ἀσθενής ἐστι· τῶν ἐπιληπτικῶν ὅθεν ἐστὶ ἐκτὸς φλέγματος τὸ
πάθος· ἄνισος· ἀργός· καὶ ἀραιός· ὅθεν δὲ ἀπὸ χολῆς μελαίνης καὶ σκληρὸς
καὶ μικρός· τῆς δὲ πολυφαγίας καὶ πολυποσίας διὰ τὸ ποιεῖν βάρος ἐναντιώσεις
ἔχει ταχὺς καὶ πυκνός· [197ᵛ] καὶ ἀραιὸς καὶ μικρός· ψευδῆ φαντασίαν ἔχων· ἡ   415
δὲ σύμμετρος βρῶσις καὶ πόσις διὰ τὸ λαμβάνειν τὸ ψυχικὸν πνεῦμα δύναμιν
ἀπὸ τῆς πέψεως καὶ βοήθειαν γίνεται ὁ σφυγμὸς μέγας καὶ σφοδρὸς καὶ ταχὺς
τῶν δὲ ὀλιγοσιτιζομένων ὁ σφυγμὸς κατὰ τὸ μέτρον τῆς δυνάμεώς ἐστιν εἰς
ὅσον λαμβάνουσιν τῶν δὲ παχέων ἀνθρώπων ὁ σφυγμὸς ὅταν φάγωσι τινὰ τῶν
θερμαινόντων ἀσθενὴς γίνεται ὅτι ἡ κρᾶσις αὐτῶν θερμοτέρα γίνεται καὶ τίκτει   420
δυσκρασίαν ἡ δὲ δυσκρασία φέρει ἀσθένειαν τοῦ σφυγμοῦ· διότι ἡ δυσκρασία
αὐτῶν γίνεται θερμοτέρα καὶ ἡ χρεία τοῦ ἀέρος περισσοτέρα γίνεται· καὶ ἡ πολλὴ
χρεία ταχύτατον ποιεῖ τὸν σφυγμὸν ἢ πυκνότατον· εἰ δὲ μετὰ λάβουσι τὰ τῶν
ψυχόντων ἀνάγκη γίνεται ἵνα ἡ κρᾶσις αὐτῶν γένηται σύμμετρος τὸν αὐτὸν οὖν
τρόπον καὶ οἱ λεπτοὶ ἄνθρωποι· εἰ φάγωσί τι τῶν ψυχόντων δυσκρασία ψυχρὰ   425
τήκτεται· καὶ ὁ σφυγμὸς αὐτῶν μικρὸς καὶ ἀσθενὴς καὶ βραδὺς γίνεται· εἰ δὲ
φάγωσι τι τῶν θερμαινόντων ὁ σφυγμὸς εἰς συμμετρίαν τρέπεται καὶ γίνεται ὁ
σφυγμὸς σφοδρός· εἰ δὲ μεταλάβοι τι τῶν μοχθηρῶν ἢ τῶν χρηστῶν κατ' αὐτῶν
τῶν ληφθέντων ἀλλοιοῦται ὁ σφυγμός· καὶ κατὰ τὴν βλάβην καὶ ὠφέλειαν τῶν
ληφθέντων· διὰ τοῦτο χρὴ τὸν ἰατρὸν ἐπιτηρεῖν ἑκάστου τῶν μετὰ λαμβανόντων   430
τὰ διαφορὰς καὶ ζητεῖν τὸν ὄντα σφυγμόν· πόσιν δὲ ἐνταῦθα τὸν οἶνον λέγουσι·
καὶ ἡ ἄμετρος πόσις αὐτοὺς τοὺς σφυγμοὺς τρέπει διὰ τὸ βάρος ὥσπερ καὶ
τὸ πλῆθος τῆς βρώσεως· ἀλλ' ἡ ἐναντίωσις τῆς βρώσεως οὐκ ἔστι κατὰ τὴν
ἐναντίωσιν τοῦ οἴνου· ὅτι ἡ οὐσία τοῦ οἴνου λεπτή ἐστι καὶ ἐλαφρὰ καὶ ὁ πολὺς
οἶνος πληρεῖ τὰς φλέβας καὶ ἔστι φόβος ἵνα μὴ ἀποπνιγῇ καὶ τὸ ἔμφυτον θερμὸν   435
εἰς τὸ βάθος· καὶ φθαρεῖ ἀνὰ μέσον τῆς μέσης ὁ ἄνθρωπος· ἀλλ' ὁ οἶνος ὁ ἔχων

About the Authenticity of Galen's Περὶ ἀλυπίας in Medieval Hebrew, Compared to the Recently Found Greek Text[1]

Mauro Zonta

It is known that in the Middle Ages, and in European Jewish culture in particular, there were cases of texts ascribed to Galen, which were partially or totally the fruit of an anonymous Medieval Jewish writer. Among the Hebrew sources here examined, there is a text which is apparently identical, or very similar at least, to another text by Galen: Περὶ ἀλυπίας.[2]

The short philosophical treatise Περὶ ἀλυπίας (Latin *De indolentia*, English *Avoiding Distress*) was written by Galen at the beginning of year 193. He wrote it as a reply to a letter he had just received from an anonymous friend dealing with that subject. The first part of the treatise deals with the fire in Galen's house, which had happened in the spring of 192, when Galen's library was destroyed. The purpose of this article is to show how the study of Περὶ ἀλυπίας can be of interest for the general textual history of Medieval Hebrew versions of Galen's works, whether complete or partial, and maybe even for some aspects of their formation.

The original Greek text of Περὶ ἀλυπίας was believed to be totally lost until the beginning of this century. Therefore, during the twentieth century some scholars tried to collect and even to reconstruct parts of the lost text, since they were not available in Greek, but only in Arabic and Hebrew. The best two attempts at reconstructing the Περὶ ἀλυπίας were made by Abraham S. Halkin and by the present author. Halkin, in a 1944 article about the Greek and Arabic sources of a Medieval Judeo-Arabic scientific-philosophical work, the *Ṭibb al-nufūs* (*Medicine of souls*) by Yosef Ibn ʿAqnīn (1200 ca.), published, translated into English and studied some passages of Galen's work, which he had discovered in Ibn ʿAqnīn's text.[3] In his turn, in a 1995 book on Galen as a philosopher as quoted in Shem Tov Ibn Falaquera's Hebrew works (1250–1290 ca.), I pointed out that not only

---

[1] Unfortunately, Mauro Zonta died before being able to revise this paper for publication. We [the editors] are grateful to Tzvi Langermann for correcting some errors, but have otherwise left the paper in the condition in which it was submitted for publication, other than updating some bibliographical information.

[2] I am grateful to Tzvi Langermann and the participants in the *Galen Conference*, Safed (Israel), November 27th, 2012, in which the contents of this article were first presented and discussed.

[3] Abraham S. Halkin, 'Classical and Arabic Material in Ibn ʿAḵnīn's "Hygiene of the Soul"', *Proceedings of the American Academy for Jewish Research*, 14, 1944, pp. 25–147.

the three passages found in Arabic in Ibn ʿAqnīn's work, but also at least another five passages, were quoted by Falaquera in his consolatory work, *Ṣeri ha-yagon* (*The Balm for Sorrow*).[4] In this text, of which a critical edition (without any attempt at identifying the relevant passages) had been made by Roberta Klugman Barkan in 1974, Falaquera ascribed the three plus five passages to an anonymous 'sage';[5] I suggested this sage ought to be identified with Galen himself. Only in 2005 did Véronique Boudon-Millot and Antoine Pietrobelli rediscover in a Greek MS (Thessalonica, Vlatadon, n. 14, folios 10v–14v) what was apparently the original text of Galen's work.[6] Unfortunately, as the discoverers of the text correctly pointed out, the Thessalonica MS was so badly flawed that the tentative reconstruction of the original text needed some years of work. An *editio princeps* was published in 2007 by Boudon-Millot in a collective volume.[7] But over the next five years, four tentative critical editions, and a 'modern critical translation', of Galen's work were made, as follows:

1. that by Boudon-Millot, together with Jacques Jouanna and Antoine Pietrobelli, as published in 2010 in Paris, in the Collection des Universités de France (Les Belles Lettres).[8] It includes a long introduction, a French translation facing the Greek text, and a long and detailed commentary;

2. that by Paraskevi Kotzia and Panagiotis Sotiroudis, published in 2010 in the review 'Hellenika', in Thessalonica.[9] The Greek text also includes a Modern Greek translation and a commentary;

3. that by Ivan Garofalo and Alessandro Lami, published in 2012 in Milan.[10] This too, like the French edition, includes a philosophical and historic-philological introduction, an Italian translation facing the Greek text, some

[4] Mauro Zonta, 'Un interprete ebreo della filosofia di Galeno. Gli scritti filosofici di Galeno nell'opera di Shem Tov Ibn Falaquera', *Eurasiatica* 39, Turin, 1995, pp. 113–123.

[5] Roberta Klugman Barkan, *Shem Tov ben Joseph Ibn Falaquera's 'Sori Yagon' or 'Balm for Assuaging Grief', its Literary Sources and Traditions*, unpublished Ph.D. Thesis, Columbia University, 1974; see Zonta, 'Un interprete ebreo della filosofia di Galeno' (n. 4 above), p. 114.

[6] Véronique Boudon-Millot – Antoine Pietrobelli, 'De l'arabe au grec: un nouveau témoin du texte de Galien (le manuscript Vlatadon 14)', *CRAI* 149-2, 2005, pp. 497–534.

[7] Véronique Boudon-Millot, 'Un traité perdu de Galien miraculeusement retrouvé, le *Sur l'inutilité de se chagriner*: texte grec et traduction française', in Véronique Boudon-Millot, Alessia Guardasole, Caroline Magdelaine (eds.), *La science médicale antique. Nouveaux regards*, Paris, 2007, pp. 72–123.

[8] Véronique Boudon-Millot, Jacques Jouanna, Antoine Pietrobelli (eds.), *Galien. Tome IV: Ne pas se chagriner, édition critique et traduction*, Collection des Universités de France, Paris, 2010.

[9] Paraskevi Kotzia and Panagiotis Sotiroudis (eds.), Γαληνοῦ Περὶ ἀλυπίας, *Hellenika*, 60 (2010), pp. 63–150.

[10] Ivan Garofalo and Alessandro Lami (eds.), *Galeno, L'anima e il dolore. De indolentia. De propriis placitis*, Biblioteca Universale Rizzoli, Rizzoli, Milan, 2012.

notes about the contents of the work and, finally, a very interesting comparison of the emendations of the Greek which are found in the three already published editions;

4. that by Mario Vegetti, published in 2013 in Rome in an Italian translation and the original Greek (which corresponds to Boudon-Millot's text);[11]

5. that by Vivian Nutton, which appeared in 2014 in English translation only.[12]

The four already published editions of Galen's work seem to have given no importance to Falaquera's quotations of the work. Kotzia and Sotiroudis do not mention them at all; Boudon-Millot, Jouanna and Pietrobelli only mention the three quotations of the Greek text shared by Ibn ʿAqnīn and Falaquera;[13] and in this they are followed by Garofalo and Lami,[14] and Nutton.[15] So, a reassessment of the paternity of this text in the Medieval Hebrew tradition, and in Falaquera's quotations in particular, is needed. One should try to re-examine the eight Hebrew passages ascribed to the 'sage' in order to arrive at some new tentative conclusions.

Let us start with a provisional English translation of these Hebrew passages.

14)[16] Said the sage: 'He who will have to live should prepare a strong soul in the face of misfortunes'.

He also said: 'Man needs to despise his life and be convinced that all things are sometimes good and sometimes bad, and (sometimes) contrary to what should be. Because of this, it is necessary that the individual, who is on his guard and intelligent, does not rejoice when he is successful and does not become sad when he is not successful, since all this is well known and life is short'.

---

[11] Mario Vegetti (ed.), *Galeno, Nuovi scritti autobiografici*, Rome, 2013, pp. 261–303.

[12] P. N. Singer (ed.), *Galen: Psychological Writings. Avoiding Distress, Character Traits, The Diagnosis and Treatment of the Affections and Errors Peculiar to Each Person's Soul, The Capacities of the Soul Depend on the Mixtures of the Body*, Cambridge, 2014, pp. 43–105.

[13] Boudon-Millot *et alii*, *Galien, tome IV*(note 8 as above), pp. 85–86. According to these editors, in Ibn ʿAqnīn's work there are not only the three passages which are partially or totally found in Falaquera as well (§§ 41, l. 22ff.; 42, l. 8–45, l. 4; 66), but also three other ones (§§ 4; 61, ll. 14–16; 79b, l. 14–82, l. 14). As a matter of fact, some of these passages (§§ 4, 41, and 42–45 in particular) seem to be free interpretations of the original Greek text: see the references of three of them as 'cf. Ibn ʿAqnīn' in the editorial notes of this edition.

[14] Garofalo – Lami, *Galeno, L'anima e il dolore* (note 10 as above), pp. XV–XVI. There is apparently no mention of Falaquera's quotations in Vegetti's work.

[15] In Singer, *Galen: Psychological Writings* (note 12 as above), p. 72.

[16] The numbering corresponds to that in Shem Tov Ibn Falaquera, *Ṣeri ha-yagon*, ed. Klugman-Barkan.

15) Said the sage: 'Misfortunes are easier to be tolerated if one knows that corruption (progressive degeneration) dominates one's existence'.

He also said: 'All that has a beginning should have an end too. The sage always remembers what might happen to him, but the fool, who is different from a wild animal since he does not get rest like the animals, is not worried about knowing man's conditions, with regard to what might happen to him every day'.

16) 'The man who thinks he has lost substantial and precious things, does not cease from his worry and his troubling thoughts, but the man who thinks that he has lost bad and inferior things, is not worried'.

17) 'It is said that a philosopher benefited from four villages; he happened to lose one of them, and three of them remained. A fellow citizen met him and showed his own grief for the loss. The philosopher laughed at him, and said: 'Why do you grieve for me? I have three villages and you do not have even one, but I do not grieve for you''.

18) 'Men are foolish. If one of them manages to have three villages, he says: 'Why don't I have thirty of them?''.

19) Said the sage: 'He who knows that generation and corruption follow on from each other in everything, is not sorry that misfortunes happen to him, since it is not possible to avoid them, and he tolerates them easily, since he has no way of driving them away'.

He also said: 'Time generates and corrupts, and the corruption of something is the cause of the generation of another thing'.

He said: 'Some misfortunes are difficult to be tolerated: he who is afflicted and tolerates them, shows his magnanimity. Others are easy to be tolerated: he who is afflicted and is not (able to) tolerate them, shows the cowardice of his soul'.

22) Said the sage: 'Like life, also joy and sorrow are not lasting so much, and worry about what is past is (a sign) of a diminished intelligence'.

He said: 'To be afraid of misfortune before it occurs is (a sign) of weakness of nature'.

23) Said the sage: 'There is no intelligence in worry'.

Now, let us study the table below. It includes the above three passages, nn. 16–18, which the French and Italian editors have accepted as Hebrew quotations of Galen's work. The present author will show similarities and differences, if any, among the quotations with respect to their Arabic version and to the original Greek texts. He also examines the other eight passages found in Falaquera's

Hebrew work only, in order to compare them to similar passages in Greek. The variant readings which have been put in the notes to the Greek text refer to the different versions of the text, as they are found in the three already published editions by Boudon-Millot, Jouanna and Pietrobelli, by Kotzia and Sotiroudis, and by Garofalo, as well as by Nutton in his English translation.[17]

	Galen, Περὶ ἀλυπίας, original Greek text, ed. Boudon-Millot, Jouanna and Pietrobelli	Galen, *Psychological Writings*, Greek-to-English transl. Nutton (adapted for the sake of parallelism)	Shem Tov Ibn Falaquera, Hebrew quotations from 'the Sage', in his *Ṣeri ha-yagon*, ed. Klugman-Barkan
	§ 52, ll. 4–5	p. 93, ll. 1–2	Passage n. 14, first quotation
1	Ἐγὼ δὲ παρὰ σοφοῦ τινος μαθών	As I once learned from a wise man,	:והחכם אומר
2			מי שרוצה לחיות
3	εἰς φροντίδ'ἀεὶ[18] συμφορὰς ἐβαλλόμην.	I fell to considering disasters constantly	.יכין לתלאות לב אמיץ
	§ 65, ll. 14–15, 17–19	p. 95, ll. 3–4, 6–7	Passage n. 14, second quotation
4			:ואמר
5	Ἐν τούτῳ τρεφόμενος ἀεὶ τῷ λογισμῷ	Brought up in this way of thinking,	צריך האדם שיבזה חייו
6	μικρὰ πάντα εἶναι νομίζω.	I always consider all these things as of little value.	ויאמין שמעשה העולם פעם טוב ופעם רע
7	(...)	(...)	והפך מה שירצה האדם
8	Τῷ δ'ἡγουμένῳ μικρὰ πάντα εἶναι,	And if someone regards all these as of little value,	ועל כן צריך האיש הזריז והמשכיל
9	τί ἂν ἐπὶ τούτοις	why should he worry about them,	שלא ישמח בהצליח דרכו
10	ἀπό τε αὐτῶν εἴη φροντίς;[19]	or be worried by them?	ולא ידאג שלא יצליח
11			מפני שהוא יודע שזה כולו נכרת

[17] They are based upon Garofalo's comparison as it is found in Garofalo – Lami, *Galeno, L'anima e il dolore* (note 10 as above), pp. 149–155.

[18] φροντίδ'ἀεὶ] φροντίδας νοῦν Kotzia and Sotiroudis; φροντίδας καὶ Garofalo.

[19] As pointed out by Nutton, in Singer, *Galen: Psychological Writings*, p. 95 n. 17, 'some words have been omitted and other wrongly copied over from the next line.'

	Galen, Περὶ ἀλυπίας, original Greek text, ed. Boudon-Millot, Jouanna and Pietrobelli	Galen, *Psychological Writings*, Greek-to-English transl. Nutton (adapted for the sake of parallelism)	Shem Tov Ibn Falaquera, Hebrew quotations from 'the Sage', in his *Ṣeri ha-yagon*, ed. Klugman-Barkan
12			ושהזמן קצר.
	§ 52, ll. 8–9	p. 93, ll. 5–6	Passage n. 15, first quotation
13			ואמר החכם:
14	εἴ τι	Should I ever	מי שידע
15	πάσχοιμ᾽ ὧν ἐδόξαζόν ποτε	suffer any of what I was imagining,	כי ההפסד מושל על הוויתו
16	μή μοι νεῶρες προσπεσὸν ψυχὴν δάκῃ.[20]	it might not gnaw at my soul because it was a novel arrival.	תהיינה התלאות קלות בעיניו.
	§ 53	p. 93, ll. 7–10	Passage n. 15, second quotation
17			ואמר:
18			כל מה שיש לו ראשית
19			יצריכהו ההכרח להיות לו אחרית
20	Ὁ μὲν οὖν σοφὸς ἀνὴρ ἑαυτὸν ἀναμιμνῄσκει διὰ παντὸς	The wise man constantly reminds himself of everything	והאדם החכם יזכיר לנפשו תמיד
21	ὧν ἐνδέχεται παθεῖν,	that he might possibly suffer,	מה שאיפשר שיקרהו
22	ὁ δὲ μὴ σοφὸς μέν,	and someone who is not a wise man,	אבל הסכל שהוא כבהמה
23	οὐ μὴν ὥσπερ βόσκημα ζῶν,	provided that he does not live like a domestic animal,	אלא שאינו הולך על פש(?) כמו הבהמות
24	ἐκ τῶν ὁσημέραι γινομένων ἐπεγείρεταί πως καὶ αὐτὸς	by the realities of daily life is in some way also stimulated	לא יתעורר לדעת עניני בני האדם
25	εἰς τὴν τῶν ἀνθρωπίνων πραγμάτων γνῶσιν.	to the knowledge of the human condition.	בדברים שיקרו להם בכל יום.

[20] See also Galen's passage, § 78a, about the same quotation by Euripides: μόνην γε ταύτην <ἄσκησιν> εὑρίσκω πρὸς τὰς ἀνιαρὰς περιστάσεις, 'this is the only <training> I find helpful against painful bad turns.' (Nutton, in Singer, *Galen: Psychological Writings*, p. 97, ll. 13–14). This passage, ascribed to Aristoteles, is found in Moshe Ibn ʿEzra's *Kitāb al-muḥāḍara* too: see Zonta, *Un interprete ebreo della filosofia di Galeno* (note 4 as above), p. 116.

	Galen, Περὶ ἀλυπίας, original text, ed. Boudon-Millot, Jouanna and Pietrobelli	Galen, *Psychological Writings*, Greek-to-English transl. Nutton	Ibn ʿAqnīn's quotations of Galen's Περὶ ἀλυπίας	Shem Tov Ibn Falaquera, Hebrew quotations from 'the Sage', in his *Ṣeri ha-yagon*, ed. Klugman-Barkan
	§ 66	p. 95, ll. 7–10	Passage n. 185	Passage n. 16
26	Ἀκόλουθον γὰρ ἐστι τῷ μὲν ὑπολαβόντι	It follows also that someone who supposed that	الذي يظن انه سلب	והאדם שחושב שאבד
27	μεγαλεῖα²¹ ἐστερῆσθαι,	he has been deprived of something big	امورا جسمية²² جليلة	דברים גדולים ויקרים
28	λυπεῖσθαί τε	must always be distressed	يلزمة الاغتمام	לא תסור ממנו הדאגה
29	καὶ φροντίζειν ἀεί,	and fret,	والفكر الدائمة	והמחשבה תמיד
30	τῷ δὲ σμικρῶν	unlike the person who thinks them	واما الذي يظن انه انما سلب	אבל החושב שאבד
31	ἀεὶ διὰ τέλους²³ καταφρονοῦντι,	small and continues to despise them,	امورا خسيسة دنية	דבר גרוע ופחות
32	<μηδέποτε λυπεῖσθαι>.²⁴	<who will never grieve>	فانه يلبث غير مغموم	לא ידאג
	§ 41, l. 22–§ 42, l. 7	p. 90, ll. 7–12	Passage n. 182	Passage n. 17
33	(Ἀρίστιππος [§ 39])	(Aristippus)	وحكى عن ارسطيفوس	וזכרו כי אחד הפילוסופים
34	τέσσαρας ἔχων ἀγροὺς ἐπὶ τῆς πατρίδος,	He had back home four fields,	انه كانت له اربعة قريات	היו לו ארבעה כפרים
35	ἕνα κατά τινα περίστασιν τῶν πραγμάτων ἐξ αὐτῶν	but because of some bad turn in his affairs,	فعرض عارض ذهبت منه	וקרה לו מקרה
36	ἀπήλασεν²⁵	he lost one,	بسببه واحدة منهم	שאבד הכפר האחד

²¹ μεγαλεῖα] μεγάλων Garofalo.

²² According to Garofalo, it should be corrected as جسمة.

²³ διὰ τέλους] διατελεῖν Garofalo.

²⁴ <μηδέποτε λυπεῖσθαι>] <μή> Kotzia and Sotiroudis; *om.* Garofalo.

²⁵ ἀπήλασεν] ἀπώλεσεν Garofalo.

	Galen, Περὶ ἀλυπίας, original text, ed. Boudon-Millot, Jouanna and Pietrobelli	Galen, *Psychological Writings*, Greek-to-English transl. Nutton	Ibn ʿAqnīn's quotations of Galen's Περὶ ἀλυπίας	Shem Tov Ibn Falaquera, Hebrew quotations from 'the Sage', in his *Ṣeri ha-yagon*, ed. Klugman-Barkan
37	ὡς λοιπὸν ἔχειν τρεῖς.	so that he then had three.	وبقيت له ثلاثة	וישארו לו השלשה
38	Ἀπαντήσας οὖν τις τῶν πολιτῶν	One of his fellow-citizens	فلقيه رجل من اهل مدينته	ויפגע בו אחד מבני עירו
39	οἷος²⁶ ἦν ἐπὶ τῇ ζημίᾳ	was eager to commiserate with him	وجعل يظهر له انه قد اغتم	והיה מראה לו שהיה דואג
40	συλλυπεῖσθαι·	when they met,	من اجله بما ناله من الخسارة	על מה שאבר
41	γελάσας οὖν ὁ Ἀρίστιππος	but Aristippus said with a laugh:	فضحك منه.	ויצחק ממנו הפילוסוף
42	ἔφη· τί μᾶλλον ἐμοὶ <σὺ>²⁷ συλλυπήσῃ	'Why should you commiserate with me	قال له : ما بانك انت بالاغتمام لي	ויאמר לו: מדוע אתה דואג עלי
43	τρεῖς ἀγροὺς ἔχοντι	for having three fields	وانا لي ثلاثة قريات	ויש לי עוד שלשה כפרים
44	τοιούτους οἷον <ἕνα>²⁸ μόνον αὐτὸς²⁹ ἔχεις	when you haven't even one?	ليس لك مثل واحدة منهن	ואין לך מהם אפי׳ אחד מהן
45	ἢ ἐγώ σοι συλλυπήσομαι;	Or should I commiserate with you?'	ولا اكون انا المغتم لك	ואין אני דואג עליך?
	§ 42, ll. 9–11	p. 90, ll. 14–15	Passage n. 183	Passage n. 18
46			(...)	ובני אדם קוצר דעתם
47	οἱ τρεῖς ἀγροὺς	Those who have inherited	الذين ورثون	אם יגיע אחד מהם
48	δεξάμενοι τοῦ πατρὸς	three fields from their father	عن ابائهم ثلاثة قريات	שיהיו לו שלשה כפרים

²⁶ οἷος] ἕτοιμος Nutton (allegedly from Garofalo).

²⁷ <σὺ>] *omittunt* Kotzia and Sotiroudis, Garofalo.

²⁸ <ἕνα>] *omittunt* Kotzia and Sotiroudis, Garofalo, Nutton.

²⁹ + <οὐκ> Kotzia and Sotiroudis, Garofalo, Nutton.

	Galen, Περὶ ἀλυπίας, original text, ed. Boudon-Millot, Jouanna and Pietrobelli	Galen, *Psychological Writings*, Greek-to-English transl. Nutton	Ibn ʿAqnīn's quotations of Galen's Περὶ ἀλυπίας	Shem Tov Ibn Falaquera, Hebrew quotations from 'the Sage', in his *Ṣeri ha-yagon*, ed. Klugman-Barkan
49	οὐκ ἀνέξονται βλέπειν[30]	will not abide	لا يصبرون ولا يحتملون ان يكون ينظرون	ואמר בלבו:
50	ἑτέρους ἔχοντας τριάκοντα·	looking at others with thirty.	قوما لهم ثلاثون قرية	למה לא יהיו לי שלשים?

	Galen, Περὶ ἀλυπίας, original Greek text, ed. Boudon-Millot, Jouanna and Pietrobelli	Galen, *Psychological Writings*, Greek-to-English transl. Nutton	Shem Tov Ibn Falaquera, Hebrew quotations from 'the Sage', in his *Ṣeri ha-yagon*, ed. Klugman-Barkan
	§ 74, ll. 14–16	p. 96, ll. 17–19	Passage n. 19, first quotation
51			ואמר החכם:
52	ἀσκεῖν <δ> ἀξιώσας τὰς φαντασίας εἰς ἄπαν δεινόν,	And even though I have thought right to train my imagination	מי שידע כי ההויה וההפסד באים זה אחר זה על כל הדברים
53	ὡς μετρίως ἐνεγνεῖν αὐτό,	to face every disaster with moderation,	לא ידאג בבוא התלאות עליו
54	περιπεσεῖν [δὲ] οὐκ ἂν εὐξαίμην οὐδενὶ τῶν λυπῆσαί με δυναμένων.	I would never pray to meet with anything that could distress me.	כי אי אפשר מהיותן
55			ותהיינה קלות בעיניו מאחר שאין ביכולתו לדחותן.
	§ 54, ll. 1–2, 4–6	p. 93, ll. 14–15	Passage n. 19, second quotation
56			ואמר:
57	παρ' ὅλον τὸν χρόνον (...) καθ' ἑκάστην ἡμέραν κἀγὼ θεώμενος ἕκαστον αὐτῶν	[in the whole time] (...) when I saw all of these things happening daily,	והזמן מוליד ומאבד

[30] οὐκ ἀνέξονται βλέπειν] οὐκ ἀνέξοντο βλέπειν οὐκ ἀνέξονται Thessalonica MS; βλέπειν οὐκ ἀνέξονται Kotzia and Sotiroudis, Garofalo, Nutton.

	Galen, Περὶ ἀλυπίας, original Greek text, ed. Boudon-Millot, Jouanna and Pietrobelli	Galen, *Psychological Writings*, Greek-to-English transl. Nutton	Shem Tov Ibn Falaquera, Hebrew quotations from 'the Sage', in his *Ṣeri ha-yagon*, ed. Klugman-Barkan
58	ἐγύμνασά μου τὰς φαντασίας πρὸς ἀπώλειαν πάντων ὧν ἔχω	I schooled my imagination to prepare for the total loss of everything that I had.	והפסד עם אחד סבה להוית עם אחר.
	§ 50b, ll. 10 and 15–17, and § 50a, ll. 8–9	p. 92, ll. 3–4, 8, 2–3	Passage n. 19, third quotation
59			‏ויאמר:
60	τὸ πάντα μὲν ἀπολέσαντα (...)	But not to be distressed at the loss of all (...)	מקצת רוע המזל קשה לשאת אותו
61	ἐδείκνυτο[31] μὴ λυπηθῆναι γενναῖον ἤδη τοῦτο καὶ μεγαλοψυχίας ἐχόμενον ἐπίδειγμα πρῶτον. (...)	that is already a prime display of nobility and nigh on magnanimity. (...)	ובעת שיקרה לאדם וישאהו יורה על גדולת נפשו
62	οὐδὲ γὰρ οὐδὲ τοῦτο μέγα μὴ μανῆναι τὴν μανίαν πολλῶν (...)	(On the contrary,) it was no great thing to avoid the madness of most people (...)	ומקצתו קל לשאת ובעת שיקרה לאדם ולא ישאהו יורה על שפלות נפשו.
	§ 62, ll. 19–22	p. 94, ll. 15–16	Passage n. 22, first quotation
63			‏והחכם אומר:
64	τοὺς δὲ τῶν τοιούτων ἡδονῶν καταφρονοῦντας, ἀρκουμένους δὲ τῷ μήτε ἀλγεῖν μήτε λυπεῖσθαι τὴν ψυχήν, οὐδέποτε ἐπήνεσεν,[32]	But he never praised those who despise such pleasures and who are simply satisfied that their soul is never pained or distressed,	כימים לא יתמידו השמחה ולא היגון והדאגה על מה שעבר שפלות השכל.
	§ 62, l. 22–l. 1	p. 94, ll. 17–18	Passage n. 22, second quotation
65			‏ואמר:
66	ἀπομαντευόμενος μεῖζόν τι καὶ κρεῖττον <ὂν>[33] τὸ ἀγαθὸν ἰδίαν ἔχειν φύσιν,	proclaiming that the good was of its own nature something bigger and better than this,	הפחד מהתלאה קודם שתבוא עיפות מהטבע.

[31] ἐδείκνυτο] <ἂν ἐπ>ἐδείκνυτο Garofalo.

[32] ἐπήνεσεν] ἔπεισεν Thessalonika MS, Kotzia and Sotiroudis.

[33] <ὂν>] *om.* Thessalonika MS, Garofalo; <εἶναι> Kotzia and Sotiroudis.

	Galen, Περὶ ἀλυπίας, original Greek text, ed. Boudon-Millot, Jouanna and Pietrobelli	Galen, *Psychological Writings*, Greek-to-English transl. Nutton	Shem Tov Ibn Falaquera, Hebrew quotations from 'the Sage', in his *Șeri ha-yagon*, ed. Klugman-Barkan
	§ 62, ll. 1–2	p. 94, l. 18	Passage n. 23
67			וַאֲמַר הֶחָכָם:
68	οὖν ἐν μόνῳ τῷ μήτε ἀλγεῖν μήτε λυπεῖσθαι περιγραφόμενον.	not confined to being merely free from pain and distress.	אֵין עִם הַדְּאָגָה שֵׂכֶל.

The case of passage n. 15, second quotation, seems to be of some textual relevance. Falaquera's Hebrew text offers a totally different interpretation of the contents of this passage with respect to the Greek text. In the Hebrew, we find an antithesis between the sage and the not-sage (here explicitly called 'foolish'); in the Greek, the not-sage is regarded as not substantially different from the sage with regard to grief. This difference might be simply due to a negative particle; this negative particle (Hebrew *lo'*, corresponding to Greek οὐ or something similar) may come either from the lost Arabic version, or from the Greek manuscript from which the Arabic version was made.

Here one can give a first detailed comparison of the above passages in Greek, Arabic and Hebrew. One could try to make some tentative observations about them, as follows:

1. Ibn ʿAqnīn's Judeo-Arabic quotations of Galen, i.e. passages nn. 182, 183 and 185, which have been compared to the corresponding Hebrew passages nn. 16, 17 and 18, are substantially faithful in contents with respect to their source, i.e., the original Greek text of the Περὶ ἀλυπίας. However, two of them (nn. 17–18) are rather free in their literal form – something which is found in other passages of Falaquera's quotations;

2. passages nn. 14–15, and the second part of passage n. 15 in particular, apparently escaped the notice of the French, Greek and Italian editors of Galen's work. As a matter of fact, they are not found in Ibn ʿAqnīn, but they more or less correspond to passages of the Greek text, so that they might contribute – like the other three ones – to the reconstruction of the Greek text or at least to its textual history.

3. it should be pointed out that, when he explicitly quotes the 'sage', Falaquera is not clear about his source. Passages n. 14 and n. 19, first and third quotations, which are ascribed to the 'sage', are partially, but not totally, altered with respect to the Greek text; however, the alteration is in form, not in substance. Passages nn. 15–18 form a unit, whose *incipit*, 'said the sage',

seems to include all of them, and provide an even more interesting case-study: while the second quotation has no apparent correspondence to the Greek text, almost all the other passages correspond both to the Greek text and to the Judeo-Arabic quotations by Ibn ʿAqnīn – as the present author has mentioned before. Finally, passages 19 (second quotation), 22, and 23, which have the reference to the 'sage' at their beginnings, are apparently altered, but not totally different, with respect to the Greek text. Here Falaquera seems to have interpreted, in a different way, what he read in the lost Arabic text of these quotations.

From the comparison to Ibn ʿAqnīn's text which was made in 1995, the present author suggested that all these passages were apparently taken from the (then unknown) Greek text. Now, in this re-assessment, he suggests three different explanations.

The first hypothesis is that the 'sage' quoted by Falaquera in his *Seri ha-yagon* was some unknown author, probably an Arabic one, who in his turn employed Galen's Περὶ ἀλυπίας among his sources. This could explain the fact that some quotations of the 'sage' are identical to passages of the original Greek text, while others are not. However, that author was apparently not Ibn ʿAqnīn, since some of the above passages (nn. 14–15, 19, 22–23) are not found in his *Ṭibb al-nufūs*, and two of them are more or less literally found in the Greek text of the Περὶ ἀλυπίας. This can be the most economical solution, but another one might be suggested.

The second hypothesis is that Falaquera might have had at his disposal an Arabic rendering of a work by Galen, which was not totally identical to the Greek text of the Περὶ ἀλυπίας. This hypotheses may explain some facts:

1. the Arabic text quoted by Ibn ʿAqnīn has the title *Nafy al-ghamm* (*The Refusal of Affliction* or *of Anxiety*), which is different from the title of the Greek text rendered into Arabic by Hubaysh, *Fī ṣarf al-ightimām* (*About Turning away the Fact of Being Distressed*);[34]
2. Galen himself, near the end of the Greek text of the Περὶ ἀλυπίας (§ 79b, ll. 11–12) as it is found in the Thessalonica MS, tells the anonymous addressee of the work about 'the advice he has already given by writing to others about the absence of affliction' (ἃ δ᾽ἄλλοις γράφων εἰς ἀλυπίαν συνεβούλευσα), so apparently referring to another work on the same subject – which commonly occurs in Galen's works;

---

[34] As it is pointed out in Garofalo – Lami, *Galeno, L'anima e il dolore* (n. 10 as above), pp. XIV–XV.

3. in a previous passage of the same work (§ 68), Galen hints at another work by himself, Περὶ ἀοχλησίας, a treatise 'about the absence of (emotional) distress' against Epicurus.[35] Such a title seems to be very similar to that of Galen's work as quoted by Ibn 'Aqnīn.

The third hypothesis is as follows. We can explain the partial difference between Falaquera's quotations on the one hand, and the original Greek text on the other, by thinking that there are different Arabic translations of the same Greek work, as seen in other cases (e.g. for the two partially different versions of the lost Greek text of Alexander of Aphrodisias' *De principiis*),[36] Moreover, here in Galen's case this difference might be due to the difference of the original Greek texts itself, which is often difficult to be read and sometimes incomplete.

The third solution seems the most complex one, but it cannot be totally excluded. For, in some cases, Falaquera is so literal in following each word of his Arabic source, that we can employ his quotation for the textual reconstruction of a passage.[37] In other cases, on the contrary, he is more free with regard to some of his sources: he apparently adapts them to his own requirements and thought. In conclusion, all the above quotations by Falaquera of the 'sage' in his *Ṣeri ha-yagon*, in different ways, coincide with passages in Galen's Περὶ ἀλυπίας (so being a sort of '[pseudo?-] Galen'). Therefore, these should be an important source for the textual reconstruction of this important work and the history of its tradition.

---

[35] This fact is pointed out by Garofalo – Lami, *Galeno, L'anima e il dolore*, p. 44 note.

[36] See Silvia Fazzo and Mauro Zonta, 'Towards a Textual History and Reconstruction of Alexander of Aphrodisias's Treatise On the Principles of the Universe', *Journal of Semitic Studies*, 59, 2014, pp. 91–116; Silvia Fazzo and Mauro Zonta, 'Toward a "Critical Translation" of Alexander of Aphrodisias' *De principiis*, Based on the Indirect Tradition of Syriac and Arabic Sources', *Chôra. Revue d'études anciennes et médiévales*, 2015, pp. 63–101.

[37] The present author has found something similar in Falaquera's quotations of Averroes' *Middle Commentary* on Aristotle's *Metaphysics*: see Mauro Zonta, 'A Case of 'Author's Variant Readings' and the Textual History of Averroes' *Middle Commentary* on Aristotle's *Metaphysics*', in Jacqueline Hamesse – Olga Weijers (eds.), *Ecriture et réécriture des textes philosophiques médiévaux. Volume d'hommage offert à Colette Sirat*, Textes et études du Moyen Age 34, Turnhout 2006, pp. 465–483.

Pseudo-Galenic texts in the Editions of Galen, 1490–1689*

Stefania Fortuna

In the initial passage of *De libris propriis*,[1] Galen tells us that he was writing this specific text in order to list his own works and describe their content, so that they could be easily distinguished from forgeries that were sold by bookshops in the Sandalarium, in Rome. Despite Galen's effort, in Late Antiquity and the Early Middle Ages, there were more Pseudo-Galenic texts available in Latin than Galenic works, and there was no interest in their authenticity.[2] Since the eleventh century and during the Late Middle Ages, when many works of Galen were translated from Arabic and from Greek, some of the preceding Pseudo-Galenic texts continued to have the same reception as the authentic ones, and other new works were attributed to Galen and added to his *corpus* for various reasons.[3] Therefore, it is not surprising that the first complete edition of Galen published in Venice in 1490 contains seventy-nine Latin translations and texts, twenty-four of which are Pseudo-Galenic – about thirty percent. Even though the Pseudo-Galenic works account for a much lower percentage in terms of pages – because none are as vast as Galen's treatises, e.g. *Methodus medendi, De simplicium medicamentorum facultatibus, De usu partium*, and *De sanitate tuenda* – they are nonetheless a significant portion of this edition.

From 1490 to the seventeenth century, twenty-five complete editions of Galen's works were published: two Greek editions, i.e. the Aldine (1525) and the Basle edition (1538); twenty-two Latin editions, and finally a Greek-Latin edition by René Chartier, printed in 1638–89.[4] Galen's Latin editions can be divided into three groups that follow a chronological order: the first seven editions, from 1490

---

* This is a revision of a paper, first presented in the conference organized by Caroline Petit in London in 2015, then printed in the volume in honour of Klaus-Dietrich Fischer, *Medicina nei Secoli*, 32, 1, 2020, pp. 117–138.

[1] Galen, *De libris propriis* XIX, 8–9 K. = p. 134 B.

[2] On Pseudo-Galenic translations and texts from Late Antiquity and the Early Middle Ages see K.-D. Fischer, 'Die vorsalernitanischen lateinischen Galenübersetzungen', *Medicina nei Secoli*, 25, 3, 2013, pp. 673–713.

[3] On the origin of Pseudo-Galenic literature and the lack of interest in questions of authenticity in the Middle Ages see V. Nutton, 'Pseudonymity and the Critic: Authentication, and Preservation', in *Between Text and Patient. The Medical Enterprise in Medieval and Early Modern Europe*, eds F. E. Glaze and B. K. Nance, Florence, 2011, pp. 481–91.

[4] Galen's editions printed in the fifteenth and sixteenth centuries, including the complete editions, are listed by R. J. Durling, 'A Chronological Census of Renaissance Editions and Translations of Galen', *Journal of the Warburg and Courtauld Institutes*, 24, 1961, pp. 230–305. These records

to 1528, which are mainly based on medieval translations; the ten editions from 1541 to 1565, which are mainly based on humanist translations (where the four Juntines by Agostino Gadaldini collect the best philological work done on Galen in the Renaissance); and the last five editions, from 1576 to 1625, all of which are Juntines, mostly reprints of Gadaldini's 1565 edition.

This article examines the Pseudo-Galenic texts in the complete editions of Galen, particularly how many they were, which one they were, the way they were defined, evaluated, and ordered, and whether they underwent philological investigation.

Bonardo's edition, 1490

In the preface to Galen's first edition, printed by Filippo Pinzi in Venice in 1490, the editor Diomede Bonardo, a physician from Brescia, writes that it was difficult to collect Galen's works, because they were scattered in libraries all over Italy: *Tantum namque dispersa erant Galieni volumina, ut opus non leve fuerit in quam plurimis Italiae gymnasiis ea perquirere.*[5] Bonardo found seventy-nine Latin

---

will be published in the online catalogue of Latin Galen (www.galenolatino.com), which currently provides the description of about 150 translations and texts (including nearly all those mentioned in the present article), 500 manuscripts, and only the first complete edition by Diomede Bonardo, Venice, 1490. On Galen's complete Latin editions from 1490 to 1625 see S. Fortuna, 'The Latin Editions of Galen's *Opera omnia* (1490–1625) and Their Prefaces', *Early Science and Medicine*, 17, 2012, pp. 391–412; the content of the first seven editions is described in Ead., 'Galeno latino, 1490–1533', *Medicina nei Secoli*, 17, 2, 2005, pp. 469–505; see also Ead., 'Editions and Translations of Galen from 1490 to 1540', in *Brill's Companion to the Reception of Galen*, eds P. Bouras-Vallianatos and B. Zipser, Leiden/Boston, 2019, pp. 437–52. On the reception of Galen's Aldine see L. Perilli, 'A Risky Enterprise: the Aldine Edition of Galen, the Failures of the Editors, and the Shadow of Erasmus of Rotterdam', *Early Science and Medicine*, 17, 2012, pp. 446–66; on its sources see S. Fortuna, 'Niccolò Leoniceno e le edizioni *Aldine* dei medici greci', in *Ecdotica e ricezione dei testi medici greci, Atti del V Seminario internazionale (Napoli, 1–2 ottobre 2004)*, eds V. Boudon-Millot, A. Garzya, J. Jouanna and A. Roselli, Naples, 2006, pp. 443–64; A. Guardasole, 'Un nouveau modèle de l'Aldine de Galien: le manuscrit *Rosanbo 286*', in *La Science médicale antique: nouveaux regards . Études réunies en l'honneur de J. Jouanna*, eds V. Boudon-Millot, A. Guardasole and C. Magdelaine, Paris, 2008, pp. 235–47; A. Pietrobelli, 'Une nouvelle copie d'impression de l'Aldine de Galien: le *Guelferbytanus Gud. Gr.* 11 (= 4198)', *Galenos*, 9, 2013, pp. 139–51. On the Basle edition see B. Gundert, 'Zu den Quellen der Basler Galen-Ausgabe (1538)', in *Ärzte und ihre Interpreten. Medizinische Fachtexte der Antike als Forschungsgegestand der Klassischen Philologie, Fachconferenz zu Ehren von Diethard Nickel (Berlin, 14. bis 15. Mai 2004)*, eds C. W. Müller, Ch. Brockmann and C. W. Brunschön, Munich/Leipzig, 2006, pp. 81–100. On Chartier's edition see *René Chartier (1572–1654) éditeur et traducteur d'Hippocrate et de Galien*, eds V. Boudon-Millot, G. Cobolet and J. Jouanna, Paris, 2012.

[5] Galen, *Opera*, Venice, 1490, c. aa1ʳ. Many sources of this edition are lost: for some translations (e.g. Niccolò's translations of *De partibus artis medicae* and *De optima doctrina ad Favorinum*, among the genuine works) no manuscripts are extant, and for others Bonardo's edition did not

translations and texts by Galen and Pseudo-Galen dating from Late Antiquity to the Middle Ages, and published them in two volumes.

The most numerous translations in this edition are those by Niccolò da Reggio, who translated about sixty works of Galen, Pseudo-Galen, and Hippocrates at the Angevin court of King Robert I in Naples, in the first half of the fourteenth century.[6] Niccolò used very good Greek manuscripts from Southern Italy and Constantinople that seem to have been lost. However, his translations – too literal for readers who did not know Greek – did not enjoy wide circulation, as reflected by the fact that some are preserved in a small number of manuscripts and

use preserved manuscripts; see e.g. S. Fortuna, *Galeno, Sulla costituzione della medicina a Patrofilo*, CMG V 1, 3, Berlin, 1997, pp. 28–30. However, this edition seems to be close to some Italian manuscripts: the *Vat. lat.* 2376 – written in Bologna or in Padua in the first half of the 14th century – in the translations from Arabic of *De tremore, palpitatione, convulsione et rigore* and *De motiis dubiis* (see M. McVaugh, 'Translatio libri Galieni De rigore et tremore et iectigatione et spasmo', in *Arnaldi de Villanova Opera medica omnia*, eds L. García-Ballester, J. A. Paniagua and M. McVaugh, Barcelona, 1981, p. 71 n. 74; V. Nutton, *Galen, On Problematical Movements*, Cambridge, 2011, pp. 77–9); the manuscript of Cesena S XXVII 4 – written in 1392 by Febo Pace da Pergola, a professor of medicine in Perugia, acquired by Marco da Rimini, and bequeathed to Cesena library at his death in 1474 – in Niccolò's translations of *De theriaca ad Pamphilianum* and *De theriaca ad Pisonem* (see V. Boudon-Millot, 'La traduction latine de la *Thériaque à Pison* attribuée à Nicolas de Reggio', *Medicina nei Secoli*, 25, 3, 2013, pp. 979–1010). On Bonardo's sources see also N. Palmieri, 'Su alcuni marginalia del codice Malatestiano S.V.4', *Galenos*, 9, 2015, pp. 241–9; Ead., 'Le traité de la bile noire traduit par Pietro d'Abano: manuscrits et éditions imprimées', *Galenos*, 11, 2017, pp. 105–19; Ead., 'L'organisation d'une recueil galénique: le manuscrit Vatican Latin 2376', *Micrologus*, 27, 2019, pp. 281–306.

[6] On Niccolò da Reggio see V. Nutton, 'Niccolò in Context', *Medicina nei Secoli*, 25, 3, 2013, pp. 941–56; J. Chandelier, 'Niccolo da Reggio', in *Dizionario Biografico degli Italiani*, vol. 78, Rome, 2013, pp. 423–5; A. M. Urso, 'Translating Galen in the Medieval West: the Greek Latin Translations', in *Brill's Companion to the Reception of Galen* (n. 4 above), pp. 372–5; also F. Lo Parco's pioneering essay *Niccolò da Reggio antesignano del risorgimento dell'antichità ellenica nel secolo XIV da codici delle biblioteche italiane e straniere e da documenti e stampe rare*, Memoria letta alla reale Accademia di Archeologia, Lettere e Belle Arti di Napoli, Naples, 1913. On his translations see S. Fortuna, 'Il *corpus* delle traduzioni di Niccolò da Reggio', in *La medicina nel Basso Medioevo, Tradizioni e conflitti*, Centro Italiano di Studi sul Basso Medioevo, Accademia Tudertina, Todi/Spoleto, 2019, pp. 285–312. Over the past few years, some anonymous translations have been attributed to Niccolò on the basis of his translation technique, which has been further investigated after the seminal essay of I. Wille, 'Überlieferung und Übersetzung. Zur Übersetzungstechnik des Nikolaus von Rhegium in Galens Scrift *De temporibus morborum*', *Helikon*, 3, 1963, pp. 259–77; see A. M. Urso, 'Burgundio, Niccolò e il *Vind. lat.* 2328: un confronto stilistico sulla tradizione del commento di Galeno ad *Aforismi*', *Aion*, 33, 2011, pp. 145–62; S. Fortuna, 'Niccolò da Reggio e la traduzione del commento di Galeno al *Prognostico* d'Ippocrate', *Medicina nei Secoli*, 30, 2, 2018, pp. 737–68; Ead., 'Le traduzioni di Galeno di Niccolò da Reggio: nuove attribuzioni e datazioni', *Galenos*, 8, 2014, pp. 79–103; Ead. 'Niccolò da Reggio e l'*Articella*: nuova attribuzione della traduzione del *de regimen acutorum* (*Vat. lat.* 2369)', *Galenos*, 11, 2017, pp. 177–92.

others only in printed editions.[7] Bonardo published more than forty of Niccolò's translations, of which twelve are Pseudo-Galenic,[8] as follows:

- *Introductio sive medicus* (chapters 1–10);
- *De virtutibus nostrum corpus dispensantibus* (Oribasius);
- *De theriaca ad Pamphilianum;*[9]
- *De theriaca ad Pisonem;*[10]
- *An omnes partes animalis, quod procreatur, fiunt simul;*
- *De optima secta ad Thrasybulum* (chapters 1–7);
- *De vinis* (Oribasius);
- *De bonitate aquae* (Oribasius);
- *De virtute centaureae;*
- *De anatomia oculorum;*
- *De cura icteri* (Rufus of Ephesus);
- *De remediis facile paralibus* II.[11]

The translation of *De optima secta ad Trasybulum* (chapters 1–7) is preserved only in printed editions, whereas there are no extant Greek manuscripts of the translations of *De virtute centaureae, An omnes partes animalis, quod procreatur, fiunt simul,* and *De anatomia oculorum.*

Moreover, Bonardo's edition included medieval translations from Greek, and especially Arabic, that had been part of the *New Galen,* the collection of Galen's works used in universities from the thirteenth century onwards.[12] The *New Galen*

---

[7] On the reception of Niccolò's translations see M. McVaugh, 'Niccolò da Reggio's Translations of Galen and Their Reception in France', *Early Science and Medicine,* 11, 2006, pp. 275–301; T. Pesenti, *Marsilio Santasofia tra corti e università: la carriera di un monarcha medicinae del Trecento,* Treviso, 2003, pp. 88–9; I. Ventura, 'Cultura medica a Napoli nel XIV secolo', in *Boccaccio angioino. Materiali per la storia culturale di Napoli nel Trecento,* eds G. Alfano, T. D'Urso and A. Periccioli Saggese, Brussels, 2012, pp. 251–88.

[8] On Pseudo-Galenic translations and works printed in Bonardo's edition see *Appendix 1.*

[9] On *De theriaca ad Pamphilianum,* besides *De theriaca ad Pisonem* and *De virtute centaureae,* see the article by Vivian Nutton in this volume.

[10] On *De theriaca ad Pisonem* see the articles by Véronique Boudon-Millot and Vivian Nutton in this volume.

[11] On *De remediis facile paralibus* see the article by Laurence Totelin in this volume.

[12] The term *New Galen* was introduced by Luis García Ballester, in an article published in 1982, to indicate the collection of Galenic and pseudo-Galenic works that were used in the late 13th century at Montpellier medical school; see L. García Ballester, 'The New Galen: a Challenge to Latin Galenism in Thirteenth-Century Montpellier', in *Text and Tradition, Studies in Ancient Medicine and Its Transmission Presented to Jutta Kollesch,* eds K.-D. Fischer, D. Nickel and P. Potter, Leiden/Boston/Cologne, 1998, pp. 55–83 [*Galen and Galenism, Theory and Medical Practice from*

also included some Pseudo-Galenic translations and texts, of which the following are found in Bonardo's edition:

- *Liber secretorum ad Monteum*, tr. Gerard of Cremona (1114–87);
- *Compendium pulsuum*, tr. Burgundio of Pisa (1110–93);
- *De dissolutione continua*, tr. Accursio of Pistoia (1185–1263);
- *De iuvamento anhelitus* (David de Dinant).

The most popular of the latter translations is Gerard of Cremona's *Liber secretorum ad Monteum*. Gerard, who was active in Toledo in the twelfth century, was a renowned translator of scientific and philosophical works from Arabic.[13] His translations of Galen dominated European medical teaching for a long time. This is especially true of the *Ars medica* and the commentaries on Hippocrates' *Prognosticon* and *Regimen acutorum*, which were included in the *Articella*, the basic medical handbook that was compiled in the School of Salerno and was subsequently adopted by all European universities until the sixteenth century.[14] In

Antiquity to the European Renaissance, eds J. Arrizabalaga, M. Cabré, L. Cifuentes and F. Salmón, Aldershot, 2002, V]. On the *New Galen* and its circulation in European universities see Nutton, *Galen, On Problematical Movements* (n. 5 above), pp. 91–100; V. Nutton, 'The New Galen Revisited', *Galenos*, 11, 2017, pp. 73–80; M. McVaugh, 'Galen in the Medieval Universities', in *Brill's Companion to the Reception of Galen* (n. 4 above), pp. 381–92.

[13] On Gerard of Cremona see 'Gerardo da Cremona', in *Dizionario Biografico degli Italiani*, vol. 53, Rome, 2000, pp. 620–33. On his translations see J. Jacquart, 'Les traductions médicales de Gérard de Crémone', *Annali della Biblioteca Statale e Libreria Civica di Cremona*, 41, 1990, pp. 57–70; C. Burnett, 'The Coherence of the Arabic-Latin translation Program in Toledo in the Twelfth Century', *Science in Context*, 14, 2001, pp. 249–88; M. McVaugh, 'Towards Stylistic Grouping of the Translations of Gerard of Cremona', *Medieval Studies*, 71, 2009, pp. 99–112; I. Garofalo, 'La traduction arabo-latine del la *Méthode thérapeutique* attribuée à Gérard de Crémone', *Galenos*, 11, 2017, pp. 51–72; B. Long, 'Arabic-Latin Translations: Transmission and Transformation', in *Brill's Companion to the Reception of Galen* (n. 4 above), pp. 348–53.

[14] On the *Articella* see P. O. Kristeller, *Studi sulla Scuola medica salernitana*, Naples, 1986; T. Pesenti, 'Le *Articelle* di Daniele di Marsilio Santasofia (m. 1410), professore di medicina', *Studi Petrarcheschi*, new ser., 7, 1990, pp. 50–92; C. O'Boyle, *The Art of Medicine: Medical Teaching at the University of Paris, 1250-1400*, Leiden/Boston/Cologne, 1998; D. Jacquart, *La médecine médiévale dans le cadre parisien*, Paris, 1998, pp. 161–73; *L'Ars medica (Tegni) de Galien: lectures antiques et médiévales*, Actes de la Journée d'étude internationale (Saint-Étienne, 26 juin 2006), ed. N. Palmieri, Saint-Étienne, 2008; McVaugh, *Galen in the Medieval Universities* (n. 12 above). The *Articella* manuscripts have been listed by C. O'Boyle, *Thirteenth-and Fourteenth-Century Copies of the Ars Medicine, A Checklist and Contents Descriptions of the Manuscripts*, Cambridge, 1998; the editions have been listed by J. Arrizabalaga, *The* Articella *in the Early Press (c. 1476–1534)*, Cambridge, 1998. On Gerard's translations included in the *Articella* or *Ars commentata* see V. Boudon-Millot, *Galien II, Exhortation à l'étude de la médecine, Art médical*, Paris, 2000, pp. 244–50; J. Jouanna and C. Magdelaine, 'La tradition latine du *Pronostic* et son commentaire par Galien', *Medicina nei Secoli*, 25, 3, 2013, pp. 765–96; A. Pietrobelli, 'De l'histoire d'un texte à l'histoire d'un livre: le commentaire de

contrast, the literal translations from Greek by Burgundio, a judge from Pisa who held political appointments that took him as far as Constantinople, circulated only as long as there were no Arabic translations, as is the case of the *Compendium pulsuum*.[15]

Finally, Bonardo's edition included some translations and texts from the period predating the School of Salerno,[16] of which the Pseudo-Galenic ones are the following:

- *De dinamidiis* (1);
- *De passionibus mulierum*;
- *De catharticis*;
- *De simplicibus medicaminibus ad Paternianum*;
- *De podagra* (Alexander of Tralles), anon. transl.

The translation of *De podagra* is appended to the pre-Salernitan translation of *Ad Glauconem*, constituting its final chapters.

Bonardo's edition is very similar to medical manuscripts in that it lacks a title page and the text is arranged in two columns. Moreover, the works are not ordered by subject; for example, the first volume begins with *De sectis*, Galen's work on medical schools (which also opens the *Alexandrine Canon*), followed by other introductory works like *Introductio sive medicus* and *Ars medica*. Yet, not all introductory works are grouped together: for instance, *De constitutione artis medicae* and *De partibus artis medicae* are found approximately in the middle of the

Galien au *De regimine acutorum* dans les recueils de l'*Articella*', in *L'*Articella *dans les manuscrits de la Bibliothèque Municipale de Reims: entre philologie et histoire*, ed. N. Palmieri, Saint-Étienne, 2016, pp. 57–76.

[15] On Burgundio see P. Classen, *Burgundio von Pisa, Richter, Gesandter, Übersetzer*, Heidelberg, 1974; F. Liotta, 'Burgundione da Pisa', in *Dizionario Biografico degli Italiani*, vol. 15, Rome, 1973, pp. 423–8; Urso, *Translating Galen in the Medieval West* (n. 6 above), pp. 364–8. Richard Durling edited two of Burgundio's translations of Galen: *Burgundio of Pisa's Translation of Galen's* Περὶ κράσεων, De complexionibus, Berlin/New York, 1976; *Burgundio of Pisa's Translation of Galen's* Περὶ τῶν πεπονθότων τότων, De interioribus, Stuttgart, 1992. Moreover, he attributed to Burgundio two translations of Aristotle and a translation of Galen (*De elementis*) that had been transmitted anonymously in manuscripts; see P. De Lacy, *Galen, On the Elements according to Hippocrates*, CMG V 1, 2, Berlin, 1996, pp. 26–8. Over the past few years, other translations of Galen have been attributed to Burgundio; see S. Fortuna and A. M. Urso, with an appendix by P. Annese, 'Burgundio da Pisa traduttore di Galeno: nuovi contributi e prospettive', in *Sulla tradizione indiretta dei testi medici greci*, eds I. Garofalo, A. Lami and A. Roselli, Pisa, 2009, pp. 141–77; Urso, *Burgundio, Niccolò e il* Vind. lat. *2328* (n. 6 above); B. Gundert, 'The Graeco-Latin Translation of Galen, *De symptomatuum differentiis*', *Medicina nei Secoli*, 25, 3, 2013, pp. 889–926.

[16] See Fischer, *Die vorsalernitanischen lateinischen Galenübersetzungen* (n. 2 above).

first volume. Of course, the Pseudo-Galenic works are not reported in a separate section. Only two Pseudo-Galenic works are described as such in the *explicit*:

- *De dissolutione continua*: *Explicit liber de dissolutione continua qui a quibusdam attribuitur Galieno;*
- *De catharticis*: *Explicit liber de catarticis medicinarum attributus Galieno.*

It is difficult to say whether Bonardo took an original stance; however, the authenticity of these works does not seem to be questioned in any manuscript.

Bonardo's two-volume collection remained almost unchanged in the six editions that followed until 1528, whereas the 1528 Juntine is in four volumes, with two supplementary volumes being printed in 1531 and 1533. From the first edition of 1490 to the Juntine of 1528, the number of Galen's and Pseudo-Galen's works rose (especially through the addition of humanistic translations), their order changed, and the Latin texts were corrected. Similar changes are also found in the subsequent editions, including Chartier's last edition in the seventeenth century.

Addition of Pseudo-Galenic translations and texts

Galen's second edition was printed by Bernardino Benali in Venice, in 1502. In the preface, the editor, Girolamo Suriano, a physician from Rimini, narrates that he was visited in a dream by Galen himself, who asked for a new edition of his works because the one by Bonardo was full of mistakes, and gave him his own Latin manuscript. Indeed, Suriano collected Latin manuscripts to improve Bonardo's edition and added eleven translations or texts. There is a single Pseudo-Galenic translation by Niccolò da Reggio – of *De historia philosopha*, for which there is no extant manuscript – and seven Pseudo-Galenic works, all described as spurious with the exception of *De compagine membrorum*, which Suriano seems to have considered genuine:

- *De spermate*: *Explicit libellus Galieno attributus;*
- *De compagine membrorum* (Constantine the African);
- *De anatomia parva*: *Incipit liber de anatomia parva ascriptus Galieno;*
- *De anatomia vivorum*: *Incipit liber de natura vivorum Galieno attributus;*
- *De natura et ordine cuiuslibet corporis* (Vindicianus): *Incipit liber de natura et ordine uniuscuiusque corporis ascriptus Galieno;*
- *De dinamidiis*: *Incipit liber de dinamidiis Galieno medicorum principi attributus;*
- *De incantatione* (Costa ben Luca): *Incipit liber de incantatione, adiuratione et colli suspensione Galieno ascriptus.*

De spermate, which had been part of the *New Galen*, was found in the first volume, after *De semine*, without its *incipit*,[17] whereas the other new Pseudo-Galenic works were found at the end of the second volume. Suriano tried to organize Galen's works by content: the first volume includes texts on biology, anatomy, physiology, and dietetics, while the second contains tracts on pathology and therapy as well as the new works. His edition thus published the Pseudo-Galenic works printed by Bonardo in two volumes, adding readings and corrections in the margins.

Further medieval translations of Galen – of which the most important were the commentaries on Hippocrates' *Aphorisms*, *Prognosticon*, and *Regimen acutorum* found in the *Articella* – were added in the fourth edition, printed in Pavia by Giacomo Pocatela di Borgofranco in 1515–16. The editor, Antonio Rustico from Piacenza, collected them in a new, third volume. Volume three also contains a translation of Pseudo-Galen's *De oculis*, probably by Constantine the African (d. 1087), the monk of Montecassino Abbey who translated from Arabic several medical texts used by the School of Salerno.[18] Additions of medieval translations to Galen's editions then stopped, except for the Juntine of 1565, which published – for the first time – a translation of the Pseudo-Galenic *De plantis* by Grumerus, a judge from Piacenza who translated it from Arabic in Marseille in the second half of the thirteenth century.

Galen's second edition of 1502 contains a single humanist translation, that of *Ars medica*, by Lorenzo Lorenzi (c.1460–1502), a Florentine physician and a pupil of Demetrios Chalcondylas.[19] Galen's fourth edition by Rustico contains further humanist translations of Galen by Lorenzi, Niccolò Leoniceno (1428–1524), and Giorgio Valla (c. 1447–c. 1500), which were printed in the third volume together with the humanist translations of four Pseudo-Galenic works: *Praesagium experientia confirmatum*, *De urinae significatione*, *Quaesita in Hippocratis de urinis*, and *De succedaneis*, the first three by Giorgio Valla and the last by his adopted son Giovanni Pietro.

However, most humanist translations of Galen were done immediately after 1525 – when the first Greek edition was published in Venice by the heirs of Aldus Manutius – until the early 1540s, when the Juntine (1541–2) and the

---

[17] On *De spermate* see the article by Outi Merisalo in this volume.

[18] On Constantine the African see E. Kwakkel and F. Newton, *Medicine at Montecassino. Constantin the African and the Oldest Manuscript of His* Pantegni, Turnhout, 2019; M. Green, 'Gloriosissimus Galienus: Galen and Galenic Writings in the Eleventh- and Twelfth- Century Latin West', in *Brill's Companion to the Reception of Galen* (n. 4 above), pp. 319–42; Long, *Arabic-Latin Translations* (n. 13 above), pp. 344–8.

[19] On the translations by Lorenzo Lorenzi and by the other humanist physicians see Fortuna, *Editions and Translations of Galen from 1490 to 1540* (n. 4 above), with the mentioned bibliography.

Farri edition (1541–5) were printed. Over this short period, Galen's works were translated several times, both tracts that had medieval translations and works that were unknown in Latin, such as those on anatomy, ethics, and psychology, and a number of Hippocratic commentaries. The two rival Venetian editions commissioned new translations, or reviewed and reprinted existing published translations. However, the number of Pseudo-Galenic works that were translated and published for the first time was very limited:

- *An animal sit id quod est in utero*;
- *De fasciis*;
- *Definitiones medicae*;
- *De melancholia*;
- *De ponderibus*;
- *De remediis facile parabilibus* I and III;
- *De renum affectus dignotione*;
- *De urinis*;
- *Prognostica de decubitu*;
- *Quod qualitates incorporeae sint.*

This means that the two Greek editions, the Aldine (1525) and the Basle edition (1538), contained very few new Pseudo-Galenic works, whereas the Pseudo-Galenic works translated into Latin after this time, and added to the later editions, were the majority. For example, the 1565 Juntine first published the translations of four works: Galen's *Synopsis de pulsibus* and Pseudo-Galen's *De humoribus*, *De diaeta Hippocratis in morbis acutis*, and the above-mentioned *De plantis*. Galen's last edition by René Chartier (1572–1654) was the first to include three Pseudo-Galenic works: *Praeceptum de humani corporis constitutione, De pulsibus ad Antonium*, and *De urinis compendium*. Chartier found them in Greek manuscripts from the French Royal library and printed them together with their Latin translations, even though he was aware that they were not genuine.[20]

Thus, Galen's editions did not establish a canon of his works, but merely collected medical works, Galenic, Pseudo-Galenic, and even forgeries. Commentaries on Hippocrates' *De humoribus, De alimento, Epidemics* II, and *Epidemics* VI (books VII–VIII) were printed in the Juntines from 1576–7 or 1586 as newly discovered Galenic texts, but were in fact forgeries prepared by Giovanni Battista Rasario

---

[20] See S. Fortuna, 'René Chartier e le edizioni latine di Galeno', in *René Chartier (1572–1654) éditeur et traducteur d'Hippocrate et de Galien* (n. 4 above), p. 315.

(1517-78), a translator and editor of Galen, at a time when Galen the physician was attracting less interest than Galen the interpreter of Hippocrates.[21]

The order of Galen's works

Luca Antonio Giunta planned a new Latin edition of Galen based on humanist translations that was published in 1541-2 by his sons, after he died in 1538. Its editor was Agostino Gadaldini (1515–75) – a young physician and philologist whose father Antonio was a printer in Modena – who worked on the texts with several collaborators to provide new translations or correct existing printed ones. The edition was organized by Giovanni Battista Da Monte (1498–1555), a distinguished professor at Padua medical school, who laid down the order in which Galen's works would be published. He described his decisions in a long letter to Giunta that was printed in all the Juntines from 1541–2.[22] Da Monte's order of contents was based on *De constitutione artis medicae*, an introductory work where Galen describes the various medical disciplines, from biology to therapy. Da Monte thus established seven subject-based sections – biology, anatomy, and physiology; dietetics; pathology; semiotics; pharmacology; surgery; and therapy – and three sections containing respectively introductory works, *extra ordinem* works, i.e. tracts on general topics or ones that could not be included under the other sections; and spurious works.

Not all the Pseudo-Galenic tracts published in this edition were included in the section of spurious works. This was mentioned by Da Monte in his letter: he included *Oratio suasoria ad artes* and *Introductio sive medicus* among the introductory works; *De urinis* in the semiotics section; and *De remediis facile parabilibus* II, *De oculis*, and *De renum affectus dignotione* in the therapy section. Additional works explicitly defined as Pseudo-Galenic were printed together with the genuine ones, at least *Quod qualitates incorporeae sint* and *Definitiones medicae* (introductory works), *An animal sit id quod est in utero* (biology section), *De remediis facile parabilibus* III and *De incantatione* (therapy section). Da Monte explained his decision as stemming from the excellence of these works, which provided a key contribution to the various sections and ensured an exhaustive

---

[21] On Rasario's forgeries see the article by Christina Savino in this volume.

[22] On Da Monte and the order of Galen's works see D. Mugnai Carrara, 'Le epistole prefatorie sull'ordine dei libri di Galeno di Giovan Battista da Monte: esigenze di metodo e dilemmi editoriali', in *Vetustatis Indagator, Scritti offerti a Filippo Di Benedetto*, eds V. Fera and A. Guida, Messina, 1999, pp. 207–34.

approach to the subject.[23] It is not surprising, then, that the dietetics section includes a treatise by Hippocrates, *De aere, aquis et locis*. Da Monte specified that he would have printed Galen's commentary on it, but that he could not find it:[24]

> ... *liber Hippocratis De locis, aere et aqua, quem Galenus De habitationibus, aquis, temporibus et regionibus inscribi maluit, speravique hactenus me tibi super eo divina Galeni commentaria traditurum, sed ab amico id pollicente frustratus sum.*

> As for the Hippocratic work *De locis, aere et aqua* (*On Places, air and water*), for which Galen would have preferred the title *De habitationibus, aquis, temporibus et regionibus* (*On Dwellings, Waters, Times and Places*), until now I had hoped to pass on to you the divine commentary of Galen on it, but I was let down by the friend who promised it to me.

The Juntine of 1541–2, the first of the new series, is a comprehensive collection of medical texts by Galen and by physicians in his tradition.

As regards the spurious works, Da Monte explained that they were included only to provide an exhaustive collection, but that they added nothing to medicine or simply repeated what Galen had said; in sum, they were useless and superfluous:[25]

> *Sunt vero et alii quidam libri, partim ex Arabia partim ex Graecia delati, non spurii tantum, sed etiam magna ex parte supervacui, quoniam in eis vel nihil tractatur quod ad artem medicam spectet, vel, si tractatur, totum illud a legitimis libris decerptum est, ut ibi frustra repetatur quod alibi copiose explicatum meminimus. Ne tamen et illos (varii enim gustus hominum sunt) omissos aliqui conquerantur, voluimus eos omnes separatim in unum corpus colligere, ut scirent qui id curae haberent et facile invenire quod quaererent, et inventum simul cognoscere non esse inter Galeni monumenta connumerandum.*

---

[23] G. B. Da Monte, *Ep.* to Luca Antonio Giunta, printed in Galen, *Omnia opera*, Venice, 1541–2, c. 6ᵛ: '*deinde liber De urinis, qui licet Galeni non sit, haud importune tamen sub hoc ordine statuitur*' (*De urinis*); c. 7ʳ: '*alter, qui ad Solonem inscribitur, me iudice spurius est, cum in eo tamen quam plurima lectione digna observentur, non reijciendum putavi*' (*De remediis facile parabilibus* II); '*horum ego neutrum Galeni esse puto, et quamvis librum De curatione oculorum a se scriptum quartodecimo therapeuticae methodi Galenus affirmet, non is tamen ordo doctrinae aut ea dicendi phrasis in hoc ipso qui extat agnoscitur, ut propterea sit ne [lege ne sit] Galeni aliqua mihi suspicio suboriatur. Utrosque tamen reliquis proxime positis subnectendos iudicavi, cum inde nihilo peior doctrina futura sit*' (*De renum affectus dignotione* and *De oculis*); 7ᵛ: '*Sunt praeterea quae Galeni quidem non esse scimus, sicut liber est qui Introductio ad medicinam inscribitur, ea tamen rei commoditate persuasi, minime reijcienda iudicavimus. Ante igitur libros omnes seriatim locatos Introductorij hoc modo extra aciem disponentur, Oratio suasoria ad bonas artes, quae non ad Galenum nostrum Niconis architecti, sed alium Menodoti filium refertur*' (*Introductio sive medicus* and *Oratio suasoria ad artes*).

[24] *Ibi*, c. 6ʳ.

[25] *Ibi*, c. 7ʳ.

There are in turn other books, some coming from Arabia, some from Greece, which are not only inauthentic but also in great part superfluous, for either nothing in them concerns the medical art, or, if something concerns the medical art, it is all extracted from authentic works, so that it is here repeated in vain what we remember to have been abundantly explained elsewhere. Nevertheless, so that nobody blames us for omitting those (for the tastes of men are many), we decided to gather all them in a separate volume, so that those who are interested could easily find what they are looking for, and once it is found, at the same time they could know that it should not be counted among the works of Galen.

The section *ascripti libri* of the Juntine of 1541–2 contains thirty-one works, most of which had already been published in the first four editions of Galen.[26] Two are actually genuine works by Galen – *De partibus artis medicae* translated by Niccolò da Reggio and *De motibus dubiis* translated by Mark of Toledo – that were considered as spurious, probably because they were preserved only in Latin. The section also contains Latin texts from Late Antiquity and the Middle Ages, and medieval translations from Arabic and Greek, of which seven are by Niccolò da Reggio. There are also humanist translations: the three translations by Giorgio Valla printed in the fourth edition of 1515–16 (*Praesagium experentia confirmatum*, *De urinae significatione*, and *Quaesita in Hippocratis de urinis*) and three humanist translations that had never been published in any previous complete edition. These are *Prognostica de decubitu* by Joseph Struthius (1510–69) and *De historia philosopha* and *De melancholia* by Marziano Rota, who edited the 1528 Juntine and the supplementary volumes of 1531 and 1533.[27] The latter three translations had used the Greek texts found in the fourth volume of the Aldine, where they were printed in a new special section of spurious works.

The order of Galen's works followed in the first Juntine edited by Da Monte was substantially preserved in the later editions: the subsequent eight Juntines until the final one of 1625, the three Froben editions from 1542 to 1561–2, and the Frellon edition of 1549–51. Only three editions followed a different order, those by Agostino Ricci (1541–45), Giovanni Battista Rasario (1562–3), and René Chartier (1638–89), all of whom justified their decisions: however, Ricci's text is not extant and may have never been published.[28] Rasario divided Galen's works into eight

---

[26] See *Appendix 2*.

[27] These very rare volumes have been described in S. Fortuna, 'Galeno a Sarnano: le Giuntine del 1531 e del 1533', *Italia Medioevale e Umanistica*, 37, 1994, pp. 241–50.

[28] Rasario wrote the *Liber, in quo ratio ordinis, quo Galeni libri dispositi sunt, redditur*, printed in his edition; see C. Savino, 'Dare ordine a Galeno. L'edizione di Giovanni Battista Rasario (1562–1563)', in *Sulla tradizione indiretta dei testi medici greci* (n. 15 above), pp. 139–52; Ead., 'Giovanni Battista Rasario and the 1562–63 Edition of Galen. Research, Exchanges and Forgeries', *Early Science*

sections based on the *De partibus artis medicae* which, like Ricci before him, he considered genuine and printed among the *libri extra ordinem*. He explained his choice in the *Liber in quo ratio ordinis, quo Galeni libri dispositi sunt, redditur*, which was published in the initial part of Galen's edition printed by Vincenzo Valgrisi in Venice in 1562–3.

Rasario wrote that it was very important to keep the spurious works apart from the genuine: *minime par est rivulos fontibus admiscere.*[29] He posed as a philologist but, as noted above, he was also an extraordinary forger. The section *ascripti libri* of his edition included as many as forty-one works. Though ostensibly a large number, it is actually the sum of the works published in the Juntines as spurious and of those defined as spurious but not printed there. In sum, Rasario did not make original decisions, but closely followed the Juntines and the Farri edition.[30] Indeed, Galen's collection printed by Farri in Venice in 1541–5 and edited by Agostino Ricci (1512–64) already placed all spurious works in a separate section. Ricci's and Rasario's editions are almost identical; the main difference is the *Oratio suasoria in artes*, which Ricci considered genuine but Rasario – following Da Monte – attributed to a different Galen, the son of Menodotus, based on the title printed in the Aldine. Of course, Ricci was right.

The spurious works do not seem to have been the subject of much philological interest after Suriano's edition.[31] This is probably due not so much to the fact that they were disregarded by Da Monte and others, but rather to the fact that collations and textual corrections in the Farri edition and in Gadaldini's Juntines were based on Greek manuscripts, and no Greek manuscripts were available for many of these spurious works, transmitted only in Latin.

A small number of works included by Da Monte among spurious works were translated again:

- *De historia philosopha*, tr. Niccolò da Reggio;
  Marziano Rota;
  Andrea Laguna;

---

and Medicine, 17, 2012, pp. 413–45. Chartier wrote a similar text entitled *Pro Graeco-Latina editione operum Hippocratis et Galeni Oratio*; see Fortuna, *René Chartier e le edizioni latine di Galeno* (n. 20 above), pp. 309–13.

[29] Rasario, *Liber, in quo ratio ordinis, quo Galeni libri dispositi sunt, redditur* (n. 28 above), c. *4r.

[30] Rasario relies on both the Juntines and the Farri edition for the surgical illustrations; see S. Fortuna, 'Le illustrazioni nei testi medici: le edizioni latine di Galeno del XVI–XVII sec.', in *Scienza antica in età moderna. Teoria e immagini*, ed. V. Maraglino, Bari, 2012, pp. 311–37.

[31] See Nutton, *Galen, On Problematical Movements* (n. 5 above), pp. 80–81; and the article by Outi Merisalo in this volume.

Giovanni Battista Rasario;
- *Prognostica de decubitu*, tr. Joseph Struthius;
Giacomo Marescotti;
- *De melancholia*, tr. Marziano Rota;
Janus Cornarius;
Giovanni Battista Rasario;
- *De bonitate aquae*, tr. Niccolò da Reggio;
Agostino Gadaldini;
- *De vinis*, tr. Niccolò da Reggio;
Agostino Gadaldini;
Giovanni Battista Rasario;
- *De partibus artis medicae*, tr. Niccolò da Reggio;
Vittore Trincavelli.

The Greek text of all these works is extant except for *De partibus artis medicae*, which is preserved only in Latin. Trincavelli based his new translation on the one by Niccolò da Reggio. However, as noted above, this is a special treatise that Ricci considered genuine.

If Da Monte's order was preserved in many editions of Galen, the debate on the authenticity of some works continued for several years. For instance, *De partibus artis medicae* was published as a spurious work in the first Juntine of 1541–2, but in the later Juntines Gadaldini added the following sentence under the title: 'Liber qui, nisi Galeni fuerit, eo tamen auctore dignus videtur'.[32] Conrad Gesner (1516– 65) shared Gadaldini's opinion and reported the same words in his catalogue of Galenic works, which was included in Galen's third edition printed in Basle in 1561–2: 'Liber est paulo maior charta qui, nisi Galeni fuerit, eo tamen autore dignus videtur'.[33]

De motibus dubiis was included among spurious works in every edition, but in the 1550 Juntine Gadaldini added the following sentence under the title: 'Liber traductoris magis quam autoris culpa mendis scatens, in quo multa Galeni doctrinam sapiunt, licet quaedam quoque insint ab eius dicendi consuetudine aliena.'[34] Conrad Gesner also reported these words in his bibliography, and pointed out that there is a reference to *De motibus dubiis* in Galen's *De dissectione musculorum*:

---

[32] Galen, *Omnia quae extant opera*, Venice, 1550, *ascripti libri*, p. 16^r.

[33] C. Gesner, 'Catalogus primus, sive enumeratio librorum Galeni, eo ordine, quo excusi sunt, ex Io. Baptista Montani fere sententia', in Galen, *Omnia quae extant*, Basle, 1562, vol. 1, c. B+1^v.

[34] Galen, *Omnia quae extant opera* (n. 32 above), c. 66^r.

Galenus quidem in libro de musculorum dissectione testatur se scripsisse librum de motibus oscuris, qui an hic ipse sit considerandum. Scatet hic quidem mendis, sed interpretis (ut apparet) culpa. Multa in eo Galeni doctrina sapiunt, licet quaedam quoque insint ab eius dicendi consuetudine aliena.[35]

In the Juntine of 1565, Gadaldini summarized his and Gesner's considerations as follows: '*Galenus huius libri sui saepius mentionem facit, et in hoc etiam multos suos libros citat, ob varias tamen translationes aliquae mendae in eum irrepserunt*'.[36]

The *Oratio suasoria ad artes* has a different history.[37] The Juntine of 1541–2 reported it at the beginning of the section containing the introductory works, but attributed it to Galen the son of Menodotus, in line with Da Monte's interpretation of its title. Even though Galen's authorship was affirmed by Ricci, Cornarius, and Gesner, the Juntines continued to report this information.

Finally, *De theriaca ad Pamphilianum* and *De theriaca ad Pisonem* were generally included among the genuine works, in the section devoted to pharmacology. Cornarius, in his edition, disagreed and wrote of the former treatise '*sed non est genuinus hic libellus*'.[38] Gesner shared his view,[39] whereas Gadaldini did not change his mind until the Juntine of 1565, where he called into question the authenticity of both works, writing '*Sed etiam qui opinentur et hunc non esse Galeni librum*' of the former, and '*Sunt qui negent hunc librum esse Galeni, nec sine causa*' of the latter.[40]

Later on, Galen's editions became collections of ancient medical texts more and more often. In the seventeenth century René Chartier was proud to publish Hippocrates' and Galen's works side by side together with medical texts from Late Antiquity and the Middle Ages. In the nine volumes of this edition Galenic and Pseudo-Galenic works were subdivided into thirteen sections. There was no separate section for spurious works, which was introduced in the Greek edition of 1525 and was subsequently found in all of Galen's Latin editions from the 1540s onwards.[41] Chartier was more interested in finding unpublished medical

---

[35] Gesner, *Catalogus primus, sive enumeratio librorum Galeni* (n. 33 above), c. B+2^r.

[36] Galen, *Omnia quae extant opera*, Venice, 1565, c. 66^r.

[37] See Boudon-Millot, *Galien II, Exhortation à l'étude de la médecine* (n. 14 above), pp. 38–42.

[38] Galen, *Opera quae ad nos extant*, Basel, 1549, vol. 5, p. 371.

[39] Gesner, *Catalogus primus, sive enumeratio librorum Galeni* (n. 33 above), c. A+5^r: '*De usu theriacae ad Pamphilianum non genuinus Galeni*'.

[40] Galen, *Omnia quae extant opera* (n. 36 above), cl. V, cc. 89^v and 97^r.

[41] On Pseudo-Galenic works in Chartier's edition, see C. Petit, 'René Chartier et l'autenticité des traités galéniques', in *René Chartier (1572–1654) éditeur et traducteur d'Hippocrate et de Galien* (n. 4 above), pp. 287–300.

Greek works, and in integrating the existing ones with newly discovered sources, than in distinguishing between genuine and spurious texts, which, in his opinion, belonged to the same tradition anyway. Therefore, even though Chartier's edition was a monumental enterprise, the best philological work on Galen's writings was produced by the generation of Da Monte, Gadaldini, Ricci, Cornarius and Gesner.

Appendix

Pseudo-Galen's works in Diomede Bonardo's edition, 1490

INTRODUCTIO SIVE MEDICUS, tr. Niccolò da Reggio

DE IUVAMENTO ANHELITUS (David de Dinant)

DE VIRTUTIBUS NOSTRUM CORPUS DISPENSANTIBUS (Oribasius),
    tr. Niccolò da Reggio

COMPENDIUM PULSUUM, tr. Burgundio of Pisa

DE THERIACA AD PAMPHILIANUM, tr. Niccolò da Reggio

DE THERIACA AD PISONEM, tr. Niccolò da Reggio

AN OMNES PARTES ANIMALIS, QUOD PROCREATUR, FIUNT SIMUL,
    tr. Niccolò da Reggio

DE OPTIMA SECTA AD THRASYBULUM, tr. Niccolò da Reggio

DE VINIS (Oribasius), tr. Niccolò da Reggio

DE BONITATE AQUAE (Oribasius), tr. Niccolò da Reggio

DE MOTU THORACIS ET PULMONIS (Oribasius), an. transl.

DE VIRTUTE CENTAUREAE, tr. Niccolò da Reggio

DE DINAMIDIIS (1)

DE PASSIONIBUS MULIERUM

DE ANATOMIA OCULORUM, tr. Niccolò da Reggio

DE DISSOLUTIONE CONTINUA, tr. Accursio of Pistoia

DE CURA LAPIDIS (Avenzoar ibn Zuhr), an. transl.

DE CURA ICTERI (Rufus of Ephesus), tr. Niccolò da Reggio

DE CATHARTICIS

DE REMEDIIS FACILE PARALIBUS II, tr. Niccolò da Reggio

LIBER SECRETORUM AD MONTEUM, tr. Gerard of Cremona

DE MEDICINA EXPERTIS, tr. Farag ibn Salim

DE SIMPLICIBUS MEDICAMINIBUS AD PATERNIANUM

DE PODAGRA (Alexander of Tralles), an. transl.

Section of spurious works in the Juntine of 1541–2

DE HISTORIA PHILOSOPHA, tr. Marziano Rota

PROGNOSTICA DE DECUBITU, tr. Joseph Struthius

DE PARTIBUS ARTIS MEDICAE, tr. Niccolò da Reggio

DE DINAMIDIIS (1)

DE DINAMIDIIS (2)

DE SPERMATE

DE NATURA ET ORDINE CUIUSLIBET CORPORIS (Vindicianus)

DE ANATOMIA PARVA

DE ANATOMIA VIVORUM

DE ANATOMIA OCULORUM, tr. Niccolò da Reggio

DE COMPAGINE MEMBRORUM (Constantine the African)

DE VIRTUTIBUS NOSTRUM CORPUS DISPENSANTIBUS (Oribasius),
    tr. Niccolò da Reggio

DE VOCE ET ANHELITU, an. transl.

DE IUVAMENTO ANHELITUS (David de Dinant)

COMPENDIUM PULSUUM, tr. Burgundio of Pisa

DE MOTIBUS DUBIIS, tr. Mark of Toledo

DE DISSOLUTIONE CONTINUA, tr. Accursio of Pistoia

DE VINIS (Oribasius), tr. Niccolò da Reggio

DE BONITATE AQUAE (Oribasius), tr. Niccolò da Reggio

PRAESAGIUM EXPERENTIA CONFIRMATUM, tr. Giorgio Valla

DE URINAE SIGNIFICATIONE, tr. Giorgio Valla

DE SIMPLICIBUS MEDICAMINIBUS AD PATERNIANUM

DE VIRTUTE CENTAUREAE, tr. Niccolò da Reggio

DE CATHARTICIS

DE PASSIONIBUS MULIERUM

LIBER SECRETORUM AD MONTEUM, tr. Gerard of Cremona

DE MEDICINIS EXPERTIS, tr. Farag ibn Salim

DE MELANCHOLIA, tr. Marziano Rota

DE CURA ICTERI (Rufus of Ephesus), tr. Niccolò da Reggio

DE CURA LAPIDIS (Avenzoar ibn Zuhr), an. transl.

QUAESITA IN HIPPOCRATIS DE URINIS, tr. Giorgio Valla

Alessandro Achillini and the 1502 Galen *Opera Omnia*: The Influence of Pseudo-Galenic Sources in Early Sixteenth Century Anatomy

R. Allen Shotwell

In 1520 Alessandro Achillini's *Anatomical Notes* was published, posthumously.[1] Achillini compiled the notes as part of his teaching duties at Bologna in the early sixteenth century, and he included in them a remarkable set of references to Galenic and Pseudo-Galenic works. There is a close parallel between Achillini's sources and the 1502 edition of the collected works of Galen in Latin, especially in his use of the Pseudo-Galenic *De anatomia vivorum* written in the thirteenth century but appearing in print for the first time in the 1502 Galen. *De anatomia vivorum*'s influence on anatomical writing had been minimal before 1502. After 1502, however, first Achillini and then his contemporary at Bologna, Berengario da Carpi, made active use of it, citing it as the source for various pieces of information in conjunction with the anatomy of the uterus and of the eye.

In what follows, I provide an overview of Achillini's work and its context, establishing it as a set of notes on the fourteenth century anatomical text of Mondino de Luzzi arising from Achillini's dissection experiences and his study of written anatomical sources. I then analyze the common ground between Achillini's sources and the 1502 Galen and specifically explore the material he included from *De anatomia vivorum* in describing the anatomy of the uterus and the anatomy of the eye. I also trace the use of the same material by Berengario when discussing those topics and compare the differences between Berengario and Achillini's use of *De anatomia vivorum* and Gabrielle Zerbi's, an anatomist whose book was published in 1502. Ultimately I hope to show that these various aspects of Achillini's work highlight both the impact of the Pseudo-Galenic *De anatomia vivorum* and the use of an edition of Galen's Latin *opera omnia* by anatomists in the early sixteenth-century.

Alessandro Achillini and his *Anatomical Notes*

Except for a brief stint at Padua in 1506–8, Alessandro Achillini taught at Bologna from 1484 until his death in 1512. Between 1484 and 1494 he taught philosophy and then moved to theoretical medicine, which he taught until 1497 when he

---

[1] Alessandro Achillini, *Annotationes Anatomicae*, Bologna, 1520.

returned to philosophy. Between 1501 and his death in 1512, Achillini taught both theoretical medicine and philosophy (medicine in the morning and philosophy in the afternoon). He published a number of works, many of them on logic and Aristotelian philosophy, and was an active and well-known figure in early sixteenth-century intellectual circles in Italy.[2]

During Achillini's time, Bologna had the largest medical school in Italy and produced a number of new works on anatomy. It is possible that Achillini's anatomy, which was published by his brother after his death, was printed in part in response to a growing interest in the subject. An unpublished work on anatomy was written by Girolamo Manfredi at Bologna in the late fifteenth century, the same year as the first edition of Galen's works in Latin was printed. Garbiele Zerbi (who left Bologna in 1483, when Achillini was still a student) and the Venetian physician, Alessandro Benedetti, both published anatomies in 1502, a year which also saw the second edition of Galen's works. Berengario da Carpi of Bologna published his own anatomy in 1521, one year after Achillini's *Notes* and the same year as its second edition.[3]

Published in 1520 Achillini's *Annotationes Anatomicae* consisted of a series of brief remarks on the parts of the body. As his modern translator, Lind, has pointed out, the title of Achillini's book, *Anatomical Notes*, accurately reflected its nature as a set of lecture notes. The text was organized in the way anatomy would have been presented to medical students in the form of annual demonstrations and closely followed the fourteenth-century anatomical text of Mondino de Luzzi which was read and commented upon at those demonstrations at Bologna where Achillini taught. In these demonstrations, annual dissections of bodies, reading and commenting on Mondino were the responsibility of a member of the medical faculty while actually cutting open the body was normally performed by surgeons. Anatomical demonstrations had been formally incorporated into the statutes at Bologna in the fifteenth century.[4]

---

[2] For an account of Achillini's life and career see H. S. Matsen, *Alessandro Achillini (1463–1512) and His Doctrine of 'Universals' and 'Transcendentals'. A Study in Renaissance Ockhamism*, London, 1974, pp. 21–42 as well as L.R. Lind, *Studies in Pre-Vesalian Anatomy. Biography, Translations, Documents*, Philadelphia, 1975, pp. 42–65, which is the most comprehensive discussion of his anatomy.

[3] For Bologna's medical school see P. Grendler, *The Universities of the Italian Renaissance*, Baltimore, 2002, pp. 314–51. For Manfredi's manuscript see C. Singer, 'A Study in Renaissance Anatomy with a New Text: The *Anatomia* of Hieronymo Manfredi, Transcribed and Translated by A. Mildred Westland', in *Studies in the History and Method of Science*, ed. C. Singer, New York, 1917, pp. 79–164. Zerbi, Berengario and Benedetti's work are discussed in Lind, *Pre-Vesalian* (n. 2 above), pp. 69–166.

[4] On the idea of Achillini's work as a set of notes on Mondino, see Lind, *Pre-Vesalian* (n. 2 above),

In his notes Achillini refers to observations he made in dissected bodies in 1502, 1503 and 1506, all years when he was teaching medicine at Bologna.[5] While there were other possible contexts in which Achillini could have observed dissected bodies, anatomical demonstrations seem the most likely source of these observations.[6] The connection between Achillini's work and anatomical demonstrations is reinforced in the way Achillini's text closely mirrors Mondino's in structure, recites anatomical information as it appears in Mondino, and contains elements suggesting that it was meant to be read whilst a dissection was being conducted.

Because parts of the body decayed at different rates, it was necessary to dissect some parts before others, and Mondino arranged the order of his text to match this requirement, beginning with the internal organs in the lowest part of the body and moving upward to the chest and then the head. Mondino also focused most of his discussion on the internal organs rather than other structures like bones or veins because, he said, dissection was more useful for studying them. These basic elements are also found in Achillini's text which followed the same order as Mondino and focused on the same parts of the body.[7]

Achillini also provided the same anatomical descriptions as Mondino, albeit without attributing them. His typical approach was to describe a part of the body in the same way that Mondino had and then to add to that description based on ideas derived either from observation or from other authors. While Mondino often digressed by discussing typical diseases and their cures associated with certain parts of the body, Achillini eliminated those references, although his notes contained one artefact of Mondino's description of a treatment apparently

p. 42 n. 2. On anatomical demonstrations see G. Ferrari, 'Public Anatomy Lessons and the Carnival: The Anatomy Theatre of Bologna', *Past And Present*, 17, 1987, pp. 50–106A. Carlino, *Books of the Body: Anatomical Ritual and Renaissance Learning*, trans. J. Tedeschi and A. Tedeschi, Chicago, 1999, pp. 8–68; J. Bylebyl, 'Interpreting the *Fasciculo* Anatomy Scene', *Journal of the History of Medicine and Allied Sciences*, 45, 1990, pp. 308–16 and *Statuti delle Università e dei Collegi dello Studio Bolognese*, ed. C. Malagola, Bologna, 1888, pp. 289–90.

[5] Achillini, *Annotationes* (n. 1 above), fols 5ᵛ, 12ᵛ, 13ʳ.

[6] Achillini does refer to bodies that were wonders of natures or *monstruosum* and such bodies were sometimes dissected outside of school demonstrations. On the examination of anatomical wonders see L. Daston and K. Park, *Wonders and the Order of Nature:1150–1750*, New York, 1998, pp. 200–214.

[7] Mondino de Luzzi, *Anatomia Mundini, ad vetustissimorum eorundemque aliquot manu scriptorum codicum fidem collata, justoque suo ordini restituta, per Joannem Dryandrum*, Marburg, 1541, fol. 2ʳ.

mistakenly lumped together with dissection instructions that were also included by Mondino (see below).[8]

Instructions about how to dissect and otherwise examine the parts of the body were included in many of Mondino's descriptions. Often written in the imperative, these instructions were cues for the dissector about what to do next. Many of Mondino's instructions were repeated by Achillini. For example, in the passage on the heart, Mondino provided instructions for how to cut it open. 'Cut open the right side of the heart' and 'Cut open the left ventricle [of the heart]'.[9] Achillini provided the same instructions using the same imperative construction. 'Cut open the right side of the heart' and 'Cut the left ventricle of the heart'.[10]

In one passage Achillini's notes included both Mondino's instructions for dissection and his advice for treatment in a way that suggests Achillini (or possibly whoever edited his work after his death) did not recognize that a transition between dissection instructions and treatment instructions had occurred. After describing the initial incisions in the abdomen and the examination of the layers found there, Mondino went on to describe the treatment of various conditions associated with that region of the body including the procedure to follow if a portion of the internal membrane, called the *zirbus* (or *girbus*) by Mondino, protrudes through a wound in the abdomen. Such an injury required a ligature to cut off that portion of the membrane that protruded, according to Mondino, because its contact with air caused it to putrefy.[11]

While Mondino had made a clear distinction between dissection and treatment by including the instructions about a ligature under a separate section labeled, *On the Diseases of the Mirach and Siphac and Their Cure*, Achillini's notes included the ligature step seamlessly with the dissection instructions. To paraphrase, Achillini's instructions were – cut the *siphac*, cut the *mirach*, make a lateral incision, the protruding *omentum* must be tied because it putrefies in contact with

---

[8] Achillini made very little mention of Mondino in his *Notes*. Lind, *Pre-Vesalian* (n. 2 above), p. 42 n. 2 only found three references. This was possibly because they could already be understood to be encompassing Mondino's work from their context, particularly if they were being read out in a demonstration.

[9] Mondino, *Anatomia* (n. 7 above), fols 38ᵛ and 38ʳ, 'Scinde igitur cor primo in parte dextra', '... scinde ventriculum sinistrum...'.

[10] Achillini, *Annotationes* (n. 1 above), fols 9ʳ and 10ᵛ, 'Scinde cor in parte dextra ... ', 'Scinde sinistrum cordis ventriculum habentes densos parietes'. This connection between an anatomical teaching text and specific dissection instructions can still be found in the 1530s in the work of Johann Guinter and Andreas Vesalius. See V. Nutton, *Principles of Anatomy according to the Opinion of Galen by Johann Guinter and Andreas Vesalius*, New York, 2017.

[11] Mondino, *Anatomia* (n. 7 above), fol. 10ᵛ.

the air. The last step in this series was Mondino's advice about treatment and made little sense for a dissection where the internal cavity would be exposed to air indefinitely.[12]

While Achillini repeated many of Mondino's instructions, in some places he clearly added his own, describing details of the process of examining body parts that Mondino did not. For example, Achillini included instructions for cutting open the uterus, which he advised cutting down the middle, while Mondino provided no specific dissection advice.[13] In his discussion of the brain Achillini made a first person reference to the dissection process, noting 'I cut the brain through the middle where the conjunctiva separates the right from the left', another step not mentioned by Mondino.[14]

Achillini's dissection instructions reinforce the sense that his text was an updating of Mondino, and those updates went beyond dissection methods, extending into information about anatomical structures, terminology and conflicting opinions mostly derived from other texts. When it came to those texts, Achillini made use of a number of sources that Mondino did not, including a number of Latin translations and some Pseudo-Galenic sources. While both authors referred to roughly the same number of works by Galen, they were different works, Achillini's references reflecting a change in what was available in Latin translation and the appearance of early print editions of Galen.

Achillini's Galenic References

Overall, Achillini made roughly fifty references to Galen, scattered over eleven different works. Most of them (sixty percent) were to *De anatomia vivorum* or *De usu partium*. A number of works by Galen had been translated into Latin directly from Greek by Niccolò da Reggio in the fourteenth century. One of those translations was of Galen's *De usu partium*, his most extensive account of anatomical knowledge. Niccolò's efforts did not have an immediate impact. While *De usu partium* was incorporated into medieval medicine by Guy de Chauliac in the fourteenth century, many authors still made use of a much abbreviated version of the work, *De juvamentis membrorum*, which was Mondino's main source.[15]

---

[12] Achillini, *Annotationes* (n. 1 above), fol. 3ʳ 'Scinde siphac… Lateralis incisio… Girbus exiens ligatur: post abscinditur: quia tactum ab aere statim putrefit.'

[13] Achillini, *Annotationes* (n. 1 above), fol. 6ᵛ, 'Scinde eam per medium'.

[14] Achillini, *Annotationes* (n. 1 above), fol. 12ʳ, 'Aperio cerebrum per medium ubi conjunctiva sep<ar>at dextrum a sinistro'.

[15] For the impact of Niccolò's work see V. Nutton, *John Caius and the Manuscripts of Galen*, Cambridge, 1987, pp. 19–21. For Guy de Chauliac's use of the translations of Galen, see M. McVaugh,

De anatomia vivorum, on the other hand, was a Pseudo-Galenic work. The earliest extant Latin manuscript was written in the thirteenth century.[16] It was considerably shorter than *De usu partium*. Despite its reference to sources, like Avicenna, that made it clear it could not have been written by Galen, *De anatomia vivorum* was included in the Latin *opera omnia* of Galen throughout the sixteenth century.[17]

Two editions of Galen's *opera omnia* in Latin were published during Achillini's lifetime. The first, assembled by Diomede Bonardo, appeared in 1490. The second, edited by Girolamo Suriano of Rimini, was printed in 1502. Neither edition included any material that was not already available in Latin, either in manuscript or in print, and there was a considerable amount of shared content in the two. However the 1502 edition did make a number of corrections to the translations in the 1490 work and also included eleven additional works not included in the first edition. Three of those works, *De usu partium*, *De anatomia vivorum*, and *De anatomia parva* formed nearly seventy percent of Achillini's citations of Galen. The other eight works by Galen referred to by Achillini (*De anatomia matricis*, *De utilitate respirationis*, *De anatomia oculorum*, *De interioribus*, *De sectis*, *De simplicium medicamentorum*, and *De juvamentis membrorum*) were included in both the 1502 edition and the 1490 edition.[18]

Although it is possible he made use of other sources for the material, the high correlation between Achillini's references to Galen and the 1502 edition and his extensive use of *De anatomia vivorum* suggest it was his source. None of the works by Galen cited by Achillini appeared in print outside of the 1490 or 1502 *opera omnia*.[19] Achillini's two most important sources, *De usu partium* and *De anatomia vivorum* first appeared in the 1502 edition. While they were both cited

'The Lost Galen', in *The Unknown Galen*, ed. V. Nutton, London, 2002, pp. 153–64. For *De juvamentis* see R. French, '*De Juvamentis Membrorum* and the Reception of Galenic Physiological Anatomy', *Isis*, 70, 1, 1979, pp. 96–109.

[16] The Latin manuscript is Durham, Cathedral Library, ms. C.IV.4. The name, *Anatomia Vivorum*, is not actually used in the Latin manuscripts themselves; the work was normally called *Anatomia Galieni* or just *Anatomia*. Many thanks to Monica Green for this information. There is also a ninth century Arabic version of the work which was translated from earlier sources and may have been the basis for the Latin (F. Sezgin, *Geschichte des arabischen Schrifttums*, 1970, p. 100 no. 23; M. Ullmann, *Die Medizin im Islam*, 1970, p. 54, no. 75). Thanks to Simon Swain for pointing this out.

[17] For *De anatomia vivorum* see G. Corner, *Anatomical Texts of the Earlier Middle Ages*, Washington, 1927, pp. 35–43.

[18] S. Fortuna, 'The Latin Editions of Galen's *Opera omnia* (1490–1625) and Their Prefaces' *Early Science and Medicine*, 17, 2012, pp. 391–412; Nutton, *John Caius* (n. 15 above), pp. 21–2.

[19] R. J. Durling, 'A Chronological Census of Renaissance Editions and Translations of Galen', *Journal of the Warburg and Courtland Institutes*, 24, 1961, pp. 230–305.

by Gabriele Zerbi and by Berengario da Carpi, publishing before (or at least in the same year) and after the 1502 edition, there were substantial differences in degree. Zerbi referred to *De usu partium* frequently, citing the information provided by the book for virtually every part of the body. He barely mentioned *De anatomia vivorum*. Berengario, whose work appeared at nearly the same time as Achillini's, made much more use of *De anatomia vivorum*.[20]

Achillini used his references to Galen to augment the information provided in Mondino in much the same way as he augmented Mondino's dissection instructions. For example, after repeating Mondino's account of the tongue, Achillini was able to add that it had nine muscles by citing *De anatomia vivorum* and to note that Galen's *De simplicium medicamentorum* said that there were six nerves connected to it. Both statements represented additional information beyond Mondino who did not count the muscles in the tongue and who only described two nerves. In another example, *De anatomia parva* was Achillini's source for the name of the nerve that goes to the ear, the *posticus*, which Mondino had not provided a name for.[21]

Achillini employed his two most important sources, *De anatomia vivorum* and *De usu partium*, in this way throughout his text, drawing from them to add to information already contained in Mondino, but there were differences in the anatomical details in the two works as well as between them and Mondino and his main source, *De juvamentis membrorum*. When those differences could be interpreted as additional facts (like the number of muscles in the tongue), then Achillini added them without comment, but when the information in different sources conflicted in more complex ways, he had to take a different approach.

Achillini's use of *De anatomia vivorum* in particular is especially apparent in two subjects of importance in the early sixteenth century, generation and vision. Generation and reproduction were of increasing interest to male physicians beginning in the Middle Ages, and by the early sixteenth century these issues involved a variety of anatomical questions including some focused on the structure of the uterus. Achillini clearly tried to bring together a wide variety of material on the uterus from both dissection and texts, and he made a number of adjustments to Mondino's account. Vision and ocular anatomy were part of two intellectual traditions, one mathematical and one anatomical, increasingly cross-connected in the sixteenth century. The study of vision rested on important, empirical investigations of the eye, and Achillini's notes show he had some

[20] For Zerbi's sources see Lind, *Pre-Vesalian* (n. 2 above), pp. 154–5. Berengario's usage of *De anatomia vivorum* is described below.

[21] Achillini, *Annotationes* (n. 1 above), fols 11^r, 13^v.

experience in closely examining eye structure by dissection as well as through textual sources.[22]

Following the pattern of the rest of his notes, Achillini's accounts of anatomical details of the uterus repeated Mondino's ideas and then added to them, but because of the differences in Mondino and *De anatomia vivorum* he made some modifications to Mondino's ideas. Mondino described the uterus as located in the middle of the body, between the rectum and the bladder, and connected to the internal structure of the body by two ligaments which, because of their size and shape, were called the horns of the uterus (*cornua matricis*). The uterus was both nervous and membranous according to Mondino. It had a long neck the end of which was about the same size as the penis and capable of expansion. It was divided into seven cells where fetuses were formed, three on the right, three on the left, and one in the middle. All of this information was repeated by Achillini with a slight modification of the wording about the horns (see below).[23]

Achillini then added to Mondino's material from other sources. Citing Galen's *De anatomia matricis* Achillini added that the neck of the uterus was located under the neck of the bladder. Citing *De anatomia vivorum* he described the neck of the bladder as resembling an inverted penis, an idea not mentioned by Mondino but one also found in *De usu partium*. Other aspects of the anatomy of the uterus given in *De anatomia vivorum* were quite different from Mondino's account and required more careful handling.[24]

Rather than describing the uterus as composed of seven cells in which fetuses were formed, *De anatomia vivorum* said it consisted of two concavities or 'horns' where the fetuses were formed and warned the reader that there were some authors who mistakenly said the uterus consisted of five or even seven cells. *De anatomia vivorum* then pointed out that, like fruit hanging from a tree, the two horns of the uterus could accommodate more than one fetus each, a suggestion apparently intended to refute the reasoning behind a uterus having more than five

---

[22] See M. Green, *Making Women's Medicine Masculine*, Oxford, 2008, pp. 250–55 and K. Park, *Secrets of Women, Gender, Generation, and the Origins of Human Dissection*, New York, 2006, pp. 121–60 for the growing interest in generation and women's bodies. For the details on the sources that contained information about the uterus see Park, *Secrets of Women* (n. 21 above), p. 105. For eye anatomy in the sixteenth century and its connections with theories of vision see T. Baker, 'Dissection, Instruction, and Debate: Visual Theory at the Anatomy Theatre in the Sixteenth Century', in *Practices of Perspective and Renaissance Cultures of Optics*, ed. S. Dupré, Turnhout, 2019, pp. 123–47.

[23] Mondino, *Anatomia* (n. 7 above), fol. 27ᵛ; Achillini, *Annotationes* (n. 1 above), fol. 7ᵛ.

[24] Achillini, *Annotationes* (n. 1 above), fol. 7ᵛ.

or seven cells since the number of cells were often considered connected to the possible number of fetuses.[25]

Achillini repeated these ideas from *De anatomia vivorum* after his description of the seven cells derived from Mondino and shortly after he made a reference to dissection. The material from *De anatomia vivorum* is slightly modified in Achillini's version and the passages are worth repeating in full together to see how Mondino, dissection and *De anatomia vivorum* interlock to form Achillini's account.

> Cut it [the uterus] down the middle [an instruction found in Achillini, but not in Mondino]. In a virgin its mouth is covered by a thin membrane, but in a violated woman this is broken. The mouth of the uterus is like that of an old tench. [All of this echoes Mondino.]
>
> There are three cells in the right side of the uterus, three on the left, and one in the middle. A cell is a cavity in the uterus in which the sperm can coagulate the menstrual blood and bind it to the orifice of the veins. [Again, this is Mondino.]
>
> However, in the book, *De anatomia vivorum*, some people who are led astray say that there are five cells; some say seven, but it must be admitted that more than one fetus can adhere to the same horn of the uterus. [While this is essentially what *De anatomia vivorum* says, the original passage was denying cells in favor of two horns and using the idea of more than one fetus on a single horn as a way of contrasting the number of cells with its own account of two horns and providing a reason why two would be sufficient].[26]

These passages suggest that Achillini tried to fit *De anatomia vivorum*'s account of the uterus into Mondino's rather than to contrast the two, but the conflict between the two sources went beyond the number of cells. Ultimately, the terminology of 'horns' employed in *De anatomia vivorum* and in Mondino differed. While in *De anatomia vivorum* horns were a reference to internal cavities where fetuses were formed, in Mondino the term referred to the ligaments that attached the uterus to the internal structure of the body. To accommodate the problem, in

---

[25] Ps Galen, *De anatomia vivorum* in, *Secunda impressio Galieni quecunq[ue] in prima [con]tinebatur apprehend*, vol. 2, ed. G. Suriano, Venice, 1502, p. 599 (there is no pagination in this work). For the seven cells of the uterus see F. Kudlien, 'The Seven Cells of the Uterus: The Doctrine and Its Roots', *Bulletin of the History of Medicine*, 39, 1965, pp. 415–23.

[26] Achillini, *Annotationes* (n. 1 above), fol. 6ᵛ, 'Scinde eam per medium. Tegitur os matricis in virgine velamine subtili, sed in corrupta est ruptum. Os eius est ut os tinche antique. Cellulae tres in dextro, tres in sinistro, et unam in medio. Cellula est concavitas in matrice in qua sperma coagulare potest sanguinem menstruum, et alligare orificiis venarum. Contra in libro de anatomia vivorum quidam decepti dicunt.v. cellulas quidam .vii. sed dicendum quod eidem cornu<i> plures possunt foetus adherere.' Here I have used the translation found in Lind, *Pre-Vesalian* (n. 2 above), p. 50, with slight modification.

a passage that preceded the ones quoted above Achillini modified Mondino's original description of the ligaments by describing them as the *external* horns, and noting there were also *internal* horns where the fetuses were formed, giving no hint that the distinction allowed him to reconcile the question of cells in later passages essentially be equating cells with internal horns.[27]

There was another issue with the structure of the uterus involving conflicting information from various Galenic sources. Mondino said the uterus was nervous and membranous, but was silent about the number of layers (or tunics) in its walls. However Galen's *De anatomia matricis* said there the uterus consisted of two tunics, while a passage in his *De usu partium* said there was only one. The conflict was discussed early in the sixteenth century by Gabriele Zerbi without reference to *De anatomia vivorum*, but like *De anatomia matricis*, *De anatomia vivorum* also described the uterus as having two tunics. Achillini's account of the tunics of the uterus notes the passage in *De usu partium* but denies its validity without much explanation, simply stating 'but, given that there are two tunics, there is a disagreement here'.[28]

The rest of Achillini's account of the tunics of the uterus then appears to be another attempt to blend ideas from different sources into a coherent whole. According to Achillini, the nervous part of the tunic (apparently a reference to Mondino's description) is the external layer within which is a part with more veins (possibly Mondino's membranous description). The internal tunic is double, however, Achillini adds, while *De anatomia vivorum* says the external tunic is fleshy and thicker and the internal, sinewy. In this picture of the uterus, the issue is that the properties of the layers are described differently by Mondino and *De anatomia vivorum* but the existence of more than one layer is not an issue.[29]

While Zerbi made no reference to *De anatomia vivorum* in his discussion of topics related to generation, Berengario da Carpi, whose book appeared shortly after Achillini's, did. Sometimes referring to it as 'a certain book attributed to Galen [*uno certo libro qui attribuitur Galeno?*]' Berengario cited *De anatomia vivorum* as an example of one of several conflicting sources on the problem of the role of the woman in the formation of the fetus, a subject on which Aristotle and Galen disagreed. Berengario also used *De anatomia vivorum* in a more extensive

---

[27] Achillini, *Annotationes* (n. 1 above), fol. 6ʳ.

[28] Achillini, *Annotationes* (n. 1 above), fol. 6ᵛ, 'sed dato quod sunt duae tunicae discordia est'.

[29] Mondino, *Anatomia* (n. 7 above), fol. 27ᵛ. G. Zerbi, *Liber anathomie corporis humani*, Venice, 1502, fol. 43ʳ. Zerbi's page numbering is complicated. His first two books have an error in pagination so some page numbers are repeated. For clarity, I have added the notation, second, for repeated page numbers in their second appearance. Achillini, *Annotationes* (n. 1 above), fol. 7ᵛ.

way in describing the eye, and in that case his account is closely connected to Achillini's.[30]

Mondino described the eye as having seven tunics and three humours, naming each and providing descriptions that included the reasons for their names. The tunic called the cornea, for example, was so named because it resembled horn and the tunic called the uvea because of its resemblance to a black grape. However, *De anatomia vivorum* described additional details, specifically that the cornea consisted of four tunics, an idea not found in Mondino but repeated by both Achillini and Berengario.[31]

According to Achillini the four layers of the cornea were difficult to separate without boiling, but he knew about them 'from experience (*[cum] experentia*)' before he read about them in *De anatomia vivorum*. It was also by boiling the eye that Achillini was able to see that another tunic, the *conjunctiva*, was outside the cornea, another idea he had found in *De anatomia vivorum* as well as in experience. Achillini's discussion hints at a careful investigation of the eye through boiling not found in the accounts of his contemporary anatomists, but the four layers of the cornea is also a useful way to identify which authors were looking at *De anatomia vivorum*.[32]

In discussing the eye Berengario followed Achillini in naming *De anatomia vivorum* as his source for the existence of four tunics of the cornea. Many of Berengario's references actually came from Gabriele Zerbi's text which he referred to frequently, but Zerbi's account of the eye did not include either the idea that the cornea had four layers or any reference to *De anatomia vivorum*. Berengario and Achillini were teaching at Bologna at the same time, and their shared interest in *De anatomia vivorum* as a source for the anatomy of the eye suggests some common ground, possibly the interest generated by the 1502 Galen.[33]

The next printed works on anatomy after Berengario did not refer to *De anatomia vivorum* nor to anatomical facts (like the four layers of the cornea) that seemed to originate with it. These works came after the appearance of three more *opera omnia* editions, perhaps even more importantly, by 1536 when books by Niccoló Massa and Johannes Winter appeared, two Latin translations of

---

[30] Berengario, *Commentaria*, fols 240ᵛ, 7ʳ, 403ᵛ.

[31] Mondino, *Anatomia* (n. 7 above), fols 58ʳ–59ᵛ; Ps Galen, *De anatomia vivorum* (n. 24 above), p. 595.

[32] Achillini, *Annotationes* (n. 1 above), fols 14ʳ, 15ᵛ.

[33] Berengario, *Commentaria* (n. 29 above), fols 470ʳ, 472ᵛ, 461ᵛ; Zerbi, *Liber anathomie* (n. 28 above), fols 122ʳ–126ʳ (second). For Zerbi and Berengario see R. French, *Dissection and Vivisection in the European Renaissance*, Burlington, VT, 1999, pp. 78–85.

Galen's *On Anatomical Procedures* were published, the first by Berengario nearly a decade after his own anatomical text and the second, translated and published by Johannes Winter in Paris. *On Anatomical Procedures* was cited regularly and used extensively by both Massa and Winter and continued to be influential for later anatomists, like Andreas Vesalius, while *De anatomia vivorum* seems to have been confined to the authors who published in the 1520s.[34]

Achillini's *Anatomical Notes* offer some interesting suggestions about the influence of Galen in early sixteenth century anatomy. It seems clear, that the 1502 edition of Galen's works in Latin had an influence on Achillini. While it did not provide anything new in the way of Latins sources, it served to highlight key works and render them more easily available. Achillini was clearly influenced by Galen's *De usu partium*, but he was also very much interested in the Pseudo-Galenic *De anatomia vivorum*, a work with a number of idiosyncratic anatomical ideas that he sought to incorporate into his reading of Mondino. But Achillini did not confine himself to books. He made active investigations into the body itself, and combined that information with the ideas he found in *De anatomia vivorum*. A comparison between the anatomy of Gabrielle Zerbi, which came before Achillini and in the same year as the 1502 Galen, and the anatomy of Berengario da Carpi, which appeared shortly after Achillini's book, reinforces this idea that *De anatomia vivorum* and the 1502 Galen impacted anatomical study at Bologna in the early years of the sixteenth century.

---

[34] Fortuna, 'Latin Editions' (n. 17 above), p. 395; Durling, 'Chronological' (n. 18 above), pp. 256–7.

Commentariis in Hippocratis librum Epidemiarum II uti non licet: G.B. Rasario and the false 'Galenic' commentary on Epidemics II *

Christina Savino

Galen's commentaries on Hippocrates enjoyed great success in the Renaissance, when the Galenic medical system declined due to new discoveries, especially in the anatomical field. As a result, Galen became more appreciated as a commentator on the Hippocratics rather than as an author himself, and medical humanists insistently sought out as many commentaries as possible.

The publication of unknown and newly rediscovered commentaries in the Renaissance editions was a philological enterprise, which editors were proud to triumphantly announce and praise in their prefaces. This is the case with the editor of the fifth Juntine of Galen, Girolamo Mercuriale (1530–1606), who recalls his emotional state in publishing fragments of two new commentaries in the preface,[1] that is, a few fragments of the *Commentary* on *De alimento* and a short fragment of the second book of the *Commentary* on *Epidemics* II.[2] As a matter of fact, we do know nowadays that the fragments of the *Commentary* on *De alimento*, which had been provided by the well-known physician and humanist Giovanni Battista Rasario (1517–78),[3] were forgeries made by Rasario himself.[4] Rasario had

* I would like to thank the Humboldt University of Berlin, Department of Classical Philology, and particularly Philip van der Eijk, for providing both financial and intellectual support and giving the opportunity of developing this research. I owe a very special thanks to Stefania Fortuna for reading my manuscript at an early stage and offering suggestions and Caroline Petit for improving my paper both linguistically and technically.

[1] See S. Fortuna, 'Girolamo Mercuriale editore di Galeno', in *Girolamo Mercuriale. Medicina e cultura nell'Europa del Cinquecento*, eds A. Arcangeli and V. Nutton, Florence, 2008, pp. 217–31, who reports the passage of the preface where Mercuriale praises the new commentaries.

[2] R. J. Durling, 'A Chronological Census of Renaissance Editions and Translations of Galen', *Journal of the Warburg and Courtauld Institutes*, 24, 1961, pp. 230–305, and in particular p. 294 n. 150 and n. 152 (2).

[3] C. Savino, 'Giovanni Battista Rasario and the 1562–1563 Edition of Galen. Research, Exchanges and Forgeries', *Early Science and Medicine*, 17, 4, 2012, pp. 413–45; and also C. Savino, "Galenic' Forgeries of the Renaissance: An Overview on Commentaries Falsely Attributed to Galen', in *Brill's Companion to the Reception of Galen*, eds P. Bouras Vallianatos and B. Zipser, Leiden/Boston, 2019, pp. 453–71; C. Savino, *Il medico di Utopia. Giovanni Battista Rasario (1517–1578) traduttore e falsario di testi medici greci*, Udine, 2020.

[4] See above all K. Deichgräber, *Pseudhippokrates Über die Nahrung. Text, Kommentar und Würdigung einer stoisch-heraklitisierenden Schrift aus der Zeit um Christi Geburt*, Wiesbaden, 1973,

falsely attributed to Galen also other commentaries – namely the *Commentary on De Humoribus*;[5] the fragment of the *Commentary* on *Epidemics* VI supposedly belonging to the seventh, the eighth and the very end of the sixth book;[6] and the fragment of the *Commentary* on Plato's *Timaeus*,[7] all of them published in Rasario's edition of Galen's *Opera omnia* printed by Valgrisi, in Venice, in 1562–3.[8] Nevertheless, he never turned out to be involved in the falsification of the *Commentary* on *Epidemics* II, although it is well known that the work published by Mercuriale was a Renaissance forgery as well.[9]

Galen's *Commentary* on *Epidemics* II was already incomplete at Ḥunayn ibn Isḥāq's's time, when it was translated into Arabic.[10] Subsequently the original

pp. 12–13 n. 12; D. Manetti and A. Roselli, 'Galeno commentatore di Ippocrate', in *Aufstieg und Niedergang der römischen Welt*, eds H. Temporini and W. Haase, 2.37.2. Berlin/New York, 1994, pp. 1529–1635 (p. 1570); T. Raiola, 'Alle origini di un falso galenico: il *Commento* al *De alimento* e una citazione di Sabino', *Aion*, 32, 2010, pp. 101–10; I. Garofalo, 'Il commento di Galeno al *De alimento* e gli estratti di 'Alî ibn Ridwân', *Galenos*, 6, 2013, pp. 123–64.

[5] Durling, 'Chronological Census' (n. 2 above), p. 295 n. 154; K. Deichgräber, *Hippokrates De humoribus in der Geschichte der griechischen Medizin*, Wiesbaden, 1972, pp. 39–40; Manetti and Roselli, 'Galeno commentatore' (n. 4 above), p. 1532 n. 3; I. Garofalo, 'Galen's commentary on Hippocrates' *De humoribus*', in *Hippocrates in Context*, ed. P. van der Eijk, Leiden/Boston, 2005, pp. 445–56 (447 n. 17), and 'Il falso commento di Galeno al 'De humoribus' e un saggio di edizione del vero', in *Sulla tradizione indiretta dei testi medici greci*, eds I. Garofalo, A. Lami and A. Roselli, Pisa/Roma, 2009, pp. 201–18.

[6] Durling, 'Chronological Census' (n. 2 above), p. 295 n. 152 (4) e, f; see also E. Wenkebach, *Beiträge zur Textgeschichte der Epidemienkommentare Galens*, 2 vols, Berlin, 1928, and *Galeni in Hippocratis Epidemiarum librum VI commentaria I-VI; commentaria VI-VIII ...* (CMG V 10, 2, 2), Leipzig, Berlin, 1956, pp. xxiii–iv.

[7] Durling, 'Chronological Census' (n. 2 above), p. 293 n. 132 b; see also O. Schröder, *Galeni In Platonis Timaeum commentarii fragmenta*, Leipzig/Berlin, 1934 (CMG Suppl. I), pp. xxii and Appendix I, pp. 85 ff.

[8] Savino, 'Giovanni Battista Rasario' (n. 3 above).

[9] Durling, 'Chronological Census' (n. 2 above), n. 152 (2); E. Wenkebach, 'Pseudogalenische Kommentare zu den Epidemien des Hippokrates', *Abh. d. Königl. Preß. Akad. d. Wiss.: Königlich Preussische Akademie der Wissenschaften zu Berlin*, Berlin, 1917, pp. 23–52; and 'Untersuchungen über Galens Kommentare zu den Epidemien des Hippokrates', *Abh. d. Königl. Preß. Akad. d. Wiss.: Königlich Preussische Akademie der Wissenschaften zu Berlin*, 1925, pp. 18 ff.; Manetti and Roselli, 'Galeno commentatore' (n. 4 above), p. 1548 n. 67; on this see also the recent critical edition of the Arabic version of the *Commentary on Epidemics II*, U. Vagelpohl, *Galeni in Hippocratis Epidemiarum librum II commentaria I–VI, versionem arabicam* (CMG Suppl. Or. V 2), Berlin, 2016, pp. 15 ff.

[10] On this see R. Alessi, 'Un exemple de l'utilité du commentaire de Galien pour l'établissement et l'interprétation du texte du deuxième livre des Épidémies d'Hippocrate: Épidémies II, 1, c. 1–2', in *Hommage au doyen Weiss*, eds M. Dubrocard and C. Kirchner, Nice, 1996, pp. 39–59; 'The Arabic Version of Galen's Commentary on Hippocrates' Epidemics, Book Two, as a source for the Hippocratic Text: First Remarks', in *Epidemics in Context: Greek Commentaries on Hippocrates in the Arabic Tradition*, ed. P. E. Pormann, Berlin, 2012, pp. 71–92; I. Garofalo, 'I lemmi ippocratici

Greek was completely lost. It seemed to have suddenly made its reappearance in the Renaissance, as Mercuriale published the small fragment that we have mentioned. The fragment was preserved only in one Greek manuscript, which had been provided by Agostino Gadaldini.[11] Mercuriale published the text of the manuscript, which represented the final part of the second book of the *Commentary*, together with his own translation, in two synoptical columns.[12] This was published as the only extant text of Galen's genuine commentary on *Epidemics* II. A somewhat larger fragment, though, was published for the first time in the sixth Juntine, edited in Venice in 1586 by Giovanni Costeo (1528–1603). This text, which was reprinted in all later Juntines until 1625,[13] had been translated by Rasario. In 1617 a new Latin translation of the *Commentary* was published, together with the Greek text, which was hitherto unknown, by the Cypriot scholar Joannes Sozomenos (1578–1633).[14] This text was reprinted in Chartier's edition;[15] hence it came to Kühn, who merely reprinted his predecessor's edition.[16]

However, while consulting the *Index librorum*, in the twentieth and last volume of Kühn's reprinted edition, one reads the following warning: *Commentariis in Hippocratis scripta De alimento, Epidemiarum II, De humoribus uti non licet, quos falsarii saeculi XVI compilaverint.* This note was written by Professor Konrad Schubring, who rebuilt the research activities of the *Corpus Medicorum Graecorum* (CMG) after the Second World War from 1946 to 1961 and revised Kühn's work.[17] What happened in between?

di Epidemie II e la traduzione araba del commento di Galeno', in *Officina Hippocratica*, eds C. Brockmann, K.-D. Fischer, L. Perilli and A. Roselli, Berlin, 2011, pp. 57–75. The Arabic translation has been now edited by the CMG, see Vagelpohl, CMG Suppl. Or. V 2 (n. 9 above), pp. 45 ff. (on the translation); pp. 76–967 (for the critical text with the English translation).

[11] *Galeni omnia quae extant opera*, I, f. AVr.

[12] Stefania Fortuna has communicated to me that it had actually already been published in Latin by Gadaldini, in the Juntine of 1556, as a supplement to Galen's treatise *On the affected parts* IV.3, which in turn contains a long quotation from *Epidemics* II (fol. 23ᵛ). Herein the fragment had been attributed to Galen, but it is surely not authentic, as it does not match with the extant Arabic translation. Its origin may be connected with a group of manuscripts of the *On the affected parts* that contain *scholia*. Most likely Mercuriale back-translated it into Greek.

[13] Durling, 'Chronological Census' (n. 2 above), n. 152 (2).

[14] J. Sozomenos, *Commentarius in secundum Epidemiorum Hippocratis [cum textu], nunc primum e graeco in latinum sermonem translatus*, Venice, 1617. This translation does not feature in Durling's Census inasmuch later than 1599.

[15] R. Chartier, *Hippocratis Coi, et Claudii Galeni ... Opera*, IX, Paris, 1689, pp. 123–83.

[16] C. G. Kühn, *Claudii Galeni opera omnia*, Leipzig, 1828, XVII A, 303–479 K.

[17] C. G. Kühn, *Claudii Galeni opera omnia*, repr. Hildesheim, 1960, vol. XX: *Continens indicem in Galeni libros auctore Fr. Guil. Assmanno epilogum et notas bibliographicas adiecit K. Schubring*, see in particular pp. xvii–lxii.

Since the early decades of the 1900s the text of the *Commentary* on *Epidemics* was intensively investigated with the purpose of completing a critical edition for the CMG. Ernst Wenkebach, who was the scholar in charge of editing the text, wrote two articles of *prolegomena* in which he claimed that the *Commentary* printed by Kühn could not have been authentic.[18] In the first article, published in 1917, Wenkebach classified the *Commentary* as a forgery of the Renaissance, based on the retroversion of the commentary on Hippocrates' *Epidemics* II written by Anuce Foes (1528–91), which had been published in 1560.[19] Concerning the origin of the forgery, Wenkebach assumed that it had been made by Sozomenos himself. Thus in the second article, published in 1925, Wenkebach strengthened his position and aimed to demonstrate his hypothesis through a textual analysis of selected sample passages. His arguments were based on a philological investigation of the Greek and the Latin text, but his conclusions were partially incorrect, as he failed to consider Rasario's text – even if he did know it and quoted it in his articles.

As already stated, Rasario's translation was published in the sixth Juntine, which was edited by Giovanni Costeo in 1586. This new text, whose title was *Commentarius secundus Galeni in librum vulgarium morborum Hippocratis secundum, nunquam alias vel graece, vel latine impressus*, was introduced on the frontispiece of the first volume together with another novelty that I have mentioned above, namely the *Commentary* on *De Humoribus*, or *Galeni in libros Hippocratis de Humoribus commentarii tres, in prioribus editionibus nostris desiderati*, which had not been printed in the Juntines yet, with the words *accesserunt nunc etiam*.

The order of the Galenic writings in the sixth Juntine is that established by Giovanni Battista Montano for the Juntine of 1541.[20] Therefore, the two novelties are included in the third class,[21] which is devoted to pathology and gathers several treatises of this medical branch – such as *De differentiis* and *De causis*

---

[18] See n. 9.

[19] A. Foes, *Liber secundus de morbis vulgaribus, difficillimus & pulcherrimus: olim à Galeno Commentarijs illustratus, qui temporis iniuria interciderunt: nunc verò penè in integrum restitutus, commentarijs sex & Latinitate donatus* … , Basel, 1560.

[20] On this order see D. Mugnai Carrara, 'Le epistole prefatorie sull'ordine dei libri di Galeno di Giovan Battista da Monte: esigenze di metodo e dilemmi editoriali', in *Vetustatis indagator. Scritti offerti a Filippo Di Benedetto*, eds V. Fera and A. Guida, Messina/Firenze, 1999, pp. 207–34. In general on the order of Galen's writings see also C. Domingues, 'Les éditions grecques et latines des œuvres de Galien', in *Lire les médecins grecs à la Renaissance: aux origines de l'édition médicale*, eds V. Boudon-Millot and G. Cobolet, Paris, 2004, pp. 169–85.

[21] Mugnai Carrara, 'Le epistole' (n. 20 above), pp. 224–8.

morborum, De marasmo, De marcore, and *De tumoribus praeter naturam* – followed by commentaries.

The table of contents of the third class displays the books of the *Commentary* presented in accordance with Hippocrates' *Epidemics,* that is, first the *Commentary* on *Epidemics* I translated by Herman Croeser, or *Cruserius,* and revised by Gadaldini; followed by the 'new' *Commentary* on *Epidemics* II, here presented as follows: *In secundum Hippocratis de morbis vulgaribus librum Commentarius secundus, novissime repertus & a Io. Baptista Rasario e Graeco in Latinum sermonem translatus;*[22] then the *Commentary* on *Epidemics* III, also translated by Croeser; and finally the *Commentary* on *Epidemics* VI translated by Giunio Paolo Grassi. This order, however, does not reflect the actual very sequence of the books of the *Commentary* in this edition, since the *Commentary* on *Epidemics* II (f. 198) does not follow that on *Epidemics* I, but the *Commentary* as a whole, that is, as it had circulated before the publication of the new books, namely *Commentary* on *Epidemics* I (f. 100), III (f. 127) and VI (f. 152); afterwards, we find the fragments remaining from books 6, 7 and 8 of the *Commentary* on *Epidemics* VI, also translated by Rasario (fols 212ᵛ–225ʳ); and finally the (false) *Commentary* on *Humors,* which had already been published by Rasario himself together with the extant fragments of the *Commentary* on *Epidemics* VI in 1562.[23]

The *Commentary* on *Epidemics* II looks defective, as it contains only the second book (fols 198ʳ–204ᵛ) and the third (fols 204ᵛ–212ʳ). Moreover, the text appears marked with asterisks, which are intended to indicate *lacunae* or illegible elements in the source. I have attempted to analyse this text by taking the sample passages considered by Wenkebach as a starting point. In his articles, these were compared with Foes's commentary and Sozomenos's text. My aim is to put Rasario's Latin translation into the frame again.

1. The first passage selected by Wenkebach[24] comes from the very beginning of the third book of the *Commentary* on *Epidemics* II 1 (cf. XVII A, 385.11 f. K.), which contains a description of the climatic condition in Perinthos and related pathological symptoms.

---

[22] After this title the following note is found: *graecus codex apud nos est, quem iustis de causis nunc una cum Latino non impressimus.*

[23] *In Hippocratis librum de humoribus, commentarii tres: Eiusdem reliquum sexti commentarii in sextum de vulgaribus morbis: itemque septimus, & octavus: nuper in lucem editi, ac latinitate donati: Io. Baptista Rasario interprete,* Venice, 1562. On this publication see also Savino, 'Giovanni Battista Rasario' (n. 3 above), pp. 415 f.

[24] Wenkebach, 'Pseudogalenische Kommentare' (n. 9 above), p. 23.

	Foes, 1560, pp. 204 ff.	Rasario, 1586, fol. 204ᵛ	Sozomenos, 1617, pp. 105 ff.
	Toto igitur anno quem describit, impense squalido et sicco, quis non febrium ardentium rabiem merito	cum igitur totus annus esset, ut ipse describit, valde squalidus, et valde siccus, ecquis non magnam febrium	totoque anni cursu, quem describit valde siccum & aridum, quisnam non praevidisset magnum ar
5	suspectabit? Cum ne ab imbribus quidem ullis, aut ventorum flatibus, tam vehementi squalori quies aut interspiratio daretur?	ardentium copiam futuram suspicaretur? Praesertim vero cum longo tempore, neque pluisset, neque venti spirassent. Praeterea vero	doris concussum futurum, praecipue vero in tanta pluviae siccitate, & diuturna respirationis carentia? Praetera vero neque vomitus
10	Unde praeter sudorum proluviem et rigoris concussationem (quae sunt febrium ardentium effugia) alvus ipsa tenuibus, spumanti	non vomebant: et alvi tenuibus, aqueis, et bile carentibus excrementis turbabantur. Hic porro annus fuit mulieribus pericu	aderant, & ventres perturbabantur ex tenuibus, aqueis minimeque biliosis. Imminebat autem praecipue hoc anno mulieribus periculum,
15	bus et aquosis proluebatur. Mulieribus autem praecipue periculum creavit hic anni status, quod temporis siccitate efferata bilis, humidam	losus maxime, quod bilis constitutionis squalore effera reddita, humidam naturam miserandum in modum exagitavit: et variis vexatam	quia nimirum bilis propter constitutionis siccitatem ferocior mirum in modum humidam naturam laedebat varieque vexabat. Unde &
20	naturam misere exagitaret aut variis modis vexatam dimitteret: unde sopores, leves etiam membrorum resolutiones ortum habuerunt.	modis dimisit: unde sopores, desipientiae, et alia huius generis orta sunt.	veternum & deliramenta, hisque similia contingebant.

From the previous synoptic table, a self-evident, remarkable similarity among the samples emerges. Looking at the very *incipit*, for instance, we could affirm that Foes, Sozomenos and Rasario basically display the same content (cf. Foes, ll. 1–3: *Toto igitur anno, quem describit, impense squalido et sicco*; Rasario, ll. 1–3: *cum igitur totus annus esset, ut ipse describit, valde squalidus, et valde siccus*; Sozomenos, ll. 1–3: *totoque anni cursu, quem describit valde siccum & aridum*). Sozomenos has clearly rephrased the text and replaced some words – for example, in the *incipit* that I have mentioned above, he employed a syntactic construction similar to that used by Foes with the addition of *cursu*, and afterwards makes the adjectives *siccum* and *aridum* agree with *quem* as predicates of the object – but he still did not distance himself significantly from his predecessors. Because of the striking similarities with Foes's commentary, Wenkebach assumed that Sozomenos's text must have depended upon it. But he overlooked Rasario's text, although Sozomenos's dependence upon Rasario is clearly demonstrated from those textual features that Wenkebach called the 'Freiheiten' of the forger

(Sozomenos) towards his model (Foes) and fill the gap between the two.[25] To turn to details, Wenkebach pointed out that Sozomenos fails to mention the *sudorum proluvies* and the *rigoris concussio*, both of them *effugia febrium ardentium* (cf. Foes, ll. 9–13), while he mentions the absence of vomit (cf. Sozomenos, ll. 8–9: *praeterea vero neque vomitus aderant*); moreover, Sozomenos omitted the qualification of 'foamy' related to excrements (cf. Foes, l. 14: *spumantibus*), adding instead that of 'poor in bile' (cf. Sozomenos, l. 11: *minimeque biliosis*).[26] If we take a look at Rasario's text, though, we realize that all these divergences were already witnessed by it (cf. Rasario, l. 8: *Praeterea vero non vomebant*; ll. 9–10: *bile carentibus excrementis*), which must have been Sozomenos's source. Moreover, it must be noticed that the peculiar elements found in Sozomenos's and Rasario's text, namely vomit and excrements poor in bile, closely recall another passage of *Epidemics* II (cf. Hipp. *Ep.* II 3,1,5–7 = L. V 100,5 f.) according to Foes's translation (cf. Foes, 1560, pp. 200, 21 f.: *nulli aderant vomitus, sed / alvi perturbationes, ex tenuibus, a- / quosis, non biliosis [et spumantibus / multis* etc...]). Most likely, this passage was also known to Rasario, who might have omitted or just left out *spumantibus*, taking *biliosis* as the endpoint, as so did Sozomenos.

2. The second passage comes from the third book of the *Commentary* on *Epidemics* II 1 as well (cf. XVII A, 388.10 f. K.).[27] In the Kühn edition the text is introduced by asterisks, which indicate damage in the model, as we find in Rasario:

	Foes, 1560, p. 208	Rasario, 1586, fols 204ᵛ ff.	Sozomenos, 1617, pp. 109 ff.
5	Istud magnam tenuium et mordacium humorum acrimoniam indicat [...]	*** quod autem ait, Quibus simile erat, quod aeri expo- nebantur; magnam tenuium, mordaciumque humorum acrimoniam significat: quaene depositis quidem excrementis, et sub dio retentis spumantem fervoris ebullitionem deponeret.	Quod vero dicit, unde & soli expositum mag- nam denotat subtilium acriumque humorum mor- dacitatem, quae expulsis eiectisque excrementis spumosum ebulitionem non deponit, quod vero dixit
10	τεθέντα] vero hic eo sen- su sumitur, quo κείμενα οὖρα πολὺν χρόνον dicit Hippocr. lib. I Epidem. ut deposita et reservata recrementa significet.	*** Illo autem verbo, Deposita, significat, cum in vase steterint, sicut in primo De morbis vulga- ribus loquitur, cum ait, Urina quae diu in matellis stetit, non subsidebat.	deposita significat iacentia ut in I. Epidem. quo loci dicit ventus diu iacens minime quiescebat.

---

[25] Wenkebach, 'Pseudogalenische Kommentare' (n. 9 above), p. 24.

[26] Wenkebach, 'Pseudogalenische Kommentare' (n. 9 above), pp. 23–4.

[27] Wenkebach, 'Pseudogalenische Kommentare' (n. 9 above), p. 24.

In this case Sozomenos's text is longer than Foes's, but corresponds to that of Rasario in significant ways. Both of them begin introducing a quotation (cf. Rasario, l. 1: *quod autem ait*; Sozomenos, l. 1: *quod vero dicit*). The following quotation corresponds once again to Hippocrates' *Epidemics* (cf. Hipp. *Ep.* II 3,1,8–9 = L. V 100,5) according to Foes's translation (cf. Foes, 1560, p. 201,1–2: *quibus sane simile erat, quod aeri exponebatur*). Sozomenos's quotation looks like a shorter, abridged version of Rasario's one and is characterized by the erroneous reading *soli* (cf. Sozomenos, l. 1) instead of *aeri* (cf. Rasario, l. 2). Thus, we have another hint that Foes was known and used by Rasario, who was in turn the model for Sozomenos. The latter also shows another significant mistake compared to his two predecessors, which can be spotted in the last passage (cf. Sozomenos, l. 11: *ventus*, against Rasario, l. 12: *urina* and Foes, l. 10: οὖρα).

3. The third passage comprises a Hippocratic lemma and related commentary, also taken from the third book of the *Commentary* on *Epidemics* II 22 (cf. XVII A, 431.7 f. K.).[28]

	Foes Comm., 1560, pp. 271 ff.	Rasario, 1586, fol. 209ʳ	Sozomenos, 1617, p. 169
5	*Podagricis humorum co-itus & tubercula dura in lingua sublevantur, & humiles calculi concrescunt, imbecillitatesque illis circa articulos fiunt. Ossium enim natura quod indurentur aut contendantur in causa est.*	*Quae in lingua* συστρέμματα *sublevabantur, et humiles calculi, et quae podagricis accidebant, imbecillitates illis ad articulos faciebant. Ossium enim natura in causa est, ut indurentur, et contendatur.*	*Quae attolluntur in linguis collectiones, & humiles calculi quae podagricis circa debiles eorum articulos, & ossium natura causa est ut haec & indurentur & distendantur.*
10	συστρέμματα καὶ συστρο-φαὶ φύματα καὶ σκληρίας *significant. Est enim humorum congeries, quae tubercula dura parit.*	συστρέμματα καὶ συστροφαί *significant tubercula, et duritias. Humorum enim congeries tubercula gignit.*	*Collectiones & convolutiones, tumores & durities significant, etenim humorum adunatio tumores parit.*

---

[28] Wenkebach, 'Pseudogalenische Kommentare' (n. 9 above), pp. 25–6.

	Foes Comm., 1560, pp. 271 ff.	Rasario, 1586, fol. 209ʳ	Sozomenos, 1617, p. 169
15	Podagrici autem cum toto nervoso genere sint imbecilles et fluxionibus obnoxii, his tamen quae ab excrementis pleno cerebro	Podagrici autem toto nervoso genere imbecilles sunt: et fluxionibus obnoxii: praecipue autem iis excrementis, quae a pleno	Podagra autem laborantes nervorum omnium infirmitates patiuntur, & catarris subiecti sunt, praecipue vero iis haec contingunt,
20	derivant, saepe tentantur. Unde non mirum est tuberculis linguae affligi, quae etiam meridianibus, et	cerebro dimanant. Unde tubercula in lingua oriuntur, quae etiam pustulae vocantur: suntque	qui excrementis repletum cerebrum habent, propterea etiam in lingua tumores adnascuntur, quos
25	vix dum cibum sumptum edormientibus, plerumque negocium facessunt. Statim enim ab exhalantibus cibis cerebro oppleto, magnus fit excrementorum proventus,	pituitae acidae, ac salsae semina.	phyctidas vocant, sunt vero hi fetus salsi, & acuti phlegmatis.
30	qui in loca vicina decumbit, linguamque et fauces salsugine et acrimonia propemodum vellicat, lancinat, convellit, et pustulis		
35	opplet, quas φλυκτίδας vocat Pollux. Et haec sunt pituitae acidae et salsae semina. Quae pro materiae aeternitate moram trahunt		
40	et sua magnitudine sunt conspicua. συστρέμματα autem, humorum coitum ex Celso verti, qui ex tuberculorum est genere. Sic enim		
45	libro quinto Hippocratis σύστρεμμα vertere videtur.		
	Calculos vero in articulorum inanitatibus fieri a crassis et viscidis humoribus certum	Calculos autem a crassis, viscidisque gigni humoribus, neminem praeterit:	Capillos (sic) autem a crassis et viscosis humoribus gigni nullum latet,
50	est, qui oppleta articulatione partes vicinas distendunt, et motum impediunt, diuturnitate vero temporis et benigni	temporis autem progressu et duritias, et callos efficiunt.	processu vero temporis & durities & tremores afferunt.
55	caloris penuria pro loci et humoris natura, duritiem et callum concipiunt.		

	Foes Comm., 1560, pp. 271 ff.	Rasario, 1586, fol. 209ʳ	Sozomenos, 1617, p. 169
	Ossium vero natura cum	Ossium vero natura cum	Ossium autem natura
	dura sit per se et inflexibilis,	ipsa per se dura, et non	cum sit dura & inflex-
	articulationibus multis	flexibilis sit, multis ar-	ibilis multis indiget ad
60	ad motum indiguit, quae	ticulationibus ad motum	motum articulationibus,
	propria sunt arthritidis	indiguit: quae propria	quae propria articularis
	conceptacula. Ossa enim	sunt doloris articulorum	potentiae vasa censentur,
	reapse terrea, humore aliquo	conceptacula. Cum enim	terrea enim cum sint ossa
	sed viscido, glutinoso et	ossa sint terrea, humorem	humorem quendam re-
65	crasso irrorantur. Quae si	aliquem, sed viscidum, et	quirunt, verum viscosum
	accessione humoris praeter	crassum expetiverunt, ut	& crassum ad hoc ut
	naturam obrigeant, tum	eo quasi irrorentur. Quod	quodam modo referiger-
	ad motum inepta sunt,	si quis humor praeter nat-	entur. Quod si & humor
	atque ipsa distensione et	uram accedat, ad motum	aliquis praeter naturam
70	affrictu humorem illum	inepta redduntur. Quibus	addatur, fiunt ad motum
	imis cavitatibus incunea-	casibus podagrici valde ob-	idonea, quibus sympto-
	tum indurant, et veluti suo	noxii sunt propter multas	matibus obnoxii valde
	affixu obfirmant. Quibus	pedum.	sunt qui podagra laborant
	casibus valde sunt obnoxii		propter multas pedum.
75	podagrici, ob numerosam		***
	pedum articulationem.		

The three texts look very similar from the beginning until the passage which is devoted to a rash on the tongue. From *unde* (cf. l. 20 ff.) on, then, Foes displays a much larger text than Rasario and Sozomenos. For instance, Rasario's text does not mention the explanation of the onset of the rash (cf. Foes, l. 21 f.), skipping directly to the definition of *pustulae*, nor does it shows any passage corresponding to that in which Foes discusses his rendering of συστρέμματα as *humorum coitus*, which derives from Celsus's work (cf. Foes, ll. 39–44). As far as Sozomenos is concerned, his text contains some other errors, such as *causa est* instead of *in causa est* in the Hippocratic lemma (cf. ll. 5–8) and *capillos* instead of *calculos* in the commentary (cf. l. 45). Moreover, he turns out not to be so familiar with the Galenic terminology by substituting *nervorum omnium* (l. 14) for *toto nervoso genere*, which is witnessed by Foes (l. 15) and Rasario (l. 14). As far as his relation to Foes is concerned, it should be noticed that in this passage they both agree on the reading *parit* (ll. 13–14) against Rasario's variant *gignit* (l. 14), and also that they both display the mention of the Greek name of the rash *phlyctidae* (cf. Foes, l. 33; Sozomenos, l. 22), which Rasario only attests in translation (cf. Rasario, l. 21: *pustulae*). This might mean that Sozomenos did know Foes and consulted his commentary independently of Rasario. On the other hand, it has to be noticed that Rasario and Sozomenos share an incomplete, lacunose sentence at the very end of the passage – whereas Foes's text displays the word *articulationem*, which makes its sense clear – and this was apparently not easy for Sozomenos to restore, as it was marked by him as defective.

4. The fourth and last passage selected by Wenkebach,[29] which is also taken from the third book of the *Commentary* on *Epidemics* II 33 (cf. XVII A, 449.14 f. K.), displays a textual transmission similar to the previous one with Rasario's and Sozomenos's final part lacking.

	Foes, 1560, pp. 296 ff.	Rasario, 1586, fol. 210ᵛ	Sozomenos, 1617, p. 191
	Ἃ δεῖ εἰδέναι ἐς τὸν	Monet Hippocrates, ut	Hortatur considerationem
	ἑπτάμηνον] rationem	partus, qui septimo, quique	habendam de eo partu,
	habendam esse septimestris	nono mense in lucem edatur,	qui septimo mense editur,
	et nonimestris partus signi-	habeamus rationem: et	& de eo qui nono. Verum
5	ficat eiusque qui hos menses	spectemus etiam eum, qui	praeterea, & de eo qui
	superat. Vitales enim sunt,	hoc tempus excedat. Si	hoc tempus excedit, vivit
	et rationem hebdomadum	quidem is vivit: et rationem	namque; hic, & computum
	Hippocraticarum subeunt.	Hippocraticarum hebdo-	Hipp. hebdomadarum ser-
	Novem autem menses,	madum servat. Novem	vat. Novem nam. menses
10	ducentorum et septuaginta	enim menses numerum	dant numerum ducentorum
	dierum numerum conficiunt,	ducentorum septuaginta	septuaginta dierum, ut
	ut indicat Hippocrates libro	dierum continent: sicut in	dedicimus (sic) ex lib. De
	Περὶ σαρκῶν. ἐννέα δὲ	libro De carnibus didicimus,	carnibus quo loci scribit.
	μηνῶν καὶ δέκα ἡμερέων	ubi scriptum est: Partus	Novem vero mensium, et
15	γόνος γίγνεται, καὶ ζῇ, καὶ	editur novem mensibus, ac	decem dierum partus fit,
	ἔχει τὸν ἀριθμὸν ἀτρεκέα ἐς	decem diebus, ac vivit: ha-	et vivit et habet numerum
	τὰς ἑβδομάδας· τέσσαρες	betque perfectum numerum	perfectum in hebdomadas.
	δεκάδες ἑβδομάδων ἡμέραι	hebdomadum. Nam quat-	Quattuor namque dec-
	εἰσὶ διηκόσιαι ὀγδοήκοντα·	tuor decades hebdomadum	ades hebdomadarum dant
20	ἐς δὲ τὴν δεκάδα τῶν ἑβδο-	dies conficiunt ducentos	numerum ducentorum oc-
	μάδων ἑβδομήκοντα ἡμέραι.	octoginta. Ad decadem	tuaginta dierum, in decade
	Quam Hippocratis opin-	autem hebdomadum dies	autem hebdomadarum sep-
	ionem sequitur Avicennas	septuaginta requiruntur.	tuaginta sunt dies *** quod
	fen. 21 tertii. Quod autem	Quod addit, Graecos menses	vero fieri Graecos menses
25	hic Graecos menses vocat	confici. ****	***
	plenos et integros, quos sol-		
	ares dicimus, intelligit: ut ex		
	Hippocraticae πραγματείας		
	numeris satis coniicere licet,		
30	quos partioni attribuit.		

---

[29] Wenkebach, 'Pseudogalenische Kommentare' (n. 9 above), p. 27.

In this case, Foes's commentary ends with a mention of Avicenna, to whom the very final sentence of the text is attributed. Such a mention would not have been suitable in a Galenic commentary and so has been left out by Rasario and Sozomenos, who both indicate a *lacuna* at this point.

Thus, the textual analysis of the passages selected by Wenkebach, reconsidered in light of Rasario's work, demonstrates that Sozomenos, who was supposed to be the forger of the *Commentary* on *Epidemics* II, represents only a further stage of the transmission of the forgery, such that the publication date of his edition, 1617, must be taken as a *terminus ante quem* for the very set-up of the text. Most likely, Sozomenos produced the Greek text backtranslating the Latin text composed by Rasario, while an independent use of Foes's commentary remains uncertain so far. Thus it would be right to say that Sozomenos was the author of deliberate falsification of the Greek version of the *Commentary*, while the primary falsification had already been made in Latin by Rasario, in the same way as other well-known fake commentaries, at the time when he worked on his complete edition of Galen.

Nevertheless, Wenkebach was right to stress the striking similarities between the forgery and Foes's commentary, except that they instead concern the relationship of Foes to Rasario.

Foes published his commentary on Hippocrates' *Epidemics* II in 1560 – even if it was written before 1558 – and Rasario was presumably working on his forgery between 1555 and 1562 – although it was printed only in 1586: this means that the two commentaries are close contemporaries and any hint of priority of one over another must be found in the text by means of a philological investigation. Let us start with a few preliminary observations.

Foes's commentary comprises the whole text of *Epidemics* II, which is divided into six sections on the basis of a philological argumentation set out by the editor in the preface. However, as already said, Rasario's Pseudo-Galenic commentary looks defective and is divided into two books, that is book II and III, which approximately correspond to section two (cf. Foes, 1560, p. 126; Rasario, 1586, p. 198^r) and three of Foes's commentary (cf. Foes, 1560, p. 197; Rasario, 1586, p. 204^v).

With regard to the ancient sources, Foes turns to Galen's writings and commentaries very frequently by quoting from them and usually openly discussing the quotations. For instance, in one passage he regrets the loss of Galen's *Commentary* on *Epidemics* II, which would have been an incredibly useful support and a guide in interpreting Hippocrates (cf. Foes, 1560, p. 8). Elsewhere he quotes sentences and interpretations from Galen's commentary on the other books of

Epidemics, namely *Commentary* on *Epidemics* I (cf. Foes, 1560, pp. 11; 29; 77; 79; 95), *Epidemics* III (cf. Foes, 1560, p. 13), *Epidemics* VI (cf. Foes, 1560, pp. 34; 55; 56; 60; 67; 73; 86), and also from many other Galenic commentaries on Hippocratics, such as the *Commentary* on *Progn.* (cf. Foes, 1560, pp. 50; 75), on *Prorrh.* (cf. Foes, 1560, pp. 37; 43; 47; 90; 95), on *Aph.* (cf. Foes, 1560, pp. 41; 57), on *De ratione victus* (cf. Foes, 1560, p. 52), on *De articulis* (cf. Foes, 1560, pp. 66; 70; 71), and on *De Fracturis* (cf. Foes, 1560, p. 67). He even acknowledges Galen as a source of inspiration for his own arguments (cf. for instance Foes, 1560, p. 43: *ex Gal. interpretati sumus*; p. 46 and 98: *ut inquit Galenus*; p. 87: *ex Gal. probavimus* etc.).

Also, when it comes to the rendering and the translation technique, Foes discusses his choices using literary parallels. In one passage, for instance, he opts for *polenta* as an equivalent to πάλην ἀλφίτων on the basis of Pliny (*ex Plinio*), who was in turn translating Dioscorides with this term, and extensively discusses his lexical choice (cf. Foes, 1560, p. 128). And it is worth mentioning that, in the corresponding passage of the Pseudo-Galenic commentary by Rasario, we find the same Latin term, except that there is no mention of a source here (cf. Rasario, 1586, p. 198ʳ). More generally, when Rasario distances himself from Foes, he encounters inconsistencies or mistakes: for instance, when Foes mentions the Hippocratic treatise *De aere* (cf. Foes, 1560, p. 152), Rasario shares the same reference, adding the words: *ac nos easdem* (scil. the passage of the *De aere*) *sumus interpretati* (cf. Rasario, 1586, fol. 200ᵛ), which allude to Galen's *Commentary* on *Airs, Waters, Places*, but, as a matter of fact, we know that this commentary is later than the genuine commentary on *Epidemics* II.[30]

In order to draw some conclusions from this study, we will consider a fifth and final passage of the two commentaries. This refers to *Epidemics* II 2,6,1 = L. V 86,7, cf. XVII A, 326.12 f. K.).

---

[30] See Manetti and Roselli, 'Galeno commentatore' (n. 4 above), and quoted bibliography.

	Foes, 1560, pp. 137; 138 ff.	Rasario, 1586, fol. 199ᵛ
	Aristaei uxoris frater, ex via delassatus incaluit: eique postea terminthi in tibia coorti sunt. Adfuit febris continua et pos- tridie sudor, qui et reliquis diebus paribus	Frater uxoris Aristaei, fessus de via, inca- luit: eique postea terminthi in tibia coorti sunt. Deinde adfuit febris continua, et pos- tridie sudor, qui et reliquis diebus paribus
5	cum febre semper subortus est. Praebebat autem suspicionem lienis aliquantulum male affecti. Sanguis ex nare sinistra cre- bro fluxit: atque ita subinde iudicatus est.	semper comitatus est. Praeterea febris adfuit, erat sublienosus. Sanguis ex nare sinistra crebro fluxit: et subinde indicatus est, postridie secundum aurem sinistram
10	Postridie secundum aurem sinistram tumor, sequentique die etiam secundum dextram subortus est, qui tamen minor erat, et inte- pescebat. Hi omnes sensim conquieverunt, nec suppurarunt. [...]	tumor: sequenti autem die, etiam secun- dum dextram, subortus est: qui tamen minor erat, et intepescebat. Hi omnes sensim conquieverunt, nec suppurarunt. *Terminthorum est apud Hippocratem men-*
15	τέρμινθοι ἐγένοντο] *Terminthi Hippoc. di- cuntur nigra quaedam in tibiis praecipue erumpentia tubercula, terebinthi fructui non absimilia, ut testatur Gal. lib. 6 Epid.*	*tio libro sexto De vulgaribus morbis, cum ait, Qui haemorroidas habent, ii neque lae- teris dolore, neque pulmonis inflammatione, neque phagedaena, neque furunculis, neque*
	τὸ τῶν τερμίνθων ὄνομα μελάνων τινῶν ἐκφυμάτων ἐν ταῖς κνήμαις μάλιστα γι-	*terminthis, corripiuntur. Eadem sententia habetur in libro De humoribus extremo. Ac*
20	νομένων ἐστὶ δηλωτικὸν ἀπὸ τῆς κατὰ σχῆμα καὶ χρόαν καὶ μέγεθος ὁμοιότητος τῷ καρπῷ τῶν <τερμίνθων> γεγονός. *Sunt etiam Galeno* τέρμινθοι: οἱ τῷ τοῦ τερμίν-	*nos eo in loco diximus, terminthorum nom- ine significari nigras quasdam pustulas, in cruribus potissimum erumpentes, a simil- itudine figurae, coloris et magnitudinis,*
25	θου καρπῷ παραπλήσιοι, κατὰ τὸ δέρμα συνιστάμενοι παρὰ φύσιν ὄγκοι. *Est et quibusdam* τέρμινθός ἀπόστημα περὶ τὴν ἐπιφάνειαν γινόμενον μετὰ φλυκταινώ- σεως, ἧς ραγείσης ἰχώρ τις ἀπορρεῖ καὶ ἡ ὑποκειμένη σάρξ κατατετρημένη φαίνεται.	*quam cum fructu ciceris gerunt. Super his pustula nigra solet eminere, qua rupta quod id subiacet, disquammato simile apparet [...] Aliis placet, terminthos esse exuperantias quasdam, in cute consistentes, rotundas, nigro et viridi colore, ciceris*
30	*Quo magis miror, Calvum huiusmodi tuber- cula per rubores tibiarum expressisse. [...] Utitur hac dictione Hipp. lib. 6 Epidem. et lib.* Περὶ χυμῶν *ad extremum. etc.*	*fructui similes. Hic autem homo cum fessus esset de via, incalavit, ac febris continua facta est etc.*

In this passage the Hippocratic text concerns the τέρμινθοι, or *terminthi*, (namely the 'terebinths', but also the 'swelling like the fruit of the terebinth-tree') which are compared to the 'the fruit of the terebinth-tree'. Once again, Foes's and Rasario's commentaries basically share the same contents and parallels, but they put them in a significantly different way Rasario substitutes chickpea for terebinth. As a premise, it should be noticed that a very similar passage occurs in the first section of *Epidemics* II, which Foes commented on, providing a list of Hippocratic parallels (cf. Foes, 1560, p. 16: *in 4 Epid. et 6 et libro* περὶ χυμῶν). In this case Foes mentions firstly the Hippocratic passage from *Epidemics* VI, without quoting it, but paraphrasing in Latin the Galenic commentary related to it (ll. 15–18: *Terminthi ... non absimilia*), then he reports the latter in Greek (ll. 18–23: τὸ τῶν τερμίνθων δ' ὄνομα ... γεγονός).[31] This first quotation is followed by a second one, which is taken from the Galenic writing *Linguarum seu dictionum exoletarum Hippocratis explicatio* (ll. 23–6: sunt etiam Galeno ... ὄγκοι).[32] Later on, Foes reports another definition of *terminthi*, introduced by the words *est et quibusdam* and quoted in Greek, which corresponds to a *scholion* preserved in some manuscripts of Erotian's lexicon (ll. 26–30: τέρμινθός ἐστιν ... φαίνεται).[33] At last, after a brief mention of the Latin edition of Hippocrates published by Marco Fabio Calvi, Foes points out that the reading *terminthi* also occurs in other Hippocratic treatises, namely *Epidemics* VI and at the very end of *De humoribus* (ll. 33–4),[34] which recalls the list of parallels given for the similar passage of *Epidemics* II 1 that I have mentioned before.

Rasario presents very similar contents, but the way he organized them is quite interesting as it reveals his dependency upon Foes. Unlike Foes, Rasario firstly quotes the Hippocratic lemma in translation, namely *Epidemics* VI 23 (ll. 15–20), immediately pointing out that the same lemma also occurs *in libro De humoribus extremo* (ll. 20–21) – and it is not by chance that a piece of marginal bibliographical information given at the very end of the commentary by Foes draws Rasario's attention before getting on the top of completing his arguments! Later on, (ll. 21–25: *ac nos eo in loco diximus ... gerunt*) Rasario writes that the Hippocratic passage mentioned above, that is *Epidemics* VI 23, has already been commented upon (*diximus*), and then he quotes in Latin the same passage from the Galenic commentary on *Epidemics* VI quoted by Foes (cf. l. 22 f.: *terminthorum ... gerunt*). In this passage Rasario made two mistakes: firstly, he goes against the chronology of Galen's writings, since the *Commentary* on *Epidemics* VI has been set up by Galen only after that on *Epidemics* II; secondly, he clearly relies upon Foes's paraphrasis *erumpentia* (l. 17) for his rendering of γινομένων (l. 20) through *erumpentes* (l. 24).

Lines 26–7 (cf. *Super his ... apparet*) closely recall the Erotian's quotation reported by Foes, or at least its second half (cf. ll. 26–30). So, *super his* must refer to the legs, on which the *pustula nigra* shows up, and the ablative absolute

---

[31] Cf. Gal. *In Hipp. Ep. VI comm.* 3.23 = XVII B, 108.13 K. = Wenkebach, CMG V 10, 2, 2, pp. 183, 4 f.

[32] Cf. Gal. *Ling. s. dict. exolet. expl.* = XIX, 145.11 f. K.

[33] Cf. E. Nachmanson, *Erotiani Vocum hippocraticarum collectio*, Gothenburg, 1918, p. 102 n. xiii.

[34] Cf. Hipp. *De hum.* 20.1 = L. V 500,9.

qua rupta must represent the rendering of the genitive absolute ἧς ῥαγείσης. However, while *rupta* refers to *pustule* in the Latin, ἧς ῥαγείσης refers to the genitive φλυκταινώσεως in Greek, which is completely omitted by Rasario, who is quoting his source erroneously.

The last part of the Pseudo-Galen's passage is introduced by the words *aliis placet* (l. 28 f.), which seem to be a *pendant* for Foes's *est et quibusdam* (l. 26 f.). Here (ll. 28–30) Rasario reports an alternative definition of *terminthi* – preferred by *aliis*, 'other physicians' – which is not in Foes's text. This definition reminds us of a passage taken from the chapter Περὶ τερμίνθου of the late compiler Paul of Aegina[35] (cf. Paul. IV 24,1,5: [Διοσκορίδης δὲ ὁ Ἀλεξανδρεύς φησιν·] τέρμινθοί εἰσιν ὑπεροχαὶ ἐπὶ τοῦ χρωτὸς συνιστάμεναι, στρογγύλαι, μελανόχλωροι, ἐοικυῖαι τερμίνθου καρπῷ). Interestingly, the same passage is echoed elsewhere, namely in the false *Commentary* on *De humoribus*: as we have said, both Foes and Rasario claim that the Hippocratic lemma on the *terminthi* also occurs in the treatise on *Humours*, and in fact, looking at the lemma and related comment in the false commentary (cf. XVI, 453 f. K.), we spot a sentence which sounds almost identical to the previous, that is: *Terminthi vero sunt eminentiae in cute consistentes, rotundae, colore ex nigro et viridi, similes ciceris fructui* (cf. XVI, 461 K.). This means that Rasario was working on the false Galenic commentaries on *Epidemics* II and on *De humoribus* at the same time, storing and inserting fitting pieces and quotations, such as that from Paul of Aegina, in the two texts he aimed at making.

In conclusion, Rasario prepared the false 'Galenic' *commentary* on *Epidemics* II, excerpting quotations and combining them as puzzle pieces. He especially relied on Galen and Hippocrates, but also took advantage of the late compilers, which were treasure troves of quotations and easy works to handle thanks to their thematic division in chapters: he may have plundered Oribasius's work, as we already know from previous investigations, but made use of Paul of Aegina as well, as this study demonstrates. He just had to build up connections between the quotations, and it was here that he turned to his contemporary, Foes. Rasario employed Fos's commentary, restyling it and scattering *lacunae* in it – in accordance with the philological method behind the making of the *Commentary* on *De humoribus*[36] – and created another Pseudo-Galenic commentary, which was going to deceive classical scholarship for ages.

[35] Paul. Med., *Epitomae medicae libri septem* IV 24 = Heiberg, CMG IX 1, Leipzig-Berlin, 1921, pp. 345, 26 f.

[36] See n. 5.

La fortune du *De spermate* dans les éditions imprimées de Galien du XVIe au XVIIe

Outi Merisalo

Le traité pseudo-galénique *De spermate* est transmis dans 48 mss. connus, datant du XIIe au XVIe s. Il n'est pas exclu qu'il s'agisse non pas d'une traduction du grec ou d'une autre langue mais d'une série de textes rédigés en latin et réunis au plus tard au milieu du XIIIe siècle.[1] L'ensemble est d'étendue variable, avec des titres variables (*Microtegni, De spermate, Liber de spermate, De .XII. portis*, etc.). Les plus anciens manuscrits, qui datent du milieu du XIIe s. et sont localisables en Angleterre et dans le Midi, comportent un traité embryologique suivi d'un traité astrologique d'étendue variée.[2] Tout à la fin du XIIe siècle, vraisemblablement en Bavière, un fragment du traité embryologique est pourvu du titre de *Microtegni* et se voit attribuer à Galien comme auteur et à Constantin Africain comme traducteur;[3] à la même époque des fragments de ce qui fera plus tard partie de la version étendue du traité d'astrologie sont attestés sans titre dans un manuscrit d'origine bavaroise.[4] L'association avec Galien garantit le succès du traité, qui

[1] Cette recherche a été financée par le projet no. 267518 (*Transmission of Knowledge in the Late Middle Ages and the Renaissance*, Académie de Finlande et Université de Jyväskylä, 2013–17), par le Fonds de la recherche scientifique (Belgique, Université de Liège 2013 et 2015) et le projet no. 307635 (*Late Medieval and Early Modern Libraries as Knowledge Repositories, Guardians of Tradition and Catalysts of Change*, Académie de Finlande et Université de Jyväskylä, 2017-2021). J'ai le plaisir de remercier Stefania Fortuna (Università Politecnica delle Marche, Ancône) pour de nombreuses discussions galéniques et autres à Recanati notamment en juin-juillet et novembre 2014, et Dominique Longrée (Université de Liège) pour d'excellentes conditions de travail en 2013 et 2015. Pour la transmission du *De spermate*, v. O. Merisalo, 'La trasmissione del *De spermate* pseudo-Galenico', *Medicina nei secoli, Arte e scienza, Journal of History of Medicine*, 25, 3, 2013, pp. 927–40. Sur la question de l'authenticité des traités attribués à Galien, v. notamment V. Nutton, 'Pseudonymity and the critic : authenticating the Medieval Galen', in *Between text and patient : the medical enterprise in Medieval & Early Modern Europe*, eds F.E. Glaze and B.K. Nance, Firenze, 2011, pp. 481–91, et C. Petit, 'René Chartier (1572–1654) et l'authenticité des traités galéniques', in *René Chartier (1572–1654), éditeur et traducteur d'Hippocrate et de Galien*, eds V. Boudon-Millot, G. Cobolet and J. Jouanna, Paris, 2012, pp. 287–300 (287–8).

[2] MS Londres, British Library, Cotton Galba E IV, fols 233vb–238va, et MS Paris, Bibliothèque Nationale de France, lat. 15114, fols 163^v–170^r, v. Merisalo, 'Trasmissione' (n. 1 above), p. 928.

[3] MS Munich, Bayerische Staatsbibliothek, clm 4622, fols 79^v–80^v, et clm 18918, fols 68^r–71^r, v. Merisalo, 'Trasmissione' (n. 1 above), p. 929.

[4] Ibid.

rejoint sa longueur maxima[5] vers le milieu du XIIIe siècle. Il circule de cette époque-là jusqu'à la première moitié du XIVe siècle dans plus de vingt gros volumes de traductions latines de Galien produits à l'intention d'étudiants de médecine avancés et médecins pratiquants.[6] Des fragments d'étendue variée circulent aussi dans d'autres contextes, entre autres avec des textes traduits par Constantin, encore à la fin du XIIIe s.[7] L'association avec Constantin disparaît dans la deuxième moitié du XIIIe s.[8] Aux XIVe et XVe s., le succès du traité, dont l'authenticité mise en doute au moins depuis le début du XIVe s., ne fait qu'augmenter, malgré la traduction du traité authentique de Galien, Περὶ σπέρματος (*De semine*) par Nicolas de Reggio vers 1320. *De spermate* survit la transition à l'imprimé. Cet article portera sur les péripéties de la transmission du texte dans les éditions galéniques des XVIe et XVIIe s.

Entre 1490 et 1625 sortent jusqu'à 22 éditions de traductions latines d'œuvres (plus ou moins complètes, nous allons le voir) de Galien.[9] Jusqu'en 1541–2, il s'agit en principe de traductions médiévales avec quelques traductions humanistiques. Après cette date, les éditions comportent un nombre toujours croissant de traductions humanistiques. Le *De spermate* pseudo-galénique figure dans la quasi-totalité des éditions.

Le premier recueil en deux tomes, publié par Diomedes Bonardus (Diomede Bonardo), médecin de Brescia en 1490,[10] comporte deux textes dont les titres rappellent ceux du *De spermate* pseudo-galénique en copies médiévales. Aux fols 10ra–15vb du premier volume figure un *Microtegni* en trois livres. Il s'agit toutefois de l'*Ars parva* de Galien. Aux fols 144rb–150va du même volume se rencontre un traité intitulé *De spermate* en deux livres. Même là, ce n'est pas le traité pseudo-galénique, mais *De semine*, la traduction du traité authentique par Nicolas de Reggio.

---

[5] Comportant les 1006 lignes du texte transmis par le MS Cotton Galba (= texte Galba), inc. *Sperma hominis descendit ex humore totius corporis* (+var.), expl. *ab humano corpore procedunt*, et les 227 lignes supplémentaires contenues dans le texte transmis par ex. dans MS Berlin, SBB-PK, fol. 638, fols 251va–252va, *inc. h(ec) mutat(i)o q(ue) fit – naturam sui corporis*.

[6] Nouveau Galien, c.-à-d. contenant des traductions postérieures à la fin du XIIe s.; Merisalo, 'Trasmissione' (n. 1 above), pp. 930–33.

[7] Merisalo, 'Trasmissione' (n. 1 above), pp. 930–31.

[8] Merisalo, 'Trasmissione' (n. 1 above), p. 935.

[9] S. Fortuna, 'The Latin Editions of Galen's *Opera omnia* (1490–1625) and Their Prefaces', *Early Science and Medicine*, 17, 2012, pp. 391–412 (391) et 'Editions and Translations of Galen from 1490 to 1540', in *Brill's Companion to the Reception of Galen*, eds P. Bouras-Vallianatos and B. Zipser, Leiden, 2019, pp. 437–52.

[10] GW 10481: Galenus : Opera, lat. Hrsg. Diomedes Bonardus. Mit Beig. von Johannes Petrus Pincius. Venedig : Philippus Pincius, 27.VIII.1490. 2°

A un premier moment, le *De spermate* pseudo-galénique courait donc le risque de ne pas survivre au passage à l'imprimé. La deuxième édition imprimée, celle publiée en deux volumes par le médecin Hieronymus Surianus (Girolamo Suriano de Rimini, mort en 1522)[11] à Venise en 1502, intitulée *Secunda impressio Galieni* [...],[12] l'intègre dans les recueils galéniques imprimés. Suriano corrige l'édition de Bonardo, ajoute 11 traductions médiévales et la traduction de l'*Ars medica* par Lorenzo Lorenzi, humaniste florentin (mort en 1502). Cette édition connaît des ré-impressions jusqu'en 1528.[13] Suriano décrit dans la préface sa rencontre avec Galien, qui lui présente l'archétype[14] de l'ensemble de ses traités latins, en lui conseillant, dans un latin parfaitement courant, de collationner et de corriger le texte à imprimer au moyen de ce volume d'une taille considérable ('libru[m] [et] q[ui]dem grande[m] cubitalis altitudinis'), d'ajouter les textes manquants ('si quid mancu[m] fuerit addere non tardabis') et d'en éliminer le *superfluum*, c.-à-d. les faux ('si q[ui]d erit superfluu[m] abradere festinabis').

L'édition Suriano comporte deux ouvrages intitulés *De spermate*, à savoir le *De semine* en deux livres (vol. 1, pp. 57a–70b), déjà contenu dans l'édition de Bonardus et la nouveauté, le *De spermate* pseudo-galénique (vol. 1, pp. 70b–78b). Le deuxième *De spermate* n'est pas signalé dans la table des traités ajoutés, peut-être parce que l'authentique *De semine*, intitulé *De spermate*, avait déjà été publié par Bonardus. Le traité pseudo-galénique débute, sans titre, immédiatement après *De semine* à la p. 70b : *inc.* 'Sperma hominis desce(n)dit ex omni corporis humore'. Le titre courant présent dès la p. 71 identifie le texte comme *Liber de spermate*. Le texte finit à la p. 78b : *expl.* 'eius siccitatis terra vertitur in humiditatem. C Explicit libellus de spermate Galieno atributus.' Le texte comporte l'intégralité du texte Galba (lignes 1–1006) suivie de 34 lignes du texte Berlin. Il présente un certain nombre de ressemblances avec MS Munich, Bayerische Staatsbibliothek, clm 4622 (cf. ci-dessus p. 189, n. 3), qui ne comporte que les lignes 1 à 144 du texte Galba, et

---

[11] Fortuna, 'Latin Editions' (n. 9 above), p. 395.

[12] Venetiae : [Bernardinus Benalius] 1502. Exemplaire utilisé : Göttingen, Niedersächsische Staats-und Universitätsbibliothek, 2 MED VET 118/53 RARA, version numérisée. J'ai le plaisir de remercier Stefania Fortuna de m'en avoir communiqué la reproduction en 2014. Dans ce qui suit, nous suivrons la pagination moderne de l'exemplaire consulté, ajouté en encre.

[13] Fortuna, 'Latin Editions' (n. 9 above), p. 396.

[14] NB les abréviations ont été résolues entre parenthèses. F. <Ai v> : *HIERO(nymus). Statimq(ue) aperto palio libru(m) (et) q(ui)dem grande(m) cubitalis altitudinis existente(m) videre me p(er)misit : ac statim fere eo aperto clausit illu(m). Ac postmodu(m) subiunxit : GAL(ienus) Hic liber est quem dicimus archetypum : omnia que condidi in se continens op(er)a : cu(m) hoc volo vt tu que imprime(n)da sunt compares : si quid ab isto dissonu(m) inueneris huic (con)cordare studebis : si quid mancu(m) fuerit addere non tardabis : ac pariformiter si q(ui)d erit superfluu(m) abradere festinabis.*

les MSS Cité du Vatican, Bibliotheca Apostolica Vaticana, Urb. lat. 246 (lignes 1 à 259 du texte Galba), Pal. lat. 1234 (lignes 1 à 144 du texte Galba) ainsi que Pal. lat. 1298 (Galba + Berlin).[15] Il ne dérive cependant d'aucun de ces témoins.

A la lumière de nos connaissances actuelles de la tradition manuscrite, le texte dans cette étendue spécifique ne se rencontre que dans la copie autographe de Hartmann Schedel (1440–1514), médecin-humaniste nurembergeois, qui la date de 1503. La copie de Hartmann est contenue dans MS Munich, Bayerische Staatsbibliothek, clm 490, fols 134^r–155^v.[16] Elle présente la division en chapitres pourvus de titres de l'édition Suriano, par ex. Suriano p. 71^a (fol. Fiij) : 'C De natura pueri s(ecundu)m quantitatem (et) qualitate(m) matricis (et)-spermatis'; Hartmann fol. 135^v : 'C De natura pueri s(ecundu)m quantitate(m) et qualitate(m) matricis et spermatis;.-'; p. 71^b : 'C De alteratione sanguinis aliorumq(ue) humorum in sperma.'; Hartmann fol. 136^v 'C De alteracione sanguinis aliorumq(ue) humorum in sperma'. Qui plus est, la copie de Hartmann comporte aussi les variantes signalées dans la marge de l'édition imprimée, par ex. Suriano p. 70b *marg.* 'al(ias) confrictio(n)e' – Munich, MS clm 490, fol. 134^r *marg.* 'al(ias) confriccione'. A part la présence d'un intitulé, absent chez Suriano, dans la copie de Hartmann (fol. 134^r : 'Libellus. de Spermate Galieno. Attributus. Foeliciter Incipit.:-'), qui semble inspiré de l'intitulé (fol. 155^v : 'C Explicit Libellus de Spermate Galieno attributus.'), les deux textes sont à peu près identiques.

Deux possibilités se présentent : soit Hartmann Schedel disposait d'un manuscrit au contenu identique à celui dont s'était servi Suriano, soit la copie manuscrite remonte à l'édition imprimée, pratique très fréquente aux débuts de l'âge du livre imprimé. En effet, la deuxième alternative n'est aucunement à exclure. Nous savons que Hartmann possédait l'édition de Bonardo (aujourd'hui, Munich, Bayerische Staatsbibliothek, 2° Inc. c.a. 2410f), mais non pas celle de Suriano.[17] Il est donc concevable qu'il ait voulu compléter sa collection par ce

---

[15] O. Merisalo, 'Il codice *Vat. Urb. lat. 246* e la tradizione testuale del *De spermate* pseudogaleniano', in *Sit liber gratus, quem servulus est operatus : Studi in onore di Alessandro Pratesi per il suo 90° compleanno* 1, eds P. Cherubini and G. Nicolaj, Città del Vaticano, 2012, pp. 579–85 (582–4).

[16] Description détaillée : O. Merisalo, 'Scripsi manu mea. Hartmann Schedel in Munich, Bayerische Staatsbibliothek, clm 490', *Ars et humanitas*, 8, 2, 2014, pp. 119–30 (123–4) (DOI : http://revije.ff.uni-lj.si/arshumanitas/article/view/3031/2708); v. Aussi *Liber Hartmanni Schedel Nurembergensis artium utriusque medicine doctoris*. Histoire de quelques textes de la bibliothèque de Hartmann Schedel de Nuremberg (1440–1514)', in *La rigueur et la passion. Mélanges en l'honneur de Pascale Bourgain*, eds D. Poirel and C. Giraud, Turnhout, 2016, pp. 821–30 (826–8).

[17] V. entre autres l'ex-libris de Hartmann sur la contre-garde ('C LIBER. DOCTORIS. HART-MANNI. SCHEDEL. DE NV°REMBERGA'), la table des matières autographe et le colophon signé 'H.S.' aux fols 2^r à 3^r. Pour les éléments paratextuels des livres possédés par Hartmann, v. Merisalo, 'Hartmann Schedel' (n. 16 above), pp. 122–5.

texte qu'il avait dû fréquenter dès ses études de médecine à Padoue, d'autant plus que l'université de Padoue semble jouer un rôle important dans la diffusion du *De spermate* pseudo-galénique.[18] Quant à Suriano, il est possible qu'il se soit servi d'un manuscrit produit dans le milieu universitaire padouan, manuscrit encore à identifier.

Le *De spermate* pseudo-galénique de l'édition Suriano est reproduit dans les éditions imprimées successives.[19] Jusqu'en 1541 (v. plus loin), notre texte suit *De semine*, soit comme traité indépendant, soit comme troisième livre du traité galénique. Par ex. l'édition de Joannes Nebriensis Rivirius, Lugdunum : Gabiano, 1528, en trois volumes,[20] présente le texte pseudo-galénique d'un côté comme traité indépendant, de l'autre comme partie intégrante du traité authentique. Au fol. lxiiij[rb], le texte commence par 'C Incipit alius liber de spermate Gal(ieno) ascript(us). Sperma ho(min)is desce(n)dit ex o(mn)i corp(or)is humore'. Dès fol. lxv[r], la marge supérieure présente cependant le titre courant 'Liber tertius Galeni De spermate'. A la fin du traité (fol. lxviij[ra]), l'explicit 'eius siccitate terra vertitur in humiditatem' est suivi de l'indication 'Explicit libellus de spermate Gal(ieno) attributus.', conformément à l'édition Suriano.

Ce sont d'une part l'édition d'Augustinus Riccus (Agostino Ricchi), Venetiae : Officina Farrea, 1541–5),[21] et les grandes éditions publiées par la maison d'édition des Giunti de Venise, préparées par Augustinus Gadaldinus (Agostino Galdadini de Modène, 1515–70) de 1541 à 1565,[22] où le traité pseudo-galénique, toujours dans la version de l'édition Suriano, avec quelques annotations et variantes marginales ajoutées, d'autres supprimées ou modifiées,[23] ainsi que quelques titres de chapitres ajoutés d'impression en impression, est regroupé parmi les textes non authentiques. Dans la quatrième édition (1565) du vol. 10 intitulé 'Galeno ascripti libri […]', le *De spermate* pseudo-galénique se trouve aux fols 36[r]–41[r]. Au

---

[18] Merisalo, '*Vat. Urb. lat. 246*' (n. 15 above), pp. 584–5; Merisalo, 'Trasmissione' (n. 1 above), pp. 932–3.

[19] Celle de Scipio Ferrarius (Scipione Ferrari, médecin de Montferrat actif à Venise), *Galeni opera*, Venetiae : Bernardinus Benalius, 1513–14, dont aucune copie n'a été conservée, est le plus probablement une ré-impression de l'édition Suriano, Fortuna, 'Latin Editions' (n. 9 above), p. 396.

[20] Pour une description de cette édition, reproduisant, avec de nouvelles traductions humanistiques, essentiellement celle de Petrus Rusticus Placentinus (Pietro Rustici de Plaisance), 3 vols, Papiae : Jacobus Pocatela, 1515–16, v. Fortuna, 'Latin Editions' (n. 9 above), p. 397.

[21] Pour cette édition, v. Fortuna, 'Latin Editions' (n. 9 above), pp. 404–5.

[22] *Galeni omnia quae extant opera* […], éd. A. Gadaldinus, 10 vols, Venetiis : Iuntae, 1541–2, 1550, 1556, 1565; pour ces éditions, v. Fortuna, 'Latin Editions' (n. 9 above), pp. 399–404.

[23] Les variantes ajoutées et modifiées sembleraient suggérer la prise en compte de quelques témoins manuscrits.

fol. 36ʳ le texte débute par le titre 'Galeno ascriptus liber De spermate', suivi d'un jugement sévère : 'Jugement. Même ce livre est plein de fautes graves et des plus importantes'.[24]

Le *De spermate* pseudo-galénique se maintiendra dans toutes les éditions successives des œuvres complètes de Galien jusqu'en 1625.[25] L'histoire imprimée de ce texte n'en finit pourtant pas là. Une nouvelle version du traité est contenue dans *Opera Hippocratis Coi et Galeni Pergameni* […], tome 3, 1638, publiée par René Chartier (1515–1654),[26] éditeur dont le rôle dans l'histoire de la transmission du Galien aussi bien grec que latin ne peut pas être sous-estimé.[27] Aux pp. 229–39 du volume 3 se trouve un traité identifié à la p. 229 comme 'Galeni De semine liber tertius, ascriptitius ac spurius' ('Le troisième livre du *De semine*, improprement attribué à Galien et faux').[28] Tout comme dans les Juntines, suit un jugement bien sévère : 'Jugement. Ce livre improprement attribué à Galien est plein de fautes graves même après l'émendation (philologique)' ('Censura. Hic liber malè Galeno ascriptus quantumuis emendatus summis erroribus scatet'). En effet, Chartier ne se contente pas de reproduire le texte de l'édition Suriano mais produit une traduction en latin classique – en tout cas d'une partie du texte. La comparaison du début de l'édition Chartier avec la copie de Hartmann Schedel, identique à l'édition Suriano, le met bien en évidence

---

[24] 'CENSVRA. Et hic quoque liber summis, & maximis erroribus refertus est.'

[25] V. Fortuna, 'Latin Editions' (n. 9 above), pp. 407–10.

[26] *Opera Hippocratis Coi, et Galeni Pergameni, medicorum omnium principum* […], ed. Renatus Charterius, 12 tomes, Lutetiae Parisiorum, 1638–79.

[27] Petit, 'René Chartier' (n. 1 above), p. 298.

[28] Cf. du Cange, et al, *Glossarium mediae et infimae latinitatis*, 1, Niort, 1883, col. 420a., s.v. 'ascriptitii', http://ducange.enc.sorbonne.fr/ASCRIPTITII, le 17 janvier 2016: 'ASCRIPTITII, dicti Coloni, Agricolæ, Villani, qui aliunde orti, in aliorum Dominorum villas et prædia pergunt, ibique eorumdem licentia, sedes suas figunt, et sub annui census conditione in cæterorum subditorum transeunt statum'.

Chartier, p. 229	Clm 490, fol. 134^r
CAPVT PRIMVM.	Libellus. de Spermate Galieno.
De ortu foetus ex semine.	Attributus. Foeliciter Incipit.:-*

SEMEN hominis ex omni humore corporis manat, qui ex tenuiore ac puriore quatuor humorum natura procreatur.	SPERMA. HOMINIS. Descendit ex omni corporis humore. Qui fit subtiliori natura quatuor humorum: hoc autem Sperma habet neruos et venas proprias attrahentes se a toto corpore ad testiculos:
Hoc autem semen habet neruos (et) venas proprias quibus ab vniuerso corpore ad testes attrahitur (et) aduehitur,	
qui nerui (et) venae masculi (et) foeminae complexu, pudendorúmque attritu, (et) calefactione illud emittunt, vt ex collisione silicis (et) chalybis elicitur ignis.	Qui nerui et vene ex fricacionis calefactione + [*marg*. al(ias) confriccione] viri et mulieris emittunt illud: sicut ex collisione ferri et petre elicitur. Ignis:

Notons d'abord la numérotation des chapitres (*caput primum*) et le titre du premier chapitre, évidemment absent dans la copie de Hartmann et chez Suriano (v. ci-dessus p. 192). Le vocabulaire a été rendu plus classique entre autre par le remplacement systématique du terme *sperma*[29] par *semen*. Le verbe *descendere*, à toute évidence à interpréter au sens de 'provenir', a été remplacé par le verbe *manare* au sens classique de 'couler'. Si le pronom relatif (peut-être utilisé de manière démonstrative) *qui*, renvoyant à *omnis humor*, a été conservé, il n'en est pas de même du prédicat. Le verbe *fieri*, dans le texte plus ancien sans doute utilisé au sens de 'commencer à exister', complété par le syntagme ablatif *subtiliori natura quatuor humorum* 'par la nature plus délicate des quatre humeurs', a été remplacé par le verbe *procreare* au passif, complété par le syntagme prépositionnel *ex tenuiore ac puriore quatuor humorum natura* 'à partir de la nature plus délicate et plus pure des quatre humeurs'. Notons l'emploi de deux adjectifs (*tenuis, purus*) au lieu de l'adjectif *subtilis*, qui contribue à préciser la sémantique de la proposition. Dans l'édition Chartier, le terme *sperma* de la proposition suivante a été encore corrigé en *semen*.

La forme réfléchie peu classique *attrahentes se*[30] a été remplacée par le doublet passif *attrahitur et aduehitur* qui n'est pas seulement classique mais contribue encore à préciser le sens de la phrase. Dans la dernière section, à *ex fricacionis calefactione viri et mulieris* ('par le réchauffement du frottement de l'homme

---

[29] Attesté chez Sulpice Sévère, *Hist. Sacr.* 1, 11, v. C. T. Lewis – C. Short, *A Latin Dictionary* [...], Oxford, 1879, s.v. 'sperma'.

[30] Pour l'emploi du réfléchi au lieu du passif morphologique dès le latin tardif, v. V. Väänänen, *Introduction au latin vulgaire*, 3e édition, Paris, 1981, p. 128.

et de la femme'), syntagme prépositionnel rempli de termes non classiques,[31] correspond la série d'ablatifs instrumentaux *masculi (et) foeminae complexu, pudendorúmque attritu, (et) calefactione* ('au moyen de l'étreinte de l'homme et de la femme, et du frottement et réchauffement des organes de reproduction'). Notons encore la multiplication de termes : *fricatio* a été remplacée par les termes classiques *complexus pudendorumque attritus*, dont *complexus* est parfaitement classique,[32] *attritus* attesté au Ier siècle apr. J.C.[33] et *pudenda* par contre tardif.[34] Seul *calefactio*, peu classique, a été conservé tel quel dans la version de Chartier. Enfin, aux termes *ferrum* 'fer' (classique) et *petra* 'pierre' (dès le Ier siècle)[35] correspondent les termes bien classiques, quoique plutôt poétiques, *silex* 'silex, caillou, rocher'[36] et *chalybs* 'acier'.[37]

Cette opération de traduction en latin classique ne regarde cependant pas l'ensemble du texte. Par ex. dans la section portant sur l'influence des humeurs sur les maladies (MS Munich, Bayerische Staatsbibliothek, clm 490, fol. 152[bisr] et l'édition Chartier p. 236b), la syntaxe du texte de départ est majoritairement conservée, les différences peu nombreuses regardant le vocabulaire. Ainsi, la terminologie humorale a été modifiée : *colera (rubea)* 'bile jaune',[38] est remplacé par *bilis flaua*, terme plus classique[39] et qui semble l'emporter aux XVIe et XVIIe, le terme *cholera* dénotant la maladie ;[40] à *flegma* du texte de départ, terme tardif,[41] correspond *pituita*.[42]

---

[31] *Fricatio*, attesté chez Celse, Vitruve, Columelle, Pline l'Ancien et des auteurs plus tardifs, v. Ae. Forcellini et al., *Lexicon totius Latinitatis*, 6 vols, 4e éd., Patavii 1864–1926 (1940), s.v. 'fricatio' ; *calefactio*, attesté chez Hermogénien (IIIe s., cité dans le *Digeste*), v. Forcellini, s.v. 'calefactio'.

[32] Attesté dès Cicéron, F. Gaffiot, *Dictionnaire latin-français*, Paris, 1934, s.v. 'complexus'.

[33] Attesté chez Sénèque et Pline le Jeune, Gaffiot, s.v. 'adtritus'.

[34] Attesté au pluriel chez Augustin, Forcellini, s.v. 'pudenda'.

[35] Attesté chez Pline l'Ancien, Curtius et des auteurs plus tardifs, Gaffiot, s.v. 'petra' et Forcellini, s.v. 'petra'.

[36] Attesté chez Gaffiot, s.v. 'silex'.

[37] Terme poétique, attesté chez Virgile et Sénèque, v. Gaffiot, s.v. 'chalybs'.

[38] Attesté chez Celse (aussi en référence à la maladie), entre autres, Gaffiot, s.v. 'cholera' et Forcellini, s.v. 'cholera'.

[39] Attesté chez Cicéron, Juvénal et Pline le Jeune, aussi au sens figuré ('mauvais humeur, colère'), Gaffiot, s.v. 'bilis'.

[40] Par ex. Daniel Sennert (1572–1637), auteur des *Institutiones Medicinae*, 2e éd., Witebergae, 1620, p. 279, distingue nettement *bilis flaua* 'bile jaune' de la maladie *cholera* ; v. aussi pp. 210–13 ('De bile').

[41] *Phlegma* est attesté entre autres dans *Mulomedicina Chironis*, Gaffiot, s.v. 'phlegma'.

[42] Terme attesté au sens de 'mucus ; humeur pituitaire' dès Catulle ; au sens de 'pus, humeur' chez Celse (v. Gaffiot, s.v. 'pituita') et utilisé entre autres par Sennert, par ex. pp. 207–10 ('De pituita').

A la fin du traité, le texte d'arrivée ne se distingue plus du texte de départ :

Chartier, p. 239[b]
remoueri a terra. Est igitur eius substan-
tia humiditas: in primis enim terra fuit
humida: (et) eius siccitate remota, (et)
frigiditate, quae est eius siccitatis, terra
vertitur in humiditatem.
FINIS.

Clm 490, fol. 155[v]
removeri a terra: Est igitur eius substancia
humiditas: In primis enim terra fuit humida: Et eius siccitate remota (et) frigiditate
Que est eius siccita<t>is terra vertitur in
hu(m)iditatem. *C* Explicit Libellus de
Spermate Galieno attributus.

Même si l'opération linguistique de Chartier s'épuise bien avant la fin du texte, elle témoigne de son intérêt vis à vis du *De spermate* pseudo-galénique, dont il a dû considérer le contenu insolite (rappelons-en notamment le système chrono-biologique raffiné permettant de prédire les caractéristiques de l'enfant jusqu'en détail, la doctrine de l'utérus aux sept cellules, et la longue section sur l'astro-médecine),[43] comme méritant d'être lu et connu de ses contemporains. Malgré les fautes qualifiées d'importantes dans le jugement initial (v. ci-dessus p. 194), Chartier voulut moderniser le texte en transformant le latin médiéval du texte en un latin du XVIIe siècle, essentiellement classique mais évidemment conforme au langage spécifique de l'érudition médicale.[44]

Conclusion

Le traité pseudo-galénique en latin intitulé entre autres *De spermate* fait son apparition sous formes différentes au XIIe siècle et atteint une étendue maxima au milieu du XIIIe siècle, circulant dans les grands volumes galéniques pour ceux qui veulent approfondir leurs connaissances médicales aux XIIIe et XIVe siècles. La transmission manuscrite se poursuit avec beaucoup de succès jusqu'au début du XVIe siècle. Le traité ne figure pas dans la toute première édition d'œuvres (plus ou moins) complètes de Galien sortie en 1490 aux bons soins de Diomedes Bonardus. Ce n'est qu'en 1502 qu'une version circulant vraisemblablement en Italie du Nord, peut-être dans le milieu universitaire padouan, est publiée dans la

[43] Pour ces aspects, v. Merisalo, 'Trasmissione' (n. 1 above) p. 928 et n. 2. Pour l'intérêt porté par Chartier à l'astro-médecine, v. Petit, 'René Chartier' (n. 1 above), pp. 296–7.

[44] De semblables opérations sont bien connues dès le XVe siècle, par ex. la modernisation du *Liber Pontificalis* par Platina dans ses *Vitae pontificum*, v. O. Merisalo, 'Platina et le Liber Pontificalis. Un humaniste devant un texte médiéval', *Arctos*, 16, 1982, pp. 73–99, et celle de *l'Orlando innamorato* de Matteo Maria Boiardo (1494) par Francesco Berni (1531), v. D. Romei, *L'*'Orlando' moralizzato dal Berni*, 1997 (2009), http://www.nuovorinascimento.org/n-rinasc/saggi/pdf/romei/orlmoral.pdf le 21 juillet 2019.

Secunda impressio Galieni de Hieronymus Surianus. Le texte de l'édition Suriano sera ré-imprimé, avec des modifications essentiellement paratextuelles (variantes marginales et titres ajoutés, modifiés et supprimés), dans toutes les éditions du Galien latin jusqu'en 1625. Dès avant le milieu du XVIᵉ siècle les éditeurs sont convaincus de l'inauthenticité de ce qui est très souvent qualifié de livre III du *De spermate*, c'est-à dire du traité authentique *De semine*. Le traité pseudo-galénique est encore inclus par Chartier dans le troisième volume de sa monumentale édition d'Hippocrate et de Galien publié en 1639. Chartier s'engage dans une opération de modernisation linguistique – transformation du latin médiéval en un latin du XVIIᵉ siècle, classique mais conforme au langage du genre médical – sans doute visant à rendre plus accessible un texte auquel il reproche d'être rempli d'erreurs importantes mais dont il a dû reconnaître l'intérêt. L'opération linguistique, qui ne se réalise qu'en partie, ne suffit pourtant à garantir la survie du traité pseudo-galénique. C'est évidemment le déclin du galénisme, déjà bien visible au XVIIᵉ siècle, qui met fin au long parcours du *De spermate* pseudo-galénique comme texte intéressant du point de vue médical. De celui de l'histoire de la médecine et de la transmission des savoirs au Moyen Âge et à la Renaissance, il garde par contre tout son intérêt.

Index codicum manuscriptorum

NB: early printed editions are included in the general index under the name of the editor.

Athos
Monê Koutloumousiou
248 (Lampros 3321): 47, 53, 57

Berlin
Staatsbibliothek
Fol. 638: 190 (n. 5)
Phillipps 1526 (gr. 122): 47, 53

Bologna
Biblioteca Universitaria
3632: 47, 58, 61, 67

Cesena
Biblioteca Malatestiana
S.V, 4 : 25 (n. 28), 145 (n. 5)
S. XXVI, 4: 25 (n. 28)
S. XXVII, 4: 25 (n. 28),
145 (n. 5)

Copenhagen
Det Kongelige Bibliotek
GKS 1648 4o: 48, 53, 56

Dresden
Sächsische Landesbibliothek – Staats-
und Universitätsbibliothek
Db 92–93: 10

Florence
Biblioteca Medicea Laurentiana
Plut. 6, 6: 56
Plut. 28, 34: 71–72
Plut. 74, 14: 48, 53–54
Plut. 75, 3: 42
Plut. 75, 7: 13–14, 27

Istanbul
Aya Sofia
3590: 14

Leiden
Universiteits Bibliotheek
Voss. gr. F. 53: 54

Leipzig
Universitätsbibliothek
gr. 52: 48, 53–54

London
British Library
Add. 11888: 48, 53–54
Cotton Galba E IV: 189 (n. 2);
190 (n. 5)
Harley 6295: 100
Wellcome Library
60: 45, 99–128
289: 48

Milan
Biblioteca Ambrosiana
B 90 sup: 48, 53–54
B 126 sup: 45
Q 94: 45
T 19 sup: 48, 53–54

Modena
Biblioteca Estense
BE α. V, 6, 12 (gr. 210): 48, 53, 55

Moscow
Gosudarstvennyj Sinod.
gr. 51: 48, 58–59, 67
gr. 508: 45

Munich
Bayerische Staatsbibliothek
clm 490: 192, 196
clm 4622: 189 (n. 3), 191
clm 18918: 189 (n. 3)
gr. 16: 55
gr. 109: 49, 53, 55
gr. 170: 55
gr. 469: 49, 58–59

Oxford
Bodleian Library

Cromwell 12: 71–72
Holkham gr. 112: 106
Orville 3 (Auct. X. 1.1.3): 49,
  53, 55

Paris
  Bibliothèque nationale de France
    gr. 1630: 76, 107 (n. 50)
    gr. 2153: 49, 51, 58–59, 61, 67
    gr. 2167: 49, 53, 55
    gr. 2175: 49, 53, 55
    gr. 2282: 49, 53, 55
    gr. 2315: 78
    gr. 2316: 78
    lat. 15114: 189 (n. 2)
    suppl. gr. 35: 49, 53, 56–57
    suppl. gr. 446: 49, 58–59, 61–62,
      65–67, 77, 79
    suppl. gr. 636: 45
    suppl. gr. 684: 45
    suppl. gr. 764: 45 (n. 62)
    suppl. gr. 1328: 50, 53, 56

Rome
  Accademia dei Lincei
    Corsini 1410: 77 (n. 24)

Thessaloniki
  Vlatadon Monastery Library
    14: 130

Vaticano (Città del)
  Barberinus gr. 147: 35, 40, 45
  Ottob. gr. 311: 50, 58, 61
  Pal. gr. 199: 50, 58, 60, 108 (n. 52)
  Pal. gr. 297: 50, 58, 60, 65–67, 98 (n. 2)
  Pal. lat. 1211: 25 (n. 28)
  Pal. lat. 1234: 192
  Pal. lat. 1298: 192
  Reg. gr. 181: 76
  Urbinas gr. 67: 35, 40, 45
  Urbinas lat. 246: 192
  Vat. gr. 175: 72
  Vat. gr. 279: 77
  Vat. gr. 292: 77
  Vat. gr. 293: 77
  Vat. gr. 1614: 50, 53, 56
  Vat. lat. 2376: 145 (n. 5)

Venice
  Biblioteca Nazionale Marciana
    gr. IV, 10 (coll. 833): 50, 57
    gr. V, 9 (coll. 1017): 51, 58, 61
    gr. Z. 521 (coll. 316): 51–53, 57–58

Vienna
  Österreichiche Nationalbibliothek
    med. gr. 16: 51, 58–59, 61, 63, 65–67
    cod. lat. 2328: 145 (n. 6)

Index

NB: a thorough concordance of titles of Galenic works in Greek, Latin, Arabic can be found in G. Fichtner, *Galen-Bibliographie*, regularly updated and downloadable from the *Corpus Medicorum Graecorum* website. Titles of Galenic works are cited in Latin or Greek in the index, and either in Latin and Greek or in modern translations by the contributors.

Abū Bakr al-Rāzī, *see* Rhazes

Accursio of Pistoia 147, 158–159

Achillini, Alessandro 161–172

Ackermann, Johan Christian Gottlieb 36, 41, 44

Actavantiis, Actavantius de 56

Actuarius (Aktouarios), John 73–74, 103

Aelianus, Meccius (Maecius) 5

Aetius of Amida 13–14, 26, 60, 65, 105

Africanus, Julius 2 (n. 7), 3, 13 (n. 3)

Agnellus of Ravenna 75

Aktouarios, *see* Actuarius

alchemy 70, 81

Aldine xi, 51–52, 55, 64, 143, 151, 154, 155

Aldus Manutius 55–56, 150

Alexander of Aphrodisias 60, 141

Alexander of Tralles 65

Alexandria 2, 7

anatomy 91, 101, 150–152, 161–172

Andromachus 2, 11, 25, 31

Angelos, Demetrios 61

Anonymus Harvardianus 56

Antipater 7, 16

Antonius 78, 99 (n. 6) (*see also* Galen/ Pseudo-Galen *Ad Antonium de pulsibus*)

Aphrahat 83–84

Apollonius 4, 10

Apollonius Mys 31

Apostolis, Aristobule 55

archiatros 5 (n. 17), 25–26, 37–39

Archigenes 20, 38–39, 97, 109–110

Argyropoulos, John 57, 115

Aristotle 64, 87

Arria 6

Articella 80, 147, 150

Asclepiades 3, 11

Askew, Anthony 100

Asia Minor 4

astrology (and astro-medicine) 70–72, 81, 197

astronomy 72

Athanasius of Nisibis 84

Athenagoras 74–75

Attalus Statilius 4, 6 n. 23

Aulus Gellius 18

authenticity (notions of) xi, 2, 90

Avicenna *see* Ibn Sīnā

Barlama (Barlaam) 43

Baladī (al-) 62

Bardaisan 83

Barlandus, Hubertus 35–36

Basel edition of Galen xi, 51–52, 143

Basil of Caesarea 85

basilisk 19

Benali, Bernardino 149

Benedetti, Alessandro 162

Berengario da Carpi 161–162, 167, 170, 172

Blemmydes, Nikephoros 106

Bologna 161–163, 171–172

Bonardo, Diomede 144–150, 158, 166, 190–192, 197

Brunfels, Otto 1

Bukhtīshū 34, 92–94

Burgundio of Pisa xii, 147–148, 158–159

Byzantium 99–128
  Byzantine Greek 43, 100, 111

Calliergis, Zacharias 54

Calvi, Marco Fabio 187

Caracalla 16

Charpentier, Simon 53

Chartier, René
  edition xi, 14–15, 35–37, 51–52, 63, 69–70, 76–81, 149, 151, 154, 157–158, 175, 194–197

centaury 4, 8–10

Cicero 10

Claudianus 40

Clement, John 55

Cleopatra 16

Colbert, Jean-Baptiste 55

Constantinus Africanus 149, 150, 159, 189–190

Constantinople 37, 57, 66, 115, 145, 148

Cop, Guillaume 53–54

Cornarius, Janus 13–14, 27, 156–158

corpus (Galenic) x–xii

Cosmas (Saint) 43

Costeo, Giovanni 175, 176

Crassus, Iunius Paulus 35–36, 177

Cratevas 11

Crete 4, 7

Crito 11

Croeser, Herman (Cruserius) 177

Cyranides 20, 28

Da Monte, Giovanni Battista (Montanus) 152–154, 156–158, 176

Damian (Saint) 43

Damilas, Démétrios 54

Damocrates 11, 25

David de Dinant 147, 158–159

Dee, John 70

Demetrios 25

Dionysius (and pseudo-Dionysius) 86

Dioscorides 22, 31, 185

doxography ix

Egypt 4, 7

emperors (Roman) 2, 16, 18, 25, 44

empiricists 90

Eparque, Andronic 56–57

Ephrem 83–84

Erotian 187

Eumenes II of Pergamon 24

Eunapius 31, 74

Euripides 8, 134 (n. 20)

eye (anatomy of) 171–172

Foes, Anuce 176–188

forgery xi–xii, 85–87
  Renaissance forgeries xii, 151–152, 154–155, 173–188

Froben editions 154

Gadaldini, Agostino 15, 144, 152, 155–158, 175, 177, 193

Galen, son of Menodotus 155, 157

Galen (and Pseudo-Galen) *passim*

Galenic works (in bold the works of which the authenticity is or has been discussed)
  περὶ ἀοχλησίας 141
  Ad Glauconem meth. med. 39, 65, 148
  ars medica (*ars parva*) xiii, 95, 147–148,

190, 191

de antidotis 21–23

de alimentorum facultatibus 32

de causis morborum 176

de causis pulsuum 107

de compositione med. sec. locos 19, 33, 39–40, 95

de compositione med. sec. genera 33, 95

de constitutione artis medicae 152

de crisibus 71

de diebus decretoriis 71

de differentiis morborum 176

de differentiis pulsuum 107, 109

de dignotione pulsuum 107

de indolentia 40 (n. 37), 63 (n. 85), 129–141

de interioribus 148 (n. 15), 166 (see also *de locis affectis*)

de juvamentis membrorum 165–167 (see also *de usu partium*)

de libris propriis (libr. propr.), ix, 69, 76, 143

de locis affectis 95, 148 (n. 15)

de marasmo 177

de marcore 177

de methodo medendi 32–33, 95, 143

de optima secta ad Thrasybulum 92, 146, 158–159

de ordine librorum propriorum (ord. libr. propr.), ix, 69

de partibus artis medicae 155, 156, 159

de praecognitione, ix n. 3

de pulsibus ad tirones 107

de sanitate tuenda 143

de semine 150, 190

de simpl. med. fac. 19–21, 29, 32–33, 89 (n. 25), 143

de symptomatum causis 95

de temperamentis 95

de tumoribus praeter naturam 177

de usu partium 143, 165–172

de utilitate respirationis 166

de victus ratione in morbis acutis ex

Hippocratis sententia 93

Glossary 187

oratio suasoria ad artes (*protrepticus*) 152, 155, 157

in Hipp. Aph. 147

in Hipp. Art. 185

in Hipp. Epid. I 185

in Hipp. Epid. III 185

in Hipp. Epid. VI 185

in Hipp. Fract. 185

in Hipp. Progn. 147, 185

in Hipp. Prorrh. 185

in Hipp. vict. acut. 185

Pseudo-Galen

περὶ οὔρων Γαληνοῦ διαίρεσις 103–106, 115–118

Ἑρμηνεία τοῦ Γαληνοῦ περὶ κλοκίου 106–107, 118

Γαληνοῦ περὶ σφυγμῶν 108–111, 118–128

Ad Antonium de pulsibus xiv, 65, 69, 77, 78–80, 99 (n. 6), 107, 110–113, 151

Ad Gaurum xii–xiii

An animal sit quod in utero est xiii (n. 16), 69, 151, 152

An omnes partes animalis, quod procreatur, fiunt simul 146, 158–159

compendium pulsuum xii, 147–148, 158–159

de anatomia parva 149, 159, 166

de anatomia matricis 166, 168, 170

de anatomia oculorum 146, 158–159, 166

de anatomia vivorum xiv, 149, 159, 165–172

de bonitate aquae 146, 156, 158–159

de catharticis 148–149, 158–159

de compagine membrorum 149, 159

de cura icteri 146, 158–159

de cura lapidis 158–159

de diaeta Hippocratis in morbis acutis 151

de dinamidiis 148, 149, 158–159

de dissolutione continua 147, 149, 158–159

de fasciis 151

de humoribus 151

de incantatione 149, 152

de iuvamento anhelitus 147, 158–159

de medicina expertis 158–159

de medicina secundum Homerum xiii

de melancholia 151, 154, 155

de motibus dubiis 1, 156–157, 159

de motu thoracis et pulmonis 158–159

de natura et ordine cuiuslibet corporis 149, 159

de oculis 150, 152

de passionibus mulierum 148, 158–159

de plantis 150–151

de podagra 148, 158–159

de ponderibus 101, 151

de remediis facile parabilibus xiv, 31–45, 93–96, 98, 146, 151, 152, 158–159

de renum affectus dignotione 151, 152

de simplicibus medicaminibus ad Paternianum 148, 158–159

de spermate xiv, 149, 150, 159, 189–198

de succedaneis 150

de theriaca ad Pamphilianum 1–11, 14, 93, 146, 157, 158–159

de theriaca ad Pisonem xii–xiii, 1–11, 13–30, 146, 157, 158–159

de urinae significatione 150, 154, 159

de urinis xiv, 69, 73–78, 105, 151, 152

de urinis compendium xiv, 69, 73–78

de urinis ex Hippocrate, Galeno aliisque 74, 105

de vinis 146, 156, 158–159

de virtutibus centaureae (virt. cent.) xii, 1–11 (*passim*), 146, 158–159

de virtutibus nostrum corpus dispensantibus 146, 158–159

de voce 1

de voce et anhelitu 159

definitiones medicae (def. med.) xiii n. 16, xiv, 47–67, 69, 77, 98, 108, 110–113, 151, 152, 154

euporista: see *de remediis parabilibus*

historia philosopha xii, 149, 154, 155, 159

in Hippocratis de foetus natura librum comm. 90–91

in Hipp. de humoribus 76, 92, 151, 174

in Hipp. de alimento 88–89, 151, 173

in Hipp. Epid. II 151, 173–188

in Hipp. Epid. VI 151, 174

in Hippocratis Sept. commentarium xi n. 12

in Plat. Timaeum 174

introductio sive medicus (introd.) x, 1, 21, 29–30, 58, 75, 98, 115, 146, 148, 158–159

liber secretorum ad Monteum 147, 158–159

Microtegni see *de spermate*

praesagium experientia confirmatum 150, 154, 159

prognostica de decubitu infirmorum ex mathematica scientia xiv, 69–72, 77, 151, 154, 156, 159

quaesita in Hippocratis de urinis 150, 154, 159

quod qualitates incorporeae sint 151, 152

synopsis de pulsibus 151

Galenism ix, xiv, 1, 11

Gerard of Cremona 147, 158–159

Gesius of Alexandria 90

Gesner, Conrad 156–158

Geta 16

Giunta, Luca Antonio 152 (*see also* Juntine editions)

Glaucon 36, 39, 65, 148

Grassi, Giunio Paulo *see* Crassus

Grimani, Domenico 57

Guinterius, Ioannes 35, 164 (n. 10), 171–172 (Winter)

Guy de Chauliac 165

gynaecology 42 (*see also* womb)

Haller, Albrecht von 36–37, 41, 44

Hamilcar 24

Hannibal 8, 24, 26

hapax legomenon 17, 111 (n. 69)

Harpocration of Alexandria 20 (n. 20)

Heraclius 72

Hermes Trismegistus 20 (n. 20), 70, 72

Herophilus 41

Hippocrates 6, 10–11, 16–17, 70, 74, 88–97, 105, 145, 147–157
    commentaries to Hippocrates 25, 77, 91, 147, 151, 173–188
    Hippocratism 2, 25

history of the book xiv (*see also* Aldine; Basel; Chartier; Kühn; Juntines)

Homer xiii, 8, 18

Hubaysh 93, 140

humanism and humanist translations xiv, 144, 149–154, 173, 190–192

Ḥunayn ibn Isḥāq xi, 3, 14, 34–35, 62, 83–97, 174

iatrosophia (Byzantine) 114

Ibn al-Jazzār 104

Ibn Aqnīn, Yosef 129–141

Ibn Falaquera, Shem Tov 129–141

Ibn Sīnā (Avicenna) 103, 166, 183–184

Imbrasius of Ephesus 71–72

Ioachos of Martyropolis 43

John of Alexandria 70, 79–80

Joly, Claude 55

julep 104–105

Juntine editions of Galen 15, 35, 144, 149–159, 173–176, 193–194

Justin I (emperor) 84

Justinian I (emperor) 84

Kral (xenon) 115

Kühn, Carl Gottlob
    edition ix–xii, 8, 36, 39, 43, 52, 60, 63–64, 69, 73–74, 77–81, 105, 175, 176, 179

Kyathos, Laurent 56

L'Aigneau, Juste 70–71

L'Aigneau, David 70

Laguna, Andrea 155

Lascaris, Janus 55–56

late antiquity x, 73, 75–81, 83–85, 89, 188

Le Pelletier, Louis-Michel (de Saint-Fargeau) 56

Leo medicus 66, 67

Leoniceno, Niccolò 56, 150

Lorenzi, Lorenzo 150, 191

Lucius of Ancona 10

magic 10, 20–21, 28–29, 41, 70

Magnus (Magnos) 11, 25

Magnus (Magnos) of Emesa 70, 74–77, 80, 102

Maimonides 20 (n. 19), 26

Manfredi, Girolamo 162

Mani 83

Marcellinus 67

Marcellus 41

Marcion 83

Marcus Aurelius 7

market ix, xiv, 91

Massa, Niccolò 171–172

Mauro de Salerno 80

Mead, Richard 100

Médicis, Pierre de 56

Menecrates 11

Mercuriale, Girolamo (Mercurialis) 15, 54, 173–175

Metrodora 42

Michael VII Doukas 104

Mithridates 8, 17

Mondino de Luzzi 161–172

Moschos, John 55

Moses ben Josua 26

Myrepsos, Nicholas 101

Nicander 11

Niccolò da Reggio, 3, 25–26, 35, 145–146, 154–156, 158–159, 165, 190

Oppianicus 10

Oribasius (and pseudo-) 31, 33, 44, 66, 146, 158–159, 188

Ovid 18

Padua 54, 76, 152, 161, 193

Palladios 60, 65, 109

Pamphilianus 4, 7, 10

Papias 4, 9–10

Paul (apostle) 86

Paul of Aegina, 14, 65, 101, 110, 188

Pellicier, Guillaume 53

Pelops 90

Pepagomenos, Demetrios 101

Pergamon (Pergamum) 1, 6, 23–24

pharmacology 1–11, 31–44, 101, 152, 157

Philagrius 34–35, 94

Philaretus 80, 107, 109

phou 22

Pinatellus 54

Pinzi, Filippo 144

Pio, Alberto (da Carpi) 55

Piso 8, 10

plague (Antonine) 5, 17

Planoudes, Maximos 106

Plato 6, 8, 18, 64

   Platonism 2

Pliny the Elder 18, 20, 185

Pocatela di Borgofranco, Giacomo 150

Porphyry xii

Priscianus, Theodorus 31

Priscus of Samos 41

prognostic 69, 77–81, 100–102, 104, 106, 115

pseudepigraphy xi, xiv, 84–87, 95, 97

pseudonymity, 2, 83–97

Ptolemy 72

Pythagoras 44

Rasario, Giovanni Battista (Rasarius) 35, 154–156, 173–188

Ricci, Agostino 154–155, 193

Rhazes (al-Rāzī) 62, 105

Ridolfi, Niccolò (cardinal) 55

Rivirius, Joannes Nebriensis 193

Rome ix–xi, 1, 4–11, 24, 54, 131, 143

Rota, Julius Martinus 154, 156

Ruel, Jean 55

Rustico, Antonio 150

Sandalarium x, 143

Schedel, Hartmann 192, 194, 195

Schubring, Konrad 175

Scoutariotes, Jean 57

Scrofa, Sebastianus 35

Septimius Severus 7, 16, 33

Sergius, 34–35, 83–97

Seth, Symeon 101, 104

Sévère, Jean (de Lacédémone) 55

Severus (of Antioch) 84

Solon 39–40

Soranus (and pseudo-Soranus) 62, 91–92, 108

Sozomenos, Joannes 175–184

Stephanus of Alexandria 60, 65, 72, 77, 109

Strategos, Cesar 57

Struthius, Josephus 70, 76, 154, 156

Suriano, Girolamo 149–150, 155, 166, 191–194

Teuthras 63

Themison 6, 8

Theon of Alexandria 72

Theophilus 60, 64, 65, 73, 101–102, 109

theriac 2, 5, 9–10

Thou, Jacques-Auguste de 55

Turriano, Gioacchino 51 (n. 39), 57

uroscopy xiv, 73–76, 99–107

uterus *see* womb

Valgrisi, Vincenzo 155, 174

Valla, Giorgio (and Giovanni Pietro) 150, 154, 159

Venice 53, 54, 143, 144, 149, 150, 155, 174, 175, 191, 193

Vesalius, Andreas 164 (n. 10), 172

Vettori, Pietro 55

viper 22–23

Wenkeback, Ernst 176, 177–184

Winter *see* Guinterius

womb (anatomy of) 167–170, 197

Xenocrates 11

Yahya ibn al Bitriq 14

Zerbi, Gabriele 161–172